Health Financing for Poor People

Health Financing for Poor People

Resource Mobilization and Risk Sharing

Editors

Alexander S. Preker and **Guy Carrin**

THE WORLD BANK

Washington, D.C.

WORLD HEALTH ORGANIZATION

Geneva

INTERNATIONAL LABOUR OFFICE

Geneva

ISBN: 0-8213-5525-2

Library of Congress Cataloging-in-Publication Data

Health financing for poor people : resource mobilization and risk sharing /
  Alexander S. Preker.
      p. cm.
   Includes bibliographical references and index.
   ISBN 0-8213-5525-2
   1. Poor--Medical care--Developing countries. 2. Public health--Developing
countries--Finance. 3. Medical economics--Developing countries. 4. Minorities--
Medical care--Developing countries. 5. Human services--Developing countries--
Finance. I. Preker, Alexander S., 1951–

RA410.53.H437   2003
338.4'33621'091724—dc21

2003057160

Contents

TABLES

Foreword

In January 2000, Dr. Gro Harlem Bruntland, the former director general of the World Health Organization (WHO), established a Commission on Macroeconomics and Health (CMH) to provide evidence on the importance of health to economic development and poverty alleviation.

This book is based on research undertaken for the Commission's Working Group 3. The mandate of Working Group 3 was to examine alternative approaches to domestic resources mobilization, risk protection against the cost of illness, and efficient use of resources by providers. Professor Alan Tait (former deputy director of Fiscal Affairs, International Monetary Fund, and currently honorary fellow at University of Kent at Canterbury and honorary fellow at Trinity College, Dublin) and Professor Kwesi Botchwey (director of Africa Research and Programs at the Harvard Center for International Development) chaired the group.

Professor Jeffrey Sachs (then chairman of the Commission and director of the Harvard Center for International Development) presented the Commission's findings in a report submitted to the WHO on December 20, 2001—*Macroeconomics and Health: Investing in Health for Economic Development.*

The Summary Report from the Commission recommended a six-pronged approach to domestic resource mobilization at low-income levels: "(a) increased mobilization of general tax revenues for health, on the order of 1 percent of GNP by 2007 and 2 percent of GNP by 2015; (b) increased donor support to finance the provision of public goods and to ensure access for the poor to essential health services; (c) conversion of current out-of-pocket expenditure into prepayment schemes, including community-financing programs supported by public funding, where feasible; (d) a deepening of the HIPC initiative, in country coverage and in the extent of debt relief (with support from the bilateral donor community); (e) effort to address existing inefficiencies in the way in which government resources are presently allocated and used in the health sector; and (f) reallocating public outlays more generally from unproductive expenditure and subsidies to social-sector programs focused on the poor."

Most community-financing schemes have evolved in the context of severe economic constraints, political instability, and lack of good governance. Usually, government taxation capacity is weak, formal mechanisms of social protection for vulnerable populations absent, and government oversight of the informal health sector lacking. In this context of both public sector failure and market failure, community involvement in the financing of health care provides a critical, *albeit* insufficient, first step in the long march toward improved access to health care by the poor and social protection against the cost of illness.

The Commission stressed that community-financing schemes are no panacea for the problems low-income countries face in resource mobilization. Instead, the Commission recommended that such community-based financing mechanisms be regarded as a complement to—not a substitute for—strong government involvement in health care financing and risk management related to the cost of illness.

The key conclusions on community financing from Working Group 3 of the Commission on Macroeconomics and Health summarized in this book make a valuable contribution to our understanding of some of the strengths, weaknesses, and policy options for securing better access for the poor to health care and financial protection against the impoverishing effects of illness, especially for rural and informal sector workers in low-income countries.

Dean T. Jamison
Professor
School of Public Health
Center for Pacific Rim Studies
University of California Los Angeles (UCLA)

Fellow
Fogarty International Center
National Institutes of Health

Preface

One of the most urgent and vexing challenges faced by many low- and middle-income countries is how to provide health care for the more than 1.3 billion poor people who live in rural areas or work in the informal sector. As pointed out by Bill Hsiao from Harvard University in the chapter on the Asia region, this population is not a homogeneous group. Their occupations range from farmers, peddlers, day laborers, taxi drivers, and employees of the informal sector to shop owners and self-employed professionals. Yet this heterogeneous group shares the same lack of access to health care that is often due to inadequate health care financing. This book focuses on how to mobilize financial resources to pay for health care for such residents of rural communities in low-income countries. It also gives some attention to mobilizing health care financing for the urban poor.

Most countries try to serve their rural populations by directly operating public clinics in rural areas, but it is often difficult to get qualified practitioners to staff them. Those who accept such postings frequently work sporadically and provide poor quality services. The facilities themselves often lack drugs and supplies. When individuals become ill, they are frequently forced to rely first on self-treatment with home remedies provided by traditional healers and pharmacists. For serious illness episodes, the majority ultimately seek care from the few public and charity hospitals located in the rural areas.

Patients often have to pay a formal copayment or informal charge when treated in hospitals, even in the public sector. As a result, many patients have to choose between bankrupting their families and purchasing needed treatment. Studies have found that higher proportions of women and children than men have to forgo medical treatments. In addition, studies consistently have found that even when the government provides free or nearly free services, poor households pay a significant part of their income in informal charges. As much as 80 percent of total health care expenditure in low-income countries comes from direct out-of-pocket payment by patients. Studies in several countries found that large medical expenditure (such as for inpatient hospital services and costly outpatient drugs) is a major cause of poverty. These observations raise three serious sets of questions:

First, do countries spend enough on health care? In many countries the answer is no, particularly in the case of health care expenditure for the poor. However, it is not always certain that governments can spend more. Most low-income countries have narrow tax bases and ineffective tax collection systems. The total amount of money mobilized through taxes is therefore limited. Competing demands for the scarce general government resources that are available often leaves little public funding for basic health care for the poor rural and urban households.

Most developed countries use general revenues and social health insurance to pay for and provide health care for citizens working in rural areas and the informal sector. As will be seen in chapter one, the feasibility of these approaches may be weak in many low-income countries, as there are several factors that can hamper the move toward universal coverage. Private health insurance frequently is not affordable to the poor. User fees are inequitable and create a high barrier to access to health care by the poor. As for foreign aid, it is often small, even in low-income countries, compared with total spending on health care.

Second, do countries have a capacity to transform the little money available into effective services for the poor living in rural areas or working in the informal sector of urban centers? In many countries in which the government intends to fund and provide free, or nearly free, services for the rural residents and the poor, the target population is not utilizing the publicly provided health services. Why is this happening? Detailed studies in low-income countries have consistently found that governments are inefficient in their funding of primary care at the village and township levels. Public funds usually support the salaries of health workers regardless of whether they are delivering satisfactory services, while funds allocated to the purchase of drugs and supplies are inadequate. Consequently, this practice creates a public employment program rather than an effective health care delivery system. It thus turns out that the so-called free services may actually become expensive, as patients have to pay for drugs and medical consumables directly out-of-pocket. Furthermore, governments, in general, do not manage or monitor public services adequately at the local level. As a result, when the poor become ill they often choose to use their limited income to consult private practitioners and buy their own drugs.

Third, is the money spent directly by households used in an efficient and cost-effective way? We know that the answer to this question, too, is often no. Out-of-pocket payment for private sector providers has some serious drawbacks. Because these resources are not channeled through collective purchasing arrangements, individual households seeking health care are frequently in a weak bargaining position against providers who can extract above-market prices due to their monopoly power. This is exacerbated at the village level, where the small population size means that the presence of multiple providers competing with each other to keep prices low is particularly unlikely.

Throughout the world, community financing has been used to mobilize resources to fund and deliver health care for the poor in rural and urban communities, in settings where governments failed to fully meet this responsibility through the public sector. Some of these community-financing schemes have successfully addressed all three issues discussed above while others are primarily income-generating schemes for providers.

KEY FINDINGS

Based on an extensive survey of the literature, the main strengths of community-financing schemes are the degree of outreach penetration achieved through community participation and the contribution to financial protection against the cost of illness for low-income rural and informal sector workers. The schemes' main weaknesses relate to both external and design factors. Often the level of revenues that can be mobilized from poor communities is low. As a result, without some form of subsidy the poorest of the poor are frequently excluded from participation in such schemes. The small size of the risk pool of many voluntary community schemes, the limited management capacity that exists in rural and low-income contexts, and the isolation of such schemes from formal health-financing mechanisms and provider networks are all major weaknesses that must be addressed. The review of the literature provided a number of insights into the policy and institutional capacity-building measures that can be used to address many of these issues.

The review of selected experiences in the Asia and Africa regions supported many of these conclusions. It emphasized the diversity of community-financing arrangements that exist there. Several of the schemes appear to improve financial protection against the cost of illness, allow better access by poor households to essential health care, and confer greater efficiency in the collection, pooling, management, and use of scarce health care resources.

The existence of risk-sharing arrangements, as well as trust and local community control over the schemes, appears to increase enrollment rates with such schemes. In particular, the literature emphasized that, although income is a key constraint to participation by the poorest of the poor, even they are often willing and able to participate if their contributions are subsidized by public or donor funds and if the benefits they receive provide access to quality services. Households were also more likely to enroll in these schemes when the households that would later use them were directly involved in their design and management. Other factors that increased the likelihood of enrollment included setting the contribution level based on an assessment of local ability and willingness to pay, and ensuring the availability of easy access to the health care providers who serve the members.

Members like broad coverage that includes basic health services for frequently encountered health problems as well as hospitalization for rarer and more expensive conditions. In the context of extreme resource constraints, this creates a tension or tradeoff between prepayment for basic services and the need for insurance coverage for more expensive, life-threatening events that may only happen once or twice in a lifetime. This observation is consistent with the experience in other areas of insurance, in which willingness to pay for rare catastrophic events (life insurance) is often significantly reduced compared with coverage for events more likely to happen at a greater frequency (crop insurance). This highlights an area of market failure relating to voluntary community involvement in health care financing that needs to be addressed by appropriate government policies, because it is precisely during hospital episodes that many of the poor become severely impoverished.

The review of selected experiences from the Asia and Africa regions also pointed to a number of measures governments could take to strengthen community financing. This included subsidizing the contributions for the poor, providing technical assistance to improve a scheme's management capacity, and establishing links with formal health care networks. Satisfaction with the scheme was often related to the nature of the direct community involvement in design and management. A critical factor was matching willingness and ability to pay with the expectation of benefits to be received at some later point. The review also highlighted areas of government actions that appear to have negative impacts on the function of community-financing schemes. Top-down interference with the design and management of the schemes appeared to have a particularly negative impact on function and sustainability.

The results of the microlevel household data analysis reinforced the conclusions from the survey of the literature and two regional reviews. Econometric analysis of household data from four countries indicated that prepayment and risk sharing through community involvement in health care financing—no matter how small—increases access by poor populations to basic health services and protects them to a limited extent against the impoverishing effects of illness. Community involvement alone is not sufficient in preventing social exclusion since the poorest of the poor often do not participate fully in these schemes. However, the analysis provided evidence that this constraint in reaching the poorest could be overcome through well-targeted design features and implementation arrangements.

Finally, the results of the macrolevel cross-country analysis presented in this book give empirical support to the hypothesis that broad risk sharing in health-financing matters in terms of impact on both the level and the distribution of health, financial fairness, and responsiveness indicators. The results even suggested that risk sharing corrects for, and may outweigh, the negative effect of overall income inequality, suggesting that financial protection against the cost of illness may be a more effective poverty alleviation strategy in some settings than direct income support.

CONCLUSIONS

The underlying causes of many of today's health problems in lower-income countries are often well known, and effective and affordable drugs, surgical procedures, and other interventions often exist. But because of a number of problems related to resource mobilization, risk sharing, and resource allocation and purchasing arrangements, as well as problems in the provision of goods and services to rural and low-income populations, potentially effective policies and programs frequently fail to reach the households and communities that need them the most.

The research on community financing undertaken for Working Group 3 of the Commission on Macroeconomics and Health emphasized the importance of general tax revenues and payroll tax-based social health insurance contributions to the financing of health care at higher income levels. These methods can be equitable and efficient in mobilizing and utilizing resources. However, most community-financing schemes have evolved in settings with severe economic constraints, political instability, lack of good public sector governance, and catastrophic out-of-pocket user charges that can lead to impoverishment. These conditions are very different from those enjoyed at higher income levels, in which public-financing instruments have been successful in financing health care.

For years, many low- and middle-income countries—with assistance from the international development community—have tried to jump from no organized financing instruments to full reliance on financing through general taxation, social health insurance, or both. In the context of large rural populations, low formal labor market participation rates, and the limited scope of the above-mentioned formal health financing methods, few have succeeded on this reform path.

This book highlights the fact that community financing provides a more incremental, first step in the transition toward improved financial protection against the cost of illness and better access to priority health services for the 1.3 billion poor people in low- and middle-income countries. Community financing is not presented as a panacea for financing health care for rural and low-income workers in the informal sector. Rather, it is one of several options that can be considered by low-income countries in expanding coverage for the poor.

The book highlights several concrete public policy measures that governments can introduce to strengthen and improve the effectiveness of community involvement in health care financing. These include (a) increased and well-targeted subsidies to pay for the contributions of low-income populations; (b) use of insurance to protect against health care costs and assessment of the feasibility of reinsurance to enlarge the effective size of small risk pools; (c) use of effective prevention and case management techniques to limit expenditure fluctuations; (d) technical support to strengthen the management capacity of local schemes; and (e) establishment and strengthening of links with the formal financing and provider networks.

Acknowledgments

This book is based on work submitted to Working Group 3 (Chairmen Alan Tait and Kwesi Botchwey) of the Commission on Macroeconomics and Health (Chairman Jeffrey D. Sachs). The authors are grateful to the World Health Organization for having provided an opportunity to contribute to the work of the Commission on Macroeconomics and Health and to the World Bank for having published the background reports on community financing as HNP discussion papers.

The following individuals contributed directly to the book: (a) preparation of the synthesis book by Alexander S. Preker, Guy Carrin, David Dror, Melitta Jakab, William C. Hsiao, and Dyna Arhin-Tenkorang; (b) survey of the literature by Melitta Jakab and Chitra Krishnan; (c) analysis of macrolevel data by Guy Carrin, Riadh Zeramdini, Philip Musgrove, Jean-Pierre Poullier, Nicole Valentine, and Ke Xu; (d) analysis of microlevel data by Melitta Jakab, Alexander S. Preker, Chitra Krishnan, Allison Gamble Kelly, Pia Schneider, François Diop, A. K. Nandakumar, Johannes Paul Jütting, Anil Gumber, M. Kent Ranson, and Siripen Supakankunti; (e) review of selected Asian and African experiences by William C. Hsiao and Dyna Arhin-Tenkorang; and (f) review of reinsurance of community schemes by David Dror and Alexander S. Preker.

Valuable guidance on methodological issues was provided by Adam Wagstaff. We are also indebted to the following individuals for data access, guidance on research methodologies, reviews, and other indirect contributions to the book: Christian Jacquier, Christian Baeaza, Michael Cichon, Chris Murray, Kei Kawabatak, Christopher Lovelace, Helen Saxenian, Davidson Gwatkin, David Peters, George Schieber, Charlie Griffin, Agnes Soucat, Abdo S. Yazbeck, Mariam Claeson, Flavia Bustreo, Steve Cummings, and Shanta Devarajan.

The authors of the book are also grateful for the access provided to parallel and ongoing research on community financing by the World Bank, the World Health Organization, and the International Labour Organization, with important input from Harvard University, the London School of Hygiene and Tropical Medicine, the University of Lyon, Abt Associates, Inc. (Partnerships for Health Reform USA), the National Council for Economic Research (India), the Center for Development Research (ZEF) (Germany), and the Chulalongkorn University Faculty of Economics (Thailand).

CHAPTER 1

Rich-Poor Differences in Health Care Financing

Alexander S. Preker, Guy Carrin, David Dror, Melitta Jakab, William C. Hsiao, and Dyna Arhin-Tenkorang

Abstract: Most community finance schemes have evolved in the context of severe economic constraints, political instability, and lack of good governance. Usually government taxation capacity is weak, formal mechanisms of social protection for vulnerable populations absent, and government oversight of the informal health sector lacking. In this context of extreme public sector failure, community involvement in financing health care provides a critical, though insufficient, first step in the long march toward improved health care access for the poor and social protection against the cost of illness. It should be regarded as a complement to—not a substitute for—strong government involvement in health care financing and risk management related to the cost of illness. Based on their extensive survey of the literature, the authors show that the main strengths of community-financing schemes are the extent of outreach penetration achieved through community participation, the contribution to financial protection against illness, and the increase in access to health care by low-income rural and informal sector workers. The schemes' main weaknesses are the low volume of revenues that can be mobilized from poor communities, the frequent exclusion of the very poorest from participation in such schemes without some form of subsidy, the small size of the risk pool, the limited management capacity existing in rural and low-income contexts, and the isolation from the more comprehensive benefits often available through more formal health-financing mechanisms and provider networks. The authors conclude by proposing concrete public policy measures that governments can introduce to strengthen and improve the effectiveness of community involvement in health care financing. These include: (a) increased and well-targeted subsidies to pay for the premiums of low-income populations; (b) use of insurance to protect against expenditure fluctuations and use of reinsurance to enlarge the effective size of small risk pools; (c) use of effective prevention and case management techniques to limit expenditure fluctuations; (d) technical support to strengthen the management capacity of local schemes; and (e) establishment and strengthening of links with the formal financing and provider networks.

This century has witnessed greater gains in health outcomes than any other time in history. These gains are partly the result of improvements in income that have been accompanied by improvements in health-enhancing social policies (housing, clean water, sanitation systems, and nutrition) and greater gender equality in education. They are also the result of new knowledge about the causes, prevention, and treatment of disease and the introduction of policies, financing, and health services that make such interventions more equitably accessible. Improving ways to finance health care and protect populations against the cost of illness has been central to this success story (see Preker, Langenbrunner, and Jakab 2002; Preker and others 2002a, 2002b).

OVERVIEW AND CONTEXT

The share of the world's population protected against the catastrophic cost of illness rose significantly during the twentieth century, with global spending on health increasing from 3 percent to 8 percent of global gross domestic product (US$2.8 trillion), or 4 percent of the GDP of developing countries (US$250 billion). At the current global growth rate for GDP of 3.5 percent, spending on health-enhancing activities will increase annually by about $98 billion a year worldwide, or $8 billion a year in low- and middle-income countries.

The Exclusion of Low-Income Rural Populations and Informal Workers

Today the populations in most industrial countries (except Mexico, Turkey, and the United States) enjoy universal access to a comprehensive range of health services that are financed through a combination of general tax revenues, social insurance, private insurance, and charges (Preker 1998).

A number of low-income countries (such as Costa Rica, Malaysia, Sri Lanka, and Zambia) have tried to follow a similar path, but the quest for financial protection against the cost of illness in low- and middle-income countries has been a bumpy ride. Many of the world's 1.3 billion poor still do not have access to effective and affordable drugs, surgeries, and other interventions because of weaknesses in the financing and delivery of health care (ILO 2000a; WHO 2000; World Bank 1993, 1997). See figure 1.1.

Although 84 percent of the world's poor shoulder 93 percent of the global burden of disease, only 11 percent of the $2.8 trillion spent on health care reaches the low- and middle-income countries. Vaccination strategies of modern health care systems have reached millions of poor. However, when ill, low-income households in rural areas continue to use home remedies, traditional healers, and local providers who are often outside the formal health system. The share of the population covered by risk-sharing arrangements is smaller at low-income levels (see figure 1.1). As a result, the rich and urban middle classes often have better access to the twenty-first century's health care advances.

Origins of Rich-Poor Differences in Financial Protection

The flow of funds through the health care system, and the public-private mix, is complex (see figure 1.2—modified from Schieber and Maeda 1997). It can be differentiated into three discrete functions: (a) collection of revenues (source of funds), (b) pooling of funds and spreading of risks across larger population groups, and (c) purchase of services from public and private providers of health services (allocation or use of funds) (see also WHO 2000). A combination of general taxation, social insurance, private health insurance, and limited out-of-pocket user charges has become the preferred health-financing instruments for

FIGURE 1.1 Less Pooling of Revenues in Low-Income Countries

Pooled health revenues as % of total

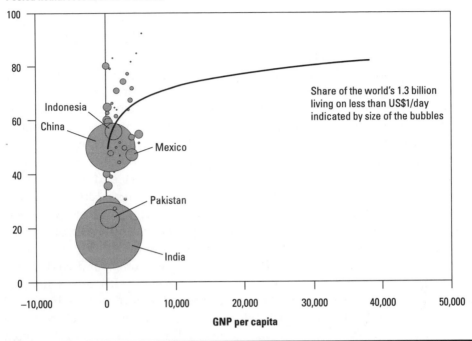

FIGURE 1.2 Flow of Funds through the System

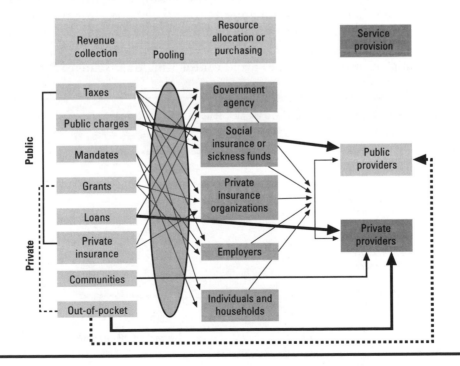

middle- and higher income countries, where income is readily identifiable and taxes or premiums can be collected at the source.

Different issues arise in the cases of public and private engagements in health care financing and service delivery. The need for collective arrangements and strong government action in health care financing is often confused with public production of services. The poor and other excluded populations frequently seek care from private providers because public services in rural and low-income urban areas are often scarce or plagued by understaffing, supply shortages, and low-quality care. Poor households and community-financing schemes therefore often turn to private providers for the care they need. Private provider engagement can still be pro-poor if there are mechanisms to exempt the poor or subsidize user fees (Preker, Harding, and Girishankar 2001) and if purchasing arrangements include coverage for the poor (Preker and others 2001).

Several factors make the policy options for financing health care at low-income levels different from financing those at higher income levels. Low-income countries often have large rural and informal sector populations, limiting the taxation capacity of their governments (see figure 1.3—modified from World Bank 1997). When a country's taxation capacity is as low as 10 percent of GDP or less, it would take 30 percent of government revenues to meet a target of 3 percent of GDP health expenditure through formal collective health care financing channels. In most countries, public expenditure on health care is much lower than this, often not surpassing 10 percent of public expenditure, which means that less than 1 percent of GDP of public resources is available for the health sector.

A related set of problems is faced during the pooling of financial resources at low-income levels. Pooling requires some transfer of resources from rich to poor, healthy to sick, and gainfully employed to inactive. In low-income countries, tax evasion by the rich and middle classes in the informal sector is widespread, allowing higher income groups to avoid contributing their share to the overall

---

FIGURE 1.3   Low-Income Countries Have Weak Capacity to Raise Revenues

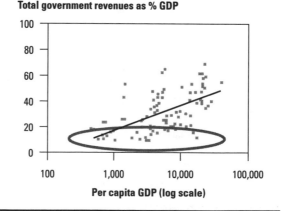

- Governments in many countries often raise less than 20% of GDP in public revenues; and

- The tax structure in many low-income countries is often regressive.

Total government revenues as % GDP

Per capita GDP (log scale)

revenue pool. Without such pooling of revenues and sharing of risks, low-income populations are exposed to serious financial hardship at times of illness (Diop, Yazbeck, and Bitran 1995). Figure 1.4 (Wagstaff, Watanabe, and van Doorslaer 2001) indicates households whose income drops below the poverty line (horizontal bar indicates poverty line) because of out-of-pocket expenditure on health care (vertical drop bars on the income distribution curve). Any pooling that does occur tends to be fragmented along income levels, preventing effective cross-subsidies between higher and lower income groups. In many poor countries, local community-financing schemes have emerged partially as an informal sector response to these shortcomings in revenue pooling at low-income levels.

Faced with overwhelming demand and very limited resources, many low-income countries use nonspecific broad expenditure caps that push rationing and resource allocation decisions to lower levels of the provider system. This often leads to serious drug shortages, equipment breakdowns, capital stock depreciation, and the lowering of hygiene standards. Such an environment also means politically and ethically difficult rationing decisions about the targeting of public expenditure to the poor. As a result of such difficulties, the rich often benefit more from public subsidies and public expenditures than the poor (figure 1.5—Peters and others 2001; see also Gwatkin 2001).

FIGURE 1.4   Out-of-Pocket (OOP) Expenditure and Poverty without Risk Sharing

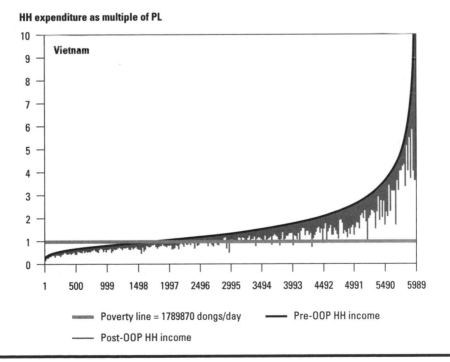

HH expenditure as multiple of PL

Vietnam

Poverty line = 1789870 dongs/day   Pre-OOP HH income

Post-OOP HH income

TABLE 1.1   Conceptual Underpinnings of Community-Financing Schemes

	Key conceptual underpinnings
Microfinance	**1. Microcredits**
	❏ Risk taking (take advantage of opportunity, avoid overcautious behavior)
	❏ Current liquidity management (smooth out consumption, increase choice)
	❏ Short-term shocks (drought, famine)
	2. Microsavings
	❏ Predictable life cycle events (education, marriage dowry, childbirth, death)
	❏ Capital formation (purchase of equipment, down payment on land, growth)
	❏ Future liquidity management (smooth consumption, increase choice)
	3. Microinsurance
	❏ Long-term income support (life and disability insurance, pensions)
	❏ Short-term income support (sick pay, unemployment insurance—not well developed)
	❏ Unpredictable health expenditure (health insurance)
	❏ Replacement of loss (fire and theft insurance)
	4. Financial intermediation
	❏ Payment and money-transfer services (facilitate trade and investments)
Social capital	**1. Community links**
	❏ Between extended families, local organizations, clubs, associations, civic groups
	2. Network links
	❏ Between similar communities (horizontal) and different communities (vertical)
	3. Institutional links
	❏ To communities' political, legal, and cultural environments
	4. Societal links
	❏ Between governments and citizens through public-private partnerships and community participation
Mainstream theories	**1. Welfare of society**
	❏ Income and growth
	2. Public finance
	❏ Taxation and social insurance
	3. Social policy
	❏ Social services and safety nets
	4. Health policy
	❏ Public health priorities and health systems

Links to Existing Microfinance Organizations

The role of microfinance in poverty alleviation for low-income groups has become a prominent theme in recent years (ADB 2000; Brown and Churchill 2000; Otero and Rhyne 1994; Zeller and Sharma 2000). Poor and rich households are equally exposed to a range of events that put them at financial risk and are beyond their immediate control. Such events range from predictable life cycle events, such as marriage, childbirth, education, and death, to less predictable events, such as droughts, fire, floods, and catastrophic illness.

The difference between poor and nonpoor households is the availability of mechanisms to cope with the financial consequences of unpredictable events. Nonpoor households take advantage of a wide range of risk-protection mechanisms that are available even in the lowest income countries. This includes savings, access to credit, insurance, and other financial intermediation mechanisms.

Until recently, few risk-protection mechanisms were accessible to the poor. It was assumed that the poor—living on less than a dollar a day—were neither willing nor able to save or contribute to insurance against the risks they faced. In sum, the poor were thought to be "unbankable" and "uninsurable" (Zeller and Sharma 2000). This led to the growth of informal risk-protection mechanisms through families, friends, and community networks. However, the past decade has witnessed a steady expansion of successful initiatives to provide the poor with savings, credit, and insurance services. Growing experience with these mechanisms suggests that the poor can be creditworthy, can save, and can buy insurance.

In particular, four microfinance instruments have been developed to improve the productive needs of low-income households. They are (a) credits that help improve the immediate human, physical, and social capital of the poor (for example, small short-term loans to help pay for training, a piece of farm equipment, and access to social networks); (b) savings to be used to build up the medium-term capital of the poor, such as education, the down payment on a piece of land, and dowry for the marriage of a daughter into a good family; (c) insurance to stave off unpredictable expenses, such as theft, loss, and illness); and (d) financial intermediation (payment systems to facilitate trade and investments).

Life, casualty, and crop insurance is often used to secure loans for low-income populations. Microfinance instruments help the poor avoid having to invest in less cost-efficient means of saving, credit, and insurance such as jewelry, livestock, and staple food, or to resort to inefficient barter systems of payment (payment in-kind). These instruments also contribute to the early transformation of barter transactions into more formal economic exchange and formalization of property rights.

The extension of such techniques to the health sector is now being observed in many microfinance and development organizations in low-income countries, especially in the case of microinsurance (Brown and Churchill 2000; Dror and Jacquier 1999; ILO 2000b, 2001). Extending microinsurance techniques to health care presents a unique set of challenges under exploration. While life and crop insurance deals mainly with the financial cost of income loss, health insurance presents an additional set of issues related to financing tangible services for which the cost is neither fully predictable nor constant. This includes the range and severity of different illnesses, the range and scope of services provided, and the behavior of patients and providers (the latter influenced particularly by the payment mechanism due to moral hazard, adverse selection, and fraud, especially in the form of supplier-induced demand).

Links to Community-Level Social Capital

Why have microfinance organizations been able to reach low-income individuals and households while more formal national systems have failed to do so? Clues to the answer come from the social capital literature of the 1990s, which can be summed up as "it is not what you know, but whom you know" (Platteau 1994; Woolcock 1998; Woolcock and Narayan 2000). When hard times strike, it is often family and friends who constitute the ultimate safety net for low-income groups.

Evidence suggests that social capital has four dimensions with potentially positive and potentially negative impacts on development. The four dimensions include:

- Community links such as those between extended families, local organizations, clubs, associations, and civic groups—people in small communities helping each other (Dordick 1997)

- Network links between similar communities (horizontal) and between different communities (vertical), such as ethnic groups, religious groups, class structures, and genders (Granovetter 1973)

- Institutional links such as those between communities' political, legal, and cultural environments (North 1990)

- Societal links between governments and their citizens through complementarity and embeddedness, such as public-private partnerships and the legal framework that protects the rights of association (for example, chambers of commerce and business groups) and community participation in public organizations (for example, community members on city councils and hospital boards) (Evans 1992, 1995, 1996).

Low-income households are likely to have greater trust in microhealth insurance programs that are linked to the community credit, savings, and insurance organizations to which they already belong and over which they feel they have some control. The people often regard national systems as impersonal and distant and think they will never benefit from those programs. This view is reinforced when the national programs ration care to focus on "global" public health priorities that—although they may have large externalities and benefits to society as a whole—often do not respond to the poor's immediate day-to-day health care needs.

Such social capital has both benefits and costs. The downside of social capital occurs when communities and networks become isolated or parochial or work at cross-purposes to societal collective interests (for example, ghettos, gangs, cartels). Intercommunity ties or bridges are needed to overcome the tendency of communities and networks to pursue narrow, sectarian interests that may run counter to broader societal goals. (Narayan 1999) Community-financing schemes are vulnerable to a number of the shortcomings associated with social capital:

- Community-financing schemes that share risk only among the poor will deprive its members of much needed cross-subsides from higher income groups.

- Community-financing schemes that remain isolated and small deprive their members of the benefits of spreading risks across a broader population.

- Community-financing schemes that are disconnected from the broader referral system and health networks deprive their members of the more comprehensive range of care available through the formal health care system.

Links to Mainstream Public Economics

Community-financing schemes—in addition to their links to microfinance and social capital—benefit from interconnectivity to the overall welfare of the society in which they exist, the system of public financing (no matter how weak it may be), and the broader social policy underpinning the prevailing national health system. Schemes that build such connections at an early stage are better able to evolve in terms of expanding the number of members covered, level of resources mobilized, size of the risk pool, and range of benefits they can cover as the local community they serve grows and evolves. Their members have more to gain through such connectivity than they would through isolation.

Principal-agent problems also explain why community-based initiatives are expected to be more successful than purely market-based institutions at providing financial protection products. These problems can be overcome in two ways: by designing incentives that align the interest of the agent (insurer) with that of the principal (member), and by designing monitoring systems that allow the principal (member) to effectively observe the actions of the agent (insurer). The proximity of community schemes (agents) to their members (principals) allows effective monitoring, which is much more difficult at the national level.

Proponents of linkage between community involvement and public finance argue their case on philosophical and technical grounds. In most societies, care for the sick and disabled is considered an expression of humanitarian and philosophical aspirations. Proponents do not, however, have to resort to moral principles or arguments about the welfare state to justify collective intervention in health. The past century is rich in examples of the failure of the private sector and market forces alone to secure efficiency and equity in the health sector. There is ample justification for such an engagement on both theoretical and practical grounds.

In the case of *efficiency,* there is ample evidence of the significant market failure that exists in the health sector—information asymmetries, public goods, positive and negative externalities, distorting or monopolistic market power of many providers and producers, absence of functioning markets in some areas, and frequent occurrence of high transaction costs (Arrow 1963; Atkinson and Stiglitz 1980; Bator 1958; Evans 1984; Musgrave and Musgrave 1984). In the case of *equity*, there is equally good evidence that on a voluntary basis individuals and families often fail to protect themselves adequately against the risks of illness and disability (Barer, Getzen, and Stoddart 1998; van Doorslaer, Wagstaff, and Rutten 1993).

METHODOLOGY FOR ASSESSING IMPACT, STRENGTHS, AND WEAKNESSES

To assess the impact, strengths, and weaknesses of community-based involvement in health care financing, we will use a modified version of the World Bank's Poverty Reduction Strategy Paper (PRSP) framework (Claeson and others 2001). According to this framework, community financing can be seen as having three independent objectives: (a) mobilizing financial resources to promote better health and to diagnose, prevent, and treat known illnesses; (b) protecting individuals and households against direct financial cost of illness when channeled through risk-sharing mechanisms; and (c) giving the poor a voice in their own destinies and making them active participants in breaking out of the social exclusion in which they are often trapped. We will not deal with the indirect impact of illness on loss of income due to interruption of employment, although this is clearly another important dimension of financial protection against the cost of illness.

This framework is consistent with the three goals of health systems emphasized by the *World Health Report 2000* (WHO 2000): financial fairness (an indicator that measures inequality of the financial contribution for health across households), disability-adjusted life expectancy (DALE, an indicator that combines life expectancy and disability measures), and responsiveness (a consumer-satisfaction indicator that combines ethical and consumer quality dimensions). This framework is also consistent with the International Development Goals (IDGs) relating to achievement of better health and protection against impoverishment by the year 2015.

The determinants of financial protection, improved health, and social inclusion are complex (see figure 1.6). The PRSP framework emphasizes the following causal links: (a) close tracking of key outcome measures relating to improved financial protection, health, and social inclusion; (b) demand and utilization patterns; (c) supply in the health system and related sectors; and (d) policy actions by governments, civil society, the private sector, and donors.

Outcome indicators. Much work is still needed to develop a meaningful set of indicators for improving health and protection against impoverishment and combating social exclusion. For this report, we have used both the financial fairness, DALE, and responsiveness indicators recommended by the World Health Organization (WHO) and several intermediate indicators (see next section for details).

Demand and utilization in influencing financial protection. There is a complex interplay between household assets (human, physical, financial, and social),

FIGURE 1.6 Determinants of Financial Protection, Health, and Social Inclusions

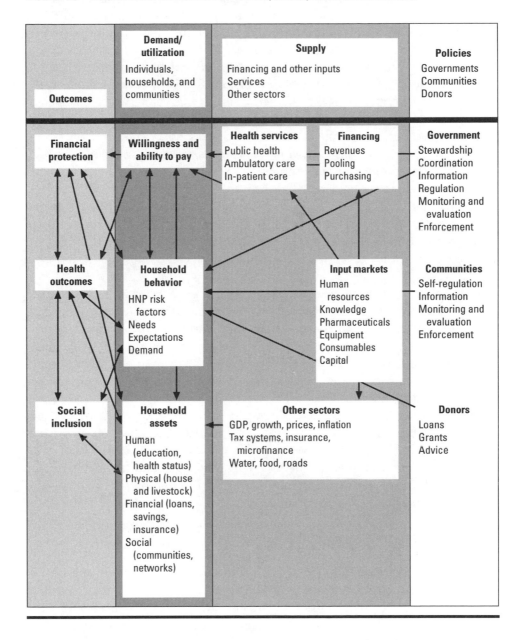

household behavior (risk factors, needs, expectations, and demands for services), ability and willingness to pay, and the availability of insurance or subsidies (Soucat and others 1997). This part of the analysis emphasizes the importance of household and community behavior in improving health and reducing the financial risks.

Supply in health system and related sectors. There is a hierarchy of interest from nonhealth sector factors in improving financial protection—such as GDP, prices, inflation, availability of insurance markets, effective tax systems, credit, and savings programs—to more traditional parts of the health system (a) preventive and curative health services, (b) health financing, (c) input markets, and (d) access to effective and quality health services (preventive, ambulatory, and in-patient). In respect to the latter, organizational and institutional factors contribute to the incentive environment of health-financing and service delivery systems in addition to the more commonly examined determinants such as management, input, throughput, and output factors (Harding and Preker 2001).

Policy actions by governments, civil society, and the private sector. Finally, through their stewardship function, governments have a variety of policy instruments that can be used to strengthen the health system, the financing of services, and the regulatory environment within which the system functions (Saltman and Ferroussier-Davis 2000). This includes regulation, contracting, subsidies, direct public production, and ensuring that information is available. In countries with weak government capacity, civil society and donors can be encouraged to play a similar role.

Four levels of analysis were used to assess the impact, strengths, and weaknesses of community involvement in financial protection against the cost of illness and improved health. They include (a) a survey of the literature on the impact, strengths, and weaknesses of different types of community involvement in health financing; (b) macrolevel cross-country analysis of the impact of different health care financing mechanisms on national health systems' performance indicators—health, financial fairness, and responsiveness; (c) microlevel household data analysis of the specific impact of community-financing schemes on overall welfare of the poor—financial protection and access to health services for the poor; and (d) regional reviews of the Asia and Africa experience of community involvement in health care financing, including different public policy options such as subsidies, reinsurance, linkages to formal public financing systems, and management-capacity building.

Methodology for Survey of Literature on Community Financing

Despite the recent growth in research on community-based health care financing, there is a paucity of systematic evidence regarding the performance of these schemes in terms of their impact on broad outcome goals such as improving health and protection against impoverishment and combating social exclusion. In particular, little is known about their effectiveness in mobilizing resources and improving access to effective and quality health care; their role in sharing risks across population groups; and their impact on addressing the problems associated with social exclusion. Despite progress made by the time the *World Health Report 2000* was published, experts are still debating which indicators best capture progress toward achieving these goals.

TABLE 1.2   Summary Statistics of the Literature Reviewed, by Publication Type

	Peer-reviewed journal articles	Published reports	Internal documents of international organizations or academic institutions	Conference proceedings
Number of studies	20	15	4	4

The review looked at any past studies whose main focus had been to examine community involvement in health care financing. Based on this broad criterion, the review comprised 43 studies. The selected papers included articles published in peer-reviewed journals, reports published in formal publication series of international organizations (such as WHO, International Labour Organisation, United Nations Children's Fund), internal unpublished documents of international organizations and academic institutions, and conference proceedings. Table 1.2 presents the breakdown of the reviewed studies, by publication type.

Of these 43 studies, 5 were conceptual papers, 7 were large-scale comparative papers (analyzing five or more community-based health financing schemes) and the remaining 31 were case studies. The regional breakdown of the case studies was 15 in Africa, 11 in Asia, and 4 in Latin America. Language barriers and time constraints created a certain selection bias—Spanish literature was not included in our search while French literature was (Jakab and Krishnan 2001).

Assessment of Performance

Since past research of community-financing schemes varies considerably in the issues examined and methodologies used, a standard set of questions were asked relating to both the review of impact assessments and the review of determinants (key strengths and weaknesses of various types of schemes). The following three questions relating to the impact of community involvement on health, financial protection, and social inclusion were asked:

Question 1: What and how robust was the evidence on the amount of resources that could be mobilized through community involvement to pay for health care and the sustainability of this source of financing?

Question 2: What and how robust was the evidence on the effectiveness of community involvement in protecting individuals against the impoverishing effects of illness?

Question 3: What and how robust was the evidence on the role that community involvement played in combating social exclusion by allowing low-income groups to have a more direct role in the financing of their health care needs and protecting them against the financial burden of illness?

A number of studies offered conclusions on resource mobilization, financial protection, and social exclusion based on the experience of authors or review of other studies but did not provide actual evidence in support of their conclusions. Our review excluded studies of performance assessments from the analysis. It also excluded studies that did not use controls from the performance evaluation. This approach yielded 11 studies for the performance assessment of the review.

Assessment of Institutional Determinants of Performance

The direct and indirect determinants of improved health, financial protection against the cost of illness, and social inclusion are complex. As described earlier by the PRSP framework, policy actions by governments, civil society, and the private sector are mediated through supply and demand factors related to both the health sector and other sectors that affect the outcome measures being examined. This would include indicators of the service delivery system (product markets), input generation (factor markets), the stewardship or government oversight function (policymaking, coordination, regulation, monitoring, evaluation), and market pressures. The current body of literature on community financing is not comprehensive so the report looked only at factors directly related to health care financing.

Table 1.3 provides a list of the core technical design, management, organizational, and institutional characteristics related to health care financing in general. Based on this framework, the study reviewed 43 assessments of community-financing schemes for their impacts, strengths, and weaknesses.

Methodology for Regional Reviews of Selected Asia and Africa Experiences

The main objective of the reviews of selected Asia and Africa experiences was to provide additional insights about several key issues from the perspective of the two regions of the world that carry the heaviest burden of mortality and morbidity, have the weakest risk-sharing arrangements to protect their populations against the impoverishing effects of illness, and have the greatest number of poor living in absolute poverty and social exclusion (Arhin-Tenkorang 2001; Hsiao 2001). In addition to contributing to an understanding about the current roles of community involvement in health care financing, the regional reviews also focused on future policy options. Key questions asked include the following:

- Using the same framework described under the survey of the literature, what are the main characteristics of existing community involvement in financing health care in the Africa and Asia regions in terms of impacts, strengths, and weaknesses of existing schemes (describe successful and unsuccessful features)?

- To what extent do community-financing schemes serve the objective of securing adequate, equitable, and sustainable financing for the low-income and rural populations served (impact on the poor)?

- What are the main challenges and obstacles to improving community arrangements to provide adequate, equitable, and sustainable financing?

TABLE 1.3   Core Characteristics of the Community-Based Financing Schemes

Key policy questions

Technical design characteristics	**1. Revenue-collection mechanisms** ❑ Level of prepayment compared with direct out-of-pocket spending ❑ Extent to which contributions are compulsory compared with voluntary ❑ Degree of progressivity of contributions ❑ Subsidies for the poor and buffer against external shocks **2. Arrangements for pooling revenues and sharing risks** ❑ Size ❑ Number ❑ Redistribution from rich to poor, healthy to sick, and gainfully employed to inactive **3. Purchasing and resource allocation** ❑ Demand (for whom to buy) ❑ Supply (what to buy and in which form, and what to exclude) ❑ Prices and incentive regime (at what price and how to pay)
Management characteristics	**1. Staff** ❑ Leadership ❑ Capacity (management skills) **2. Culture** ❑ Management style (top down or consensual) ❑ Structure (flat or hierarchical) **3. Access to information** (financial, resources, health information, behavior)
Organizational characteristics	**1. Organizational forms** (extent of economies of scale and scope, and contractual relationships) **2. Incentive regime** (extent of decision rights, market exposure, financial responsibility, accountability, and coverage of social functions) **3. Linkages** (extent of horizontal and vertical integration or fragmentation)
Institutional characteristics	**1. Stewardship** (who controls strategic and operational decisions and regulations) **2. Governance** (what are the ownership arrangements) **3. Insurance markets** (rules on revenue collection, pooling, and transfer of funds) **4. Factor and product markets** (from whom to buy, at what price, and how much)
	↓ ↓ ↓
Outcome Indicators	Health Outcomes Financial Protection Social Inclusion

- Are there other viable alternatives to community financing in the country settings where they exist today?

- In the context of these study findings, what role could the international donor community play to improve financing for rural and other low-income population groups?

TABLE 1.4   Characteristics of 5 Survey Instruments

	Name of scheme	Year of data collection	Sample size (households)	Organization associated with the survey
Rwanda	54 prepayment schemes in 3 districts of Byumba, Kabgayi, and Kabutare	2000	2,518	Partnerships for Health Reform (PHR) in collaboration with National Population Office
Senegal	3 Mutual Health Insurance Schemes (Thiés Region)	2000	346	Institute of Health and Development, Dakar in collaboration with ILO
India (1)	Self-Employed Women's Association (SEWA)	1998–99	1,200	National Council of Applied Economic Research (NCAER)
India (2)	Self-Employed Women's Association (SEWA)	1997	1,200	London School of Hygiene and Tropical Medicine
Thailand	Voluntary Health Card Scheme (HCP)	1994–95	1,005	National Statistics Office

Methodology for Microlevel Household Survey Analysis

The aim of the microlevel household survey analysis was to shed light on two questions (Jakab and others 2001): What characteristics affect the decision of households to join community-based prepayment schemes? Do community health-financing schemes provide financial protection for their members against the cost of illness?

Eleven household budget surveys, four Living Standard Measurement Surveys (LSMS), and nine Demographic and Health Surveys (DHS) were screened for community-financing data. Most of these surveys did not allow an identification of households with access to community-based health financing. Of the 11 smaller scale nonstandardized surveys that matched the requirements for the core list of variables, 5 were available for further analysis and were included in this report. Table 1.4 summarizes the key characteristics of these surveys. The remaining 6 were either not accessible for further analysis (4), data collection was incomplete (1), or authors were not available to collaborate (1).

The five household surveys identified and accessible for analysis for the purposes of this report represent nonstandardized, relatively small-scale data-collection efforts with a sample size of 346 to 1,200 households. The surveys were not nationally representative; they were a random sample of the local population. With the exception of Thailand's, all surveys are very recent.

Determinants of Inclusion

To assess the determinants of social inclusion in community-financing schemes, we assume that the choice of whether to enroll is influenced by two main determinants: individual and household characteristics, and community characteristics. Individual and household characteristics influence the cost and the benefit calculation of the rational individual decision maker.

This choice is moderated, however, through certain social characteristics of the community. The individual rational choice model of weighting costs and benefits of joining a prepayment scheme is altered by the social values and ethics of the local culture. For example, two individuals with similar individual and household characteristics (such as income, household size, assets, education level, health status) may decide differently about joining a prepayment scheme depending, for example, on encouragement from community leaders, availability of information, and ease of maneuvering unknown processes.

To estimate the weight of these determinants, a binary logit model was applied to four of the data sets, and a binary probit was applied to the Senegal data set. The model can be formally written as follows:

$$(1.1) \quad \text{Prob (membership} > 0) = X_1\beta_1 + X_2\beta_2 + \varepsilon$$

The independent variable takes on a value of 1 if the individual belongs to a community-financing scheme and 0 if he or she does not. X_1 represents a set of independent variables for characteristics of the individual and the household, such as income, gender, age, and marker on chronic illness or disability. X_2 represents a set of independent variables that approximate the social values in the communities: religion and marker on various communities where appropriate. Other variables specific to the surveys as well as interaction terms were included where appropriate. β_1 and β_2 are vectors of coefficient estimates and ε is the error term.

The two variables of primary interest are income (measure of social inclusion) and a marker for community factors (dummy variable). Control variables also included gender, age, disability or chronic illness, religion, and distance to the health center under the scheme. Some of these variables are important to control for the different probability of health care use (for example, age, health status, and distance from provider). These variables also allow us to test the presence and importance of adverse selection to which all voluntary prepayment schemes are subject. Other variables included control for the different individual and household attitudes toward investment in health at a time when illness is not necessarily present (for example, gender and religion). Literature has shown that the distance to the hospitals and local health centers and existence of outreach programs influence the decision to purchase membership to the scheme.

Determinants of Financial Protection

To empirically assess the impact of scheme membership on financial protection, a two-part model was used.[1] The first part of the model analyzes the determinants of using health care services. The second part of the model analyzes the determinants of health care expenditures for those who reported any health care use.

There are several reasons for taking this approach. First, using health expenditure alone as a predictor of financial protection does not allow capture of the lack of financial protection for people who choose not to seek health care because they cannot afford it. As the first part of the model assesses the determinants of utilization, this approach allows us to see whether membership in community financing reduces barriers to accessing health care services. Second, the distribution of health expenditures is typically not a normal distribution. Many nonspenders do not use health care in the recall period. The distribution also has a long tail due to the small number of very high spenders. To address the first cause of nonnormality, the study restricted the analysis of health expenditures to those who report any health care use. As the first part of the model assesses determinants of use, we will still be able to look into whether scheme membership removes barriers to care. To address the second part of nonnormality, a log-linear model specification is used.

Part one of the model is a binary logit model for the India, Rwanda, and Thailand data sets and a probit model in the Senegal model. The model estimates the probability of an individual visiting a health care provider. Formally, part one of the model can be written as follows:

(1.2)   Prob (visit > 0) = $X\beta + \varepsilon$.

Part two is a log-linear model that estimates the incurred level of out-of-pocket expenditures, conditioned on positive use of health care services. Formally, part two of the model can be written as follows:

Log (out-of-pocket expenditure | visit > 0) = $X\gamma + \mu$

where X represents a set of individual and household characteristics hypothesized to affect individual patterns of utilization and expenditures.

β and γ are vectors of coefficient estimates of the respective models; ε and μ are error terms.

The two variables of primary interest are scheme membership status and income. Other control variables were also included in the estimation model to control for the differences in need for health care (for example, age and gender), differences in preferences toward seeking health care (for example, gender and religion), and differences in the cost (direct and indirect) of seeking health care (for example, distance).

Methodology for Macrolevel Cross-Country Analysis

For the dependent variables of the macrolevel country analysis, the study used the standard indicators proposed by WHO for health systems performance (WHO 2000). These are the disability-adjusted life expectancy (DALE), the index of level of responsiveness (IR), the index of fairness of financial contribution (IFFC), the index of distribution of responsiveness (IRD), and the index of equality of child survival (IECS). Only the observed data for these indicators were included in the analysis.

For the independent variables of the macrolevel analysis, countries were divided into three groups based on the extent of their risk-sharing arrangements.

We assign countries to the first category, *advanced risk sharing,* when they have either a social health insurance scheme or a health-financing scheme based on general taxation, and when these two schemes are associated with the principle of universal coverage. Countries with no explicit reference to overall coverage of the population, who usually have mixed health-financing systems, with some part of the population partially covered via general taxation and specific population groups covered by health insurance schemes, are associated with the second category, *medium risk sharing.* Finally, countries with general taxation systems that incompletely cover the population are associated with the third category, *low risk sharing.* This classification system allows us to define the two main organizational dummy variables: DARS = 1 when a country belongs to the set of advanced risk-sharing systems and 0 otherwise; DMRS = 1 when a country belongs to the set of medium risk-sharing systems and 0 otherwise.

The methodology for this analysis is described by Carrin and others (2001). The objective of the analysis is to examine the degree to which risk sharing has a beneficial impact on the five indicators of health systems performance.

The analysis used the following specification for the impact of risk sharing on the level of health:

$$(1.3) \quad \mathrm{Ln}\,(80 - \mathrm{DALE}) = a_1 + b_1\,\mathrm{Ln}\,\mathrm{HEC} + c_1\,\mathrm{Ln}\,\mathrm{EDU} + d_1\,\mathrm{DARS}.$$

HEC refers to the health expenditure per capita (in U.S. dollars). EDU refers to the educational attainment in society and is measured by the primary enrollment. The dependent variable is the logarithm of the difference between the observed DALE and a maximum. Several alternative models were also tested. The hypothesis is that advanced risk sharing (among indirect determinants such as education) is associated with a better definition of the benefit package of health services to which citizens are entitled, which translates into an increased overall level of health.

The analysis used two alternative functional forms to assess the impact of risk sharing on responsiveness:

$$(1.4a) \quad \mathrm{Ln}\,(\mathrm{IR}/[1 - \mathrm{IR}]) = a_{21} + b_{21}\,\mathrm{HEC} + c_{21}\,\mathrm{EDU} + d_{21}\,\mathrm{DARS}$$

and

$$(1.4b) \quad \mathrm{Ln}\,(1 - \mathrm{IR}) = a_{22} + b_{22}\,\mathrm{LnHEC} + c_{22}\,\mathrm{Ln}\,\mathrm{EDU} + d_{22}\,\mathrm{DARS}.$$

The hypothesis to be tested is that advanced risk-sharing systems are associated with a larger degree of stewardship. The latter, in turn, is likely to positively influence the mechanisms and incentives that entail a greater responsiveness.

The analysis used three measures for distributional impact. This included an IECS, an IFFC, and an IRD.

Several models were tested. A model was developed that examined the impact of the dummy variable (DARS) on the distributional variables for health, fairness, and responsiveness. We have adopted the same functional forms as in equations (1.4a and 1.4b):

(1.5a) $\text{Ln } (I_j/[1 - I_j]) = a_{31} + b_{31} \text{ DARS}$

and

(1.5b) $\text{Ln } (1 - I_j) = a_{32} + b_{32} \text{ DARS,}$

where I_j $(j = 1,...,3)$ refers to the three above-mentioned indexes, respectively.

The effect of DARS on the indicator of *fair financing* is expected to be positive when using the logit form of the equation. The hypothesis to be tested is that in countries with advanced risk sharing, more so than in other systems, people make financial contributions according to their capacity to pay. This would be associated with a higher IFFC. In addition, systems with universal coverage generally pay more attention to the objective of equal treatment for equal need. It is therefore assumed that such systems also respond to people's expectations as to the nonmedical aspects of health care in a more equal way. Hence the effect of DARS on the distribution of *responsiveness* is anticipated to be positive as well. Finally, it is assumed that universal coverage systems are more likely to provide people with a similar benefit package than other systems, irrespective of their socioeconomic background, with a resulting positive impact on the distributional aspects of *child health*.

DISCUSSION OF MAIN FINDINGS FROM BACKGROUND REVIEWS

Based on a review of the 43 papers discussing community-based health financing, the first and foremost conclusion is that there is a paucity of systematic empirical work regarding the performance of these financing mechanisms or the determinants of good outcomes in achieving good health (Jakab and others 2001).

Discussion of Survey of Existing Literature on Community Health Financing

Although several authors have tired to create a typology for community-based schemes (Atim 1998; Bennett, Creese, and Monasch 1998; Criel, van der Stuyft, and van Lerberghe 1999; Hsiao 2001), the possibilities for variations is almost limitless, given the great diversity in objectives, design, context, and implementation arrangements. Nevertheless, the review revealed four commonly encountered and well-identifiable types of schemes. In the first type, resource mobilization relies mainly on out-of-pocket payments at the point of contact with providers, but the community is actively involved in designing these fees and managing the collection, pooling, and allocation of the funds mobilized in this way (*community cost-sharing*). In the second type, the community collects payments in advance of treatment (*prepayment*) and then manages these resources in paying for providers (*community prepayment or mutual health organization*). In the third type, providers serving a particular community collect the prepayments themselves (*community provider-based health insurance*). In the fourth type, the community acts as "agent" to reach rural and excluded populations on behalf of the formal government or social health insurance system (*government or social insurance*) via contracts or agreements.

TABLE 1.5   Types of Community-Based Financing

		Four community-based finance modalities				
Type of scheme	Government schemes: social-insurance and tax-based	**Type 4** Linked community health fund, revolving fund, or prepayment	**Type 3** Community provider-based health insurance	**Type 2** Community-based prepayment schemes	**Type 1** Community-managed user fees	Direct user fees (spot market)

Table 1.5 summarizes these four types of community-based financing schemes based on their core design features and management, organizational, and institutional characteristics.

Assessment of Impact

Following the framework presented in table 1.3, the survey of the literature looked at three indicators of performance of community-based financing schemes (Jakab and others 2001): (a) their effectiveness in mobilizing resources and improving access to effective and quality health care; (b) their role in sharing risks across population groups; and (c) their impact on addressing the problems associated with social exclusion (see table 1.6). This is followed by a discussion on the key conclusions from the performance review of the literature.

Resource Mobilization. There is good evidence from the literature that community-financing arrangements make a positive contribution to the financing of health care at low-income levels, thereby improving access to drugs, primary care, and even more advanced hospital care (Dave 1991). Such community involvement allowed rural and low-income populations to mobilize more resources to pay for health care than would have been available without this involvement (Diop, Yazbeck, and Bitran 1995; McPake, Hanson, and Mills 1993; Soucat and others 1997). But there are great variations in the volume of resources that can be mobilized this way, constrained largely by the low income of the contributing population (Atim 1998; Bennett, Creese, and Monasch 1998; Hsiao 2001; Jütting 2000—see box 1.1). This is particularly true when most members of the community

TABLE 1.6   Number of Studies that Examined Core Health-Financing Subfunctions

Financing function	Revenue collection	Pooling of revenues	Resource allocation or purchasing
Type 1	5	2	3
Type 2	6	4	9
Type 3	2	2	3
Type 4	3	3	2
Multiple	10	2	3

BOX 1.1   REVENUE MOBILIZATION

Based on data from Bennett, Creese, and Monasch (1998), this graph shows the cost recovery from prepayment of six Modality II schemes. The range is from 12 percent to 51 percent of recurrent expenditure. This shows that, for these schemes, the resources collected contribute significantly to the full recurrent costs but do not fully cover them, thereby necessitating other sources of funding, such as out-of-pocket spending, government subsidies, and donor grants.

Percent of recurrent costs from prepayment

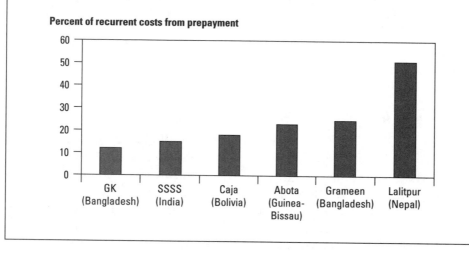

schemes are already below the poverty line. None of the studies reviewed reported the share of aggregate national resources that were mobilized through community-financing arrangements. There is an urgent need to strengthen the evidence base of community-financing arrangements through more rigorous registration, monitoring, and evaluation of the resource mobilization capacity of these schemes.

Financial Protection. Where household survey data have been analyzed, a consistent observation was that community-based health financing has been effective in reaching more low-income populations who would otherwise have no financial protection against the cost of illness (Litvack and Bodart 1992). Improved financial protection is achieved through reducing the members' out-of-pocket spending while increasing their utilization of health care services (Atim 1998; Criel, van der Stuyft, and van Lerberghe 1999; Desmet, Chowdhury, and Islam 1999, Gumber and Kulkarni 2000; Jütting 2000; Supakakunti 1997). At the same time, some of the research suggested that the poorest and socially excluded groups are often not included in community-based health-financing initiatives (Arhin-Tenkorang 1994; Criel, van der Stuyft, and van Lerberghe 1999; Jütting 2000). Those studies that compared the level of financial protection of scheme members with that of nonmembers found that belonging to some form of prepayment scheme reduced the financial burden of seeking health care (Arhin-Tenkorang 1994; Diop, Yazbeck, and Bitran 1995; DeRoeck and others 1996;

TABLE 1.7   Studies that Looked at Ways to Prevent Impoverishment

Studies that confirmed key hypothesis being tested	Utilization of members relative to nonmembers		Level of out-of-pocket expenditures of members relative to nonmembers	
	Increase	Decrease	Increase	Decrease
Type 1 Community user fees	3	1	0	1
Type 2 Community prepayment	4	≅2	0	6
Type 3 Provider prepayment	3	0	0	0
Type 4 Linked to formal system	3	0	0	2

TABLE 1.8   Studies that Looked at Ways to Combat Social Exclusion

Studies that confirmed key hypothesis being tested	Scheme reaches the poor	Poorest not covered	Inability to pay, main reason for not being covered	Rich do not participate	Distance gradient to scheme provider
Type 1 Community user fees	3	1	1	0	0
Type 2 Community prepayment	5	1	2	1	1
Type 3 Provider prepayment	2	2	1	1	1
Type 4 Linked to formal system	3	1	2	1	1

Gumber and Kulkarni 2000; see table 1.7). Two studies indicated that community financing does not eliminate the need for broader coverage in the case of catastrophic health care expenditures (Pradhan and Prescott 2000; Xing-Yuan 2000).

Combating Social Exclusion. Community-based health-financing schemes appear to extend coverage to many rural and low-income populations who would otherwise be excluded from collective arrangements to pay for health care and protect them against the cost of illness. However, the poorest are often excluded even from community-financing arrangements, and higher income groups often do not belong, thereby segmenting the revenue pool by income group (see table 1.8).

Identification of Determinants

The survey of the literature also looked at factors that would contribute to strengths and weaknesses of the schemes (Jakab and others 2001) in the following four areas: (a) technical design characteristics, (b) management characteristics, (c) organizational characteristics, and (d) institutional characteristics. The key advantages and disadvantages of community-based schemes lie in their ability to fill the policy, management, organizational, and institutional void left by extreme government failure to secure more organized financing arrangements for the poor. In this context, a number of strengths (see box 1.2) and weaknesses (see box 1.3) of community-financing schemes have been identified by various authors.

BOX 1.2   STRENGTHS OF COMMUNITY-FINANCING SCHEMES

Technical Design Characteristics

Revenue Collection Mechanisms

- Shift away from point-of-service payment to increasing prepayment and risk sharing
- Flat-rate premium, which facilitates revenue collection, reduces the scope for manipulation, and contributes to low transaction costs
- Contribution payment that accommodates the income-generating patterns of households employed in agriculture and the informal sector (irregular, often noncash)
- Modest degree of household-level affiliation
- Pro-poor orientation even at low-income levels through exemptions of premiums and subsidies, despite flat-rate contribution rate
- Some buffering against external shocks though accumulation of reserves and links to formal financing schemes

Arrangements for Pooling Revenues and Sharing Risks

- Some transfers from rich to poor, healthy to sick, and gainfully employed to inactive through some pooling of revenues and sharing of risk within community groups

Purchasing and Resource Allocation

- Most community schemes make a collective decision about who is covered through scheme, based on affiliation and direct family kinship (for whom to buy).
- Many community schemes define the benefit package to be covered in advance (what to buy, in what form, and what to exclude).
- Some community schemes engage in collective negotiations about price and payment mechanisms.

Management

- Most community schemes are established and managed by community leaders. Community involvement in management allows social controls over the behavior of members and providers that mitigates moral hazard, adverse selection, and induced demand.

- Many schemes seek external assistance in strengthening management capacity.

- The management culture tends to be consensual (high degree of democratic participation).

- Most schemes have good access to local utilization and behavior patterns.

BOX 1.2 *continued*

Organizational Structure

- Most community schemes are distributed organizational configurations that reach deep into the rural and informal sectors.

- Incentive regimes include: (a) extensive decision rights, (b) strong internal accountability arrangements to membership or parent community organization, (c) ability to accumulate limited reserves if successful but unsuccessful schemes often ask governments for bailouts, (d) mainly factor-market exposure since few overlapping schemes compete with each other in the product market, and (e) some limited coverage of indigent populations through community or government subsidies.

- Vertical integration may lead to increased efficiency and quality services. Schemes that have a durable partnership arrangement or contractual arrangement with providers able to negotiate preferential rates for their members. This in turn increases the attractiveness of the scheme to the population and contributes to sustainable membership levels.

- Better organized schemes use horizontal referral networks and vertical links to formal sector.

Institutional Environment

- Stewardship function is almost always controlled by local community, not central government or national health insurance system, which is apt to make the schemes responsive to local contexts.

- Ownership and governance arrangements (management boards or committees) are almost always directly linked to parent community schemes; freestanding health insurance schemes are rare.

- There is little competition in the product market.

- Competition is limited in factor markets and through consumer choice.

Discussion of Main Findings from Asia Regional Review

The review of selected Asia experiences emphasized the heterogeneity of community-financing schemes and the fact that their performance is highly dependent on the nature of their technical design and management, organizational, and institutional characteristics. For the purpose of this review, Hsiao (2001) classified community involvement in health care financing into five types: (a) direct subsidy to individuals (Thai Health Card and Tanzania Community Health Fund), (b) cooperative health care (Jiangsu Province and Tibet), (c) community-based third-party insurance (Rand Experiment in Sichuan Province and Dana Sehat), (d) provider sponsored insurance (Dkaha Community Hospital, Gonoshasthya and Bwamanda), and (e) producer-consumer cooperative (Grameen).

BOX 1.3   WEAKNESSES OF COMMUNITY-FINANCING SCHEMES

Technical Design Characteristics

Revenue Collection Mechanisms

- Without subsidies, resource mobilization is limited when everyone in the pool is poor.
- Many of the poorest do not join since they cannot afford premiums.
- Pro-poor orientation is undermined by regressive flat-rate contributions and by a lack of subsidies or premium exemption, which create a financial barrier for the poor.
- Community-based voluntary prepayment schemes are also prone to adverse selection.
- Few schemes have reinsurance or other mechanisms to buffer against large external shocks.

Revenue-Pooling and Risk-Sharing Arrangements

- The scope for transfers within very small pools is limited (often fewer than 1,000 members per scheme).

Purchasing and Resource Allocation

- Without subsidies, the poorest are often left out (for whom to buy).
- The benefit package is often very restricted (what to buy, in what form, and what to exclude).
- Providers can often exert monopoly power during price and payment negotiations.

Management

- Community leaders are as vulnerable to adverse incentives and corruption as national bureaucrats.

- Even with external assistance, absorptive capacity in management training is limited.

- Extensive community consultation is time consuming and can lead to conflicting advice.

- Most schemes do not use modern information management systems.

Organizational Structure

- Even widely distributed organizational configurations may have difficulty reaching deep into the rural and informal sectors.

- There are often conflicting incentives, especially among extensive decision rights, soft budget constraints at time of deficits (bailouts by governments and external sources of funding such as nongovernmental organizations), limited competitive pressures in the product markets, and lack of financing to cover the poorest population groups.

- The less-organized schemes are often cut off from formal sector networks.

BOX 1.3 *continued*

Institutional Environment

- Government stewardship and oversight function are often very weak, leading to a poor regulatory environment and lack of remedies in the case of fraud and abuse.

- Ownership and governance arrangements are often driven by nonhealth and financial protection objectives.

- Choice in strategic purchasing is limited by small number of providers in rural areas.

- True consumer choice is often limited by lack of a full insurance and product market, leading to (a) adverse selection (signing on only the better-off, working age, and healthy), (b) moral hazard (members making unnecessary claims because they have insurance coverage), (c) free-rider effect (households waiting until they think they will be sick before joining), and (d) information asymmetry (for example, concealing pre-existing conditions).

Sources: Bennett, Creese, and Monasch (1998); Carrin, Desmet, and Basaza (2001).

Based on this typology, the Asia review ranked the community-financing schemes examined according to their potential impacts on several intermediate outcome indicators (coverage, equity in financing, efficiency and cost containment in service delivery, access, quality, and degree of risk sharing). The results are summarized in table 1.9.

Based on this framework, the review made the following observations:

- Rural households and urban poor households are willing to prepay a portion of their health services. The resources that can be raised in this manner depend on both economic and social factors.

- Since the membership of many community-financing schemes consists of poor households, their ability to raise significant resources to pay for health care is limited by the community's overall income, exposure to out-of-pocket payment when not enrolled, availability and size of subsidies, and satisfaction with the services provided. The poor and near poor are more motivated to prepay if their contributions are supplemented by government or donor subsidies. For the poorest households, this subsidy has to be a large share of the total payment.

- The social factors that influence membership rates include a sense of kinship, mutual community concern, and trust and confidence in the management of the scheme.

TABLE 1.9 Potential Value Added by Types of Community-Financing Schemes

Type of community-financing scheme	Who controls use of fund	Population to be covered and raise funds	Equity in financing	Increase efficiency and reduce cost	Improve access	Improve quality	Greater risk pooling
Prepay user fees	Government	Low	Low	None	Low	Low	Low
	Individual households	Modest	Low	None	Modest	Low	Low
Cooperative health care	Local community and special purpose NGO	High	Low	High	High	High	Modest unless w/ gov't subsidy
Community-based third-party insurance	Community	Cover higher income families	Low	Low	High for those insured	Low	High
Provider-sponsored insurance	Hospitals	Cover higher income families	Low	Low	High for those insured	Low	High
Provider or consumer cooperative	Cooperatives	Cover member	Low	High	High	High	Medium

Source: Hsiao (2001).

FIGURE 1.7   Hospitalization and Impoverishment

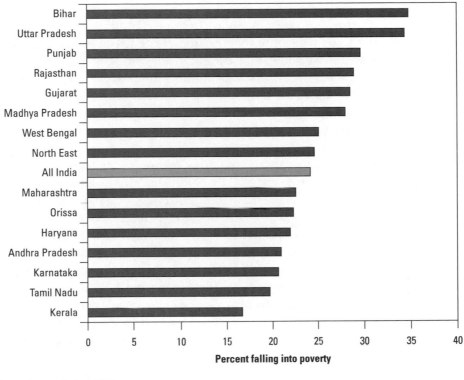

Source: Peters and others (2001).

- A major additional value of well-performing community-financing schemes is expanded access to quality services, improved efficiency of management and service delivery, and cost containment.

- Governmental and nongovernmental organizations (NGOs) often catalyzed the startup of the community-financing schemes in question and contributed to its management and sustainability.

- Finally, members appear to prefer coverage for both primary care and more expensive hospital care. Since many schemes do not mobilize sufficient resources to pay for both, a number of communities opt for primary care coverage, which they will use regularly for their basic health care needs, rather than insurance coverage for rarer and more expensive events that may only happen once or twice in a lifetime and whose concept is often poorly understood. This creates a tension or trade-off between individual needs and demands for basic care and household and community needs for financial protection (see figure 1.7).

Discussion of Main Findings from Africa Regional Review

The review of selected Africa experiences (Arhin-Tenkorang 2001) emphasized that a common feature of many of the reforms introduced during the past two decades have consisted of copayments to influence utilization patterns and direct out-of-pocket user charges to mobilize much-needed additional resources (Vogel 1990). Most of the population currently does not benefit from formal insurance coverage, and government expenditures often do not meet the basic health needs of the poor, let alone the entire population (Abel-Smith and Rawal 1994). These user charges add significantly to the financial hardship of poor households, often fully exposed to the financial risks associated with illness. This has been especially true during recent years, due to the rising incidence and prevalence of HIV/AIDS, tuberculosis, and other communicable diseases.

A central premise of the Africa review is that individuals in the informal sector of poor countries cannot access appropriate health care—particularly curative care—at the time of need partially because of lack of adequate insurance coverage (Arhin-Tenkorang 2001). Although preventive measures may have long-term payoffs in improving the overall welfare and productivity of the population, the income shock associated with seeking access to curative and palliative care has become such a great financial burden for the poor that some form of insurance coverage has to be considered an essential part of any serious poverty alleviation strategy.

The first section of the chapter conceptualizes how the interaction between several design features and institutional factors influences scheme performance in terms of risk protection and resource mobilization. In the absence of risk protection, several African studies demonstrated that poor households often deferred visits to formal health facilities until their illnesses became quite severe or used ineffective self-medication sometimes injurious to their health, leading to more severe health and financial consequences than would have been the case had care been sought earlier.

Key design features included the methodology, nature, and quality of the data used to determine contribution levels, benefit packages, and subsidy levels. The argument is that appropriate specifications require (a) data on the target population's willingness-to-pay (WTP) and ability-to-pay, often not collected or available, (b) data on projected costs of the benefits to be consumed, and (c) operational modalities that facilitate interaction between individuals in an informal environment and in a range of formal organizations. The review concludes that in an informal environment, decisions cannot rely on such written information because the needed data are usually not available in this form. To be effective and affordable, activities undertaken by community-financing schemes must be based on simple and directly observable behavior patterns with low transaction costs.

Key institutional features included the degree of congruence between the scheme's operating rules and the participating population's normal behavior patterns. They also included the degree of participating health care providers' past experience with third-party payments and contractual arrangements. The review found that these institutional factors had a significant influence on the nature and extent of community participation in any given scheme, as well as the quality of its management and monitoring of performance. The review did not examine other institutional factors, such as government regulations and laws governing insurance and health care provision.

The second part of the chapter proposes the design features of several potential "high population schemes" for Africa's informal sector and assesses their performances with respect to risk protection and resource mobilization. Potential "high population" schemes examined include the Abota Village Insurance Scheme (Guinea-Bissau); Bwamanda Hospital Insurance Scheme (Democratic Republic of Congo); Carte d'Assurance Maladie, or CAM, program (Burundi); Dangme West Health Insurance Scheme (Ghana); Nkoranza Community Financing Health Insurance Scheme (Ghana); and Community Health Fund, or CHF, (Tanzania). These schemes had large target populations and provided a comprehensive range of benefits and geographically accessible care to its members. Key factors influencing enrollment appeared to include a matching of the premium to the willingness and ability to pay, availability of government subsidies for the poor who cannot afford the basic premium; and ready access to basic care for common health problems and emergency care—both geographic proximity and availability of range of basic services appeared to significantly affect enrollment.

The final part of the chapter presents a set of policy measures that national and international health policymakers may consider implementing to increase the level of risk protection provided for informal sector populations. The financial risk protection and resource mobilization that can be achieved by any given scheme appears to be influenced by the compatibility between the way it is designed and operated and the behavior of the individuals and households from the informal sector that enroll in the schemes. The enrollment rate of a given population with such schemes appears to reflect the target population's WTP, in turn, closely related to its ATP. In most cases, some central government support in the form of fiscal transfers, budget allocations, or both is necessary, given the small volume of resources available at low-income levels in poor communities. Schemes that are operated as solidarity-based partnerships with service providers appear to create additional incentives to increase efficiency and accountability. The authors conclude that national government policies, a legal framework, and financial support for these organizations are likely to be a good investment of scarce government resources. The authors emphasize that, in the absence of established practices in the design of community-financing schemes, donor funding, procedures, and regulations supporting community financing through communities, local governments and local NGOs need further pilot testing to identify the elements that would be needed to expand the schemes or to go to scale with them.

Discussion of Main Findings from Microlevel Household Survey Analysis

Determinants of Social Inclusion in Community Financing

In terms of the determinants of social inclusion through community financing, the results from the microlevel household survey analysis are varied. Table 1.10

TABLE 1.10 Statistically Significant Determinants of Inclusion in Community Financing

	Rwanda	Senegal	India (1)	India (2)	Thailand
			Model		
	Logit	Probit	Logit	Logit	Logit
			Dependent variable		
Dependent variable	Proportion of population enrolled in 1 of 66 schemes	Proportion of population enrolled in 1 of 4 schemes	Proportion of population enrolled in SEWA-insurance	Proportion of population enrolled in SEWA-insurance	Proportion of population that purchased new health card, continued, dropped out, never purchased
		Independent variables: individual & household characteristics			
Income/assets	No	**Yes**	No	No	**Yes**
Age	No	No	**Yes**	**Yes**	No
Education	**Yes**	No	No	No	**Yes**
Gender	No	No	—	—	No
Health status	No	—	**Yes**	**Yes**	**Yes**
Household size	**Yes**	No	**Yes**	No	—
Marital status		**Yes**	No	No	No
Religion	—	**Yes**	—	No	—
Distance of household from scheme provider	**Yes**	—	—	—	—
		Independent variables: community characteristics			
Community marker for unobservable characteristics	**Yes**	**Yes**	—	—	—
Solidarity	N/A	**Yes**	N/A	N/A	N/A

Note: Yes—variable is significant at least at the 10 percent level. No—variable is not significant. (—)—not included in the particular model.

presents the determinants that were found statistically significant in the five household surveys (Gumber 2001; Jütting 2001; Ranson 2001; Schneider and Diop 2001; Supakankunti 2001).

- *Income and other socioeconomic determinants.* In Senegal and Thailand, household income was a significant determinant of being member of a prepayment scheme; in Rwanda and India income was not significant.

- *Other individual and household characteristics.* Health status was included in the analysis of the Rwanda, Thailand, and both India surveys. In all four surveys, the analysis confirmed the presence of the adverse selection that characterizes voluntary prepayment schemes. Patients with recent illness episodes or with chronic illnesses are more likely to purchase a prepayment plan. Distance of the household from the provider of the scheme was included in the Rwanda analysis. Households less than 30 minutes from the health facility of the scheme were four times more likely to belong to the prepayment scheme than households living farther away.

- *Community characteristics.* Dummy variables for community characteristics were significant predictors of the probability of enrolling in the prepayment scheme (Senegal and Rwanda).

Determinants of Financial Protection in Community Financing

The results are varied in terms of the determinants of financial protection through community financing. Table 1.11 presents the determinants found statistically significant in four of the household surveys. The household survey conducted in Thailand did not permit analysis of the determinants of out-of-pocket payments and was therefore excluded. The key findings from this part of the study include:

- *Insurance effect.* In three of the five household surveys, membership in a community-financing scheme was a significant determinant of the probability of using health care and in reducing out-of-pocket payments. This confirms our original hypothesis that even small-scale prepayment and risk pooling reduce financial barriers to health care (Rwanda, Senegal, and India).

- *Socioeconomic determinants.* The analysis indicated that even with insurance, low income remains a significant constraint to health care utilization and ability to pay out-of-pocket payments (Rwanda, Senegal, and India).

- *Other determinants.* Distance from scheme provider was a significant determinant of the likelihood of using health care (Rwanda and Senegal).

Discussion of Main Findings from Macrolevel Cross-Country Analysis

A first observation was that most routine national statistical sources do not include data on the share of overall financing channeled through either community-based or private health insurance schemes (Carrin and others 2001). The analysis therefore had to focus on the extent of collective risk sharing provided at low-income levels through different combinations of general tax revenues and social insurance.

The equations have been estimated with the ordinary least squares method, using data for the explanatory variables HEC, EDU, and PHE percents that pertain to the year 1997. The Gini index pertains to specific years, depending upon the country, in 1986–99. In this synthesis chapter, we present only the "best" regressions[2] in summary tables 1.12 and 1.13 in the appendix. Except for the functional form of the regression for DALE, we present only the results of the logit specification. The estimation results for the *basic model* presented in summary table 1.12 are discussed next.

TABLE 1.11 Summary Findings: Statistically Significant (at Least at 10 Percent) Determinants of Utilization and Out-of-Pocket Expenditure Patterns

	Rwanda		Senegal		India (1)		India (2)	
	Utilization	OOPs	Utilization	OOPs	Utilization	OOPs	Utilization	OOPs
Model								
	Logit	Log-linear conditional on (use > 0)	Logit	Log-linear conditional on (use > 0)	Logit	Log-linear conditional on (use > 0)	Logit	Log-linear conditional on (use > 0)
Dependent variable	Proportion of sample w/ at least one visit to professional health care provider	Total illness-related to out-of-pocket payment per episode of illness for the full episode	Proportion of sample w/ at least one hospitalization	Out-of-pocket spending for hospitalization	Proportion of sample reporting any health care use	Total annual direct and indirect cost of health care use	Proportion of sample w/ at least one hospitalization	Total annual out-of-pocket payment for use of hospital care
Independent variables: Insurance effect								
Scheme membership	Yes	Yes	Yes	Yes	Yes	No	No	Yes
Independent variables: Individual and household characteristics								
Income/assets	Yes	Only for poorest quartile	Only for richest terzile	Yes	No	Yes	Only for richest quintile	Only for richest quintile
Age	Yes	No	No	Yes	No	No	Only for oldest group	Only for oldest group
Education	No	No	No	No	No	—	No	Yes
Gender	No	Yes	Yes	No	No	—	—	—
Health status/severity of illness	Yes	No	—	Yes	Only for very severe	Yes	Yes	Yes
Household size	No	No	—	—	No	Only small hh size	No	Yes
Marital status	—	—	—	—	No	—	No	No
Religion	—	—	—	—	—	—	Yes	Yes
Distance of household from scheme provider	Yes	No	Yes	No	—	—	—	—

Note: Yes—variable is significant at least at the 10 percent level. No—variable is not significant. (—)—not included in the particular model. Other control variables were included in some of the studies but, as they are not discussed in the paper, we did not include them in this table.

First, concerning the *level of health (DALE)*, the effects of DARS, HEC, and EDU are as expected and are statistically significant at the 1 percent significance level.

Second, from the equation for the *level of responsiveness (IR)*, we see that HEC and EDU do not have a statistically significant impact. One major reason is likely to be that the index of responsiveness contains elements of both respect for persons and client orientation and that both are influenced differently by HEC and EDU. For instance, HEC may be important in explaining client orientation, but it may not be when explaining respect for persons. Therefore, when analyzing the determinants of the overall index of responsiveness, the effect of HEC may disappear. Notice, however, that both the coefficients of DARS and DMRS have the expected sign and are statistically significant.

Third, the explanatory power of the regression for the *index of fair financing (IFFC)* is minimal; DARS does not have a statistically significant impact on the IFFC. We submit that the major reason for this unsatisfactory result is the relatively small sample size. Moreover, the sample did not include sufficient data on countries with advanced and low risk sharing. For instance, the (full sample) data on advanced risk sharing are those of Bulgaria, Jamaica, Kyrgyz Republic, Romania, and Russia and do inadequately reflect the experience of high-income countries with either social health insurance or general taxation financing.

Fourth, in the equation for the *distribution of responsiveness (IRD)*, the coefficient of DARS is statistically significant. The impact of DSHI is statistically insignificant. Fifth, the results for the *index of equality of child survival (IECS)* show that both DARS and DMRS have statistically significant impacts.

We next present the estimation results for the *enlarged model* with the Gini index as an explanatory variable in the equations for the distributional measures. The results are presented in table 1.13 (appendix 1A). In the *fair financing equation (IFFC)*, which has very low explanatory power, the coefficient of the Gini index has the anticipated sign but is not statistically significant. The coefficient of DARS is also not statistically significant.

Related to the *distribution of responsiveness (IRD)*, the result shows significant impacts of both DARS and DMRS, as well as of the Gini index. All coefficients have the expected sign. One can conclude that these risk-sharing arrangements are efficient in counterbalancing the overall effect of income inequality. A threshold for the Gini indexes can be computed, indicating the value above which risk sharing is no longer able to counteract the effect of overall income inequality. In the case of a country with an advanced risk-sharing scheme, the threshold value is 57.9. In the case of medium risk-sharing schemes, the threshold is 26.3. From these estimates we can infer that advanced risk-sharing schemes are more effective in counteracting the effects of overall income inequality in society. For example, let us assume that a country has a Gini coefficient of 35. If this country has an advanced risk-sharing scheme, its effect will outweigh the impact of income equality: the combined effect will be +0.8588. However, if the country has a medium risk-sharing arrangement, the combined effect will be –0.3252.

In the regression result related to the *inequality of child survival (IECS),* the sign of the Gini coefficients is against our expectations. Surprisingly, the Gini coefficient is also statistically significant at the 10 percent level. The coefficient of DARS has the anticipated sign, however, and is statistically significant at the 1 percent level.

Inclusion of the *interaction variables* with PHE percent in the equations did not result in a general improvement of the estimation results. For instance, in a number of cases, the coefficients of DARS have the correct sign but are statistically insignificant. In other instances, the coefficient of DARS has a negative sign. Further estimations were done with *transformed* interaction variables. In the case of the interaction between DARS and PHE percents, the variable constructed was DARS*(PHE percent – 0.5). The coefficient associated with this variable reveals the impact of the difference between the PHE percent and a threshold of 50 percent. The results for IR, IFFC, IRD, and IECS are not satisfactory: the coefficient of the new interaction variable has the wrong sign, is not statistically significant, or both. Only in the case of DALE did we obtain a satisfactory result: both the coefficients of DARS and the interaction variable have the expected sign and are statistically significant. This result is presented in table 1.13 (appendix 1A). In other words, for advanced risk-sharing systems with a PHE percent above 50, the level of the PHE percent reinforces the "average" effect of DARS. For instance, in the case of Oman with a PHE percent of 63.31, the combined impact of DARS and DARS*(PHE percent – 0.5) becomes –0.2694. For countries with a PHE percent below 50 (Chile, Republic of Korea, Brunei Darussalam, and United Arab Emirates), the initial effect of DARS is weakened. For instance, for Chile with a PHE percent of 40.1, the combined effect of DARS and DARS*(PHE percent – 0.5) on the dependent variable becomes –0.1637.

Key conclusions can be drawn from the various estimates. A first conclusion is that the extent of advanced risk sharing, as measured by the dummy variable DARS, is significant in the equations for four of the five goal measurements. No effect could be found in the case of the index of fair financing, but we submit this is due to the small sample size. In addition, in at least two of these measurements (level of responsiveness and distribution of health), the variable DMRS also has been shown to have a statistically significant impact.

Second, when enlarging the set of explanatory variables in the models for the distributional measures with the Gini index, DARS remains statistically significant in the equations for IRD and IECS. In addition, DMRS has a statistically significant impact in the equations for IRD. An additional interpretation emerges from the results, namely that risk sharing corrects for, or may even outweigh, the negative effect of overall income inequality on the fair financing index and the index of distribution of responsiveness.

Third, using interaction terms with PHE percent leads to plausible results for DALE only: the level of PHE percent reinforces the average positive effect of advanced risk sharing.

An analysis with preliminary updated data was also undertaken; since publication of the *World Health Report 2000,* WHO has developed updated estimates for the level (HEC) and share of public health expenditure in total health expenditure (PHE percent). When using updated data for HEC in the equations for DALE and IR, similar results to those presented here are obtained (in terms of explanatory power, sign, and statistical significance of coefficients). The use of the updated PHE percent does not significantly change the estimates for the equations with the interaction terms. Estimates of the index of fair financing (IFFC) were also obtained for an additional 30 countries. Reestimation of the equations, using an enlarged sample of 50, now leads to two interesting results: the advanced risk-sharing dummy variable DARS exerts a statistically significant effect on the fair financing index; and the Gini index has a statistically significant impact on IFFC but is counterbalanced by a health-financing system characterized by advanced risk sharing. These preliminary results prove to be more in line with those obtained for the other distributional measures.

CONCLUSIONS AND RECOMMENDATIONS

Most community-financing schemes have evolved in the context of severe economic constraints, political instability, and lack of good governance. Usually, government taxation capacity is weak, formal mechanisms of social protection for vulnerable populations absent, and government oversight of the informal health sector lacking. In this context of extreme public sector failure, community involvement in the financing of health care provides a critical, though insufficient, first step in the long march toward improved access to health care for the poor and social protection against the cost of illness. It should be regarded as a complement to—not as a substitute for—strong government involvement in health care financing and risk management related to the cost of illness.

Based on an extensive survey of the literature, the main strengths of community-financing schemes are the degree of outreach penetration achieved through community participation, their contribution to financial protection against illness, and increase in access to health care by low-income rural and informal sector workers. Their main weaknesses are the low volume of revenues that can be mobilized from poor communities, the frequent exclusion of the poorest from participation in such schemes without some form of subsidy, the small size of the risk pool, the limited management capacity that exists in rural and low-income contexts, and isolation from the more comprehensive benefits often available through more formal health-financing mechanisms and provider networks.

The results of the macrolevel cross-country analysis presented in this report give empirical support to the hypothesis that risk sharing in health financing matters in terms of its impact on both the level and distribution of health, financial fairness, and responsiveness indicators. The results even suggest that risk sharing corrects for, and may outweigh, the negative effect of overall income inequality, suggesting that financial protection against the cost of illness may be a more effective poverty alleviation strategy in some settings than direct income support.

FIGURE 1.8   Stages of Financial Protection

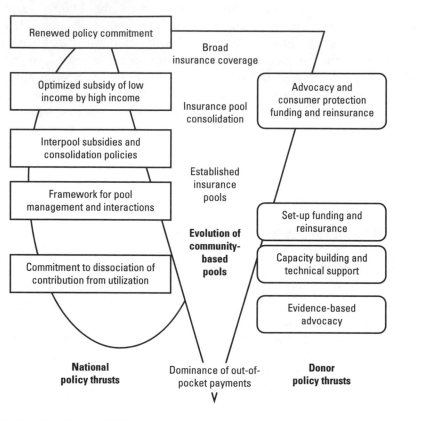

Source: Adapted from Arhin-Tenkorang (2001).

The results of the microlevel household data analysis indicate that prepayment and risk sharing through community involvement in health care financing—no matter how small—increases access by poor populations to basic health services and protects them to a limited extent against the impoverishing effects of illness. Community involvement alone is not sufficient in preventing social exclusion since the very poorest often do not participate fully in these schemes. However, the study provides evidence that this constraint in reaching the poorest could be overcome through well-targeted design features and implementation arrangements.

The Asia regional review supports many of these conclusions. In particular, the review emphasizes that, although income is a key constraint to participation by the very poorest, even they are often willing to participate if their contributions are supplemented by a government subsidy and if the benefits they receive provide access to quality services that address their most frequent health problems. In the context of extreme resource constraints, this creates a tension or trade-off between prepayment for basic services and the need for insurance coverage for rarer, more expensive, and life-threatening events that may only happen once or twice in a lifetime. This highlights an area of market failure relating to voluntary community involvement in health care financing that needs to be addressed by appropriate government policies since it is precisely during hospitalization that many of the poor become even more impoverished.

More rigorous research is still needed on understanding the institutional strengths and weaknesses of community involvement in health care financing, and in monitoring and evaluating their impacts on financial protection, increasing access to needed health care, and combating social exclusion of the poor. Yet the research for this report points to five key policies available to governments for improving the effectiveness and sustainability of community financing: (1) increased and well-targeted subsidies to pay the premiums of low-income populations, (2) insurance to protect against expenditure fluctuations and reinsurance to enlarge the effective size of small risk pools, (3) effective prevention and case-management techniques to limit expenditure fluctuations, (4) technical support to strengthen the management capacity of local schemes, and (5) establishment and strengthening of links with the formal financing and provider networks.

See page 46 for acknowledgments, notes, and references.

APPENDIX 1A. STATISTICAL DATA (SUMMARY TABLES)

TABLE 1.12   Estimation Results[a] for the Basic Models

Explanatory variables	DALE[b] Ln (80– DALE)	IR[c] (Logit)	IFFC[b] (Logit)	IRD[d] (Logit)	IECS[e] (Logit)
Constant	4.9423	−0.4896	2.2874	1.6327	0.2798
	(0.3328)	(0.2160)	(0.2786)	(0.4507)	(0.2038)
	(14.8493)	(−2.2663)	(8.2099)	(3.6228)	(1.3329)
HEC	−0.1919	0.0000			
	(0.0197)	(0.0003)			
	(−9.7498)	(0.1150)			
EDU	−0.2141	0.0032			
	(0.0834)	(0.0026)			
	(−2.5684)	(1.2540)			
DARS	−0.2963	0.7244	−0.1146	4.2257	6.6269
	(0.0654)	(0.2244)	(0.6072)	(0.8228)	(0.3868)
	(−4.5321)	(3.2275)	(−0.1888)	(5.1355)	(17.1343)
DSHI		−0.2521		−1.4049	
		(0.1987)		(0.9107)	
		(−1.2688)		(−1.5427)	
DMRS		0.2673		0.7217	1.0737
		(0.1148)		(0.5355)	(0.4202)
		(2.3294)		(1.3478)	2.5550
DMRS1					−0.1079
					(0.4607)
					(−0.2343)
DMRS2					−0.6458
					(0.3995)
					(−1.6165)
R–squared	0.7874	0.5678	0.0021	0.5749	0.8778
Adjusted R–squared	0.7821	0.4597	−0.0566	0.5276	0.8671
S.E. of regression	0.2639	0.2134	1.0791	1.1924	0.7350
Ak. Info criterion	0.2049	−0.0525	3.0894	3.3097	2.3149
Sample size	124	26	19	31	51

a. The first and second coefficients in the parentheses refer to the standard error and t-statistic, respectively.

b. Restricted samples.

c. Bulgaria is excluded from the sample.

d. Chile and Poland are excluded from the full sample.

e. Uzbekistan is excluded from the restricted sample.

TABLE 1.13   Estimation Results[a] for the Enlarged Models

Explanatory variables	IFFC[b] (Logit)	IRD (Logit)	IECS[b] (Logit)	DALE[b] Ln(80− DALE))
Constant	2.8260	3.0610	−0.7471	4.9446
	(1.3698)	(0.7956)	(0.9164)	(0.3306)
	(2.0630)	(3.8539)	(−0.8153)	(14.9580)
Gini	−0.0119	−0.0375	0.0355	
	(0.0296)	(0.0180)	(0.0206)	
	(−0.4020)	(−2.0853)	(−0.8153)	
DARS	−0.2568	2.1713	5.3537	−0.2088
	(0.7162)	(0.5222)	(0.5531)	(0.0843)
	(−0.3586)	(4.1577)	(9.6789)	(−2.4774)
DARS*[PHE percent− 0.5]				−0.4556
				(0.2798)
				(−1.6284)
DMRS		0.9873		
		(0.4637)		
		(2.1291)		
HEC				−0.1897
				(0.0196)
				−9.6837
EDU				−0.2166
				(0.0828)
				(−2.6155)
R−squared	0.0121	0.5191	0.7053	0.7920
Adjusted R−squared	−0.1114	0.4590	0.6906	0.7850
S.E. of regression	1.1067	0.9320	1.1912	0.2621
Ak. Info criterion	3.1846	2.8286	3.2550	0.1990
Sample size	19	28	43	124

a. The first and second coefficients in the parentheses refer to the standard error and t-statistic, respectively.

b. Restricted samples.

Acknowledgments: Valuable guidance on methodological issues was provided by Adam Wagstaff. We are also indebted to the following individuals for data access, guidance on research methodologies, reviews, and other indirect contributions: Christian Jacquier, Christian Baeaza, Michael Cichon, Chris Murray, Kei Kawabatak, Christopher Lovelace, Helen Saxenian, Jack Langenbrunner, David Peters, George Schieber, Charlie Griffin, Agnes Soucat, Abdo S. Yazbeck, Mariam Claeson, Flavia Bustreo, Steve Cummings, and Shanta Devarajan.

The authors are also grateful for the access provided to parallel and ongoing research on community financing by the World Bank, the World Health Organization (WHO), and the International Labour Organisation (ILO), with important inputs from Harvard University, the London School of Hygiene and Tropical Medicine, the University of Lyon, Partnerships for Health Reform—Abt Associates Inc. (USA), the National Council for Economic Research (India), the Center for Development Research (ZEF) (Germany), and Chulalongkorn University Faculty of Economics (Thailand).

The authors are grateful to WHO for having provided an opportunity to contribute to the work of the Commission on Macroeconomics and Health and to the World Bank for having published the material in this chapter as an HNP Discussion Paper.

NOTES

1. This model is similar to the two-part demand model developed as part of the Rand Health Insurance experiment to estimate demand for health care services (Duan and others 1982; Manning and others 1987). For a recent application of the model that analyzes the access impact of school health insurance in Egypt, see Yip and Berman 2001.

2. "Best" according to the adjusted R-squared and/or the Akaike criterion, as well as the theoretical consistency of the model. In addition, we present only the results using restricted samples where data points have been deleted from the "full" samples because of uncertainty in the risk-sharing classification, or restricted samples with additional deletion of influential data.

REFERENCES

Abel-Smith, B. 1988. "The Rise and Decline of the Early HMOs: Some International Experiences." *Milbank Quarterly* 66(4): 694–719.

Abel-Smith, B., and P. Rawal. 1994. "Employer's Willingness to Pay: The Case for Compulsory Health Insurance in Tanzania." *Health Policy and Planning* 9(4): 409–18.

ADB (Asian Development Bank). 2000. *Finance for the Poor: Microfinance Development Strategy.* Manilla.

Arhin-Tenkorang, D. C. 1994. "The Health Card Insurance Scheme in Burundi: A Social Asset or a Non-Viable Venture?" *Social Science and Medicine* 39(6): 861–70.

———. 1995. *Rural Health Insurance: A Viable Alternative to User Fees.* London School of Hygiene and Tropical Medicine, Discussion Paper. London.

———. 2000. "Mobilizing Resources for Health: The Case for User Fees Re-Visited." Report submitted to Working Group 3 of the Commission on Macroeconomics and Health, Jeffrey D. Sachs (Chairman). World Health Organization (WHO), Geneva.

————. 2001. "Health Insurance for the Informal Sector in Africa: Design Features, Risk Protection, and Resource Mobilization." Report submitted to Working Group 3 of the Commission on Macroeconomics and Health, Jeffrey D. Sachs (Chairman). WHO, Geneva.

Arrow, K. W. 1963. "Uncertainty and the Welfare Economics of Medical Care." *American Economic Review* 53(5): 940–73.

Atim, C. 1998. *Contribution of Mutual Health Organizations to Financing, Delivery, and Access to Health Care: Synthesis of Research in Nine West and Central African Countries.* Technical Report 18. Partnerships for Health Reform Project, Abt Associates Inc., Bethesda, Md.

————. 1999. "Social Movements and Health Insurance: A Critical Evaluation of Voluntary, Non-Profit Insurance Schemes with Case Studies from Ghana and Cameroon." *Social Science and Medicine* 48(7): 881–96.

Atkinson A. B., and J. E. Stiglitz. 1980. *Lectures on Public Economics.* Maidenhead, Berkshire: McGraw-Hill.

Barer, L. M., T. E. Getzen, and G. L. Stoddart, eds. 1998. *Health, Health Care, and Health Economics: Perspectives on Distribution.* Chichester, West Sussex: John Wiley and Sons.

Bator, F. 1958. "The Anatomy of Market Failure." *Quarterly Journal of Economics* 72(3): 351–79.

Bennett S., A. Creese, and R. Monasch. 1998. *Health Insurance Schemes for People Outside Formal Sector Employment.* ARA Paper No. 16. WHO, Geneva.

Brown, W., and C. Churchill. 2000. *Insurance Provision in Low-Income Communities: Part II—Initial Lessons from Microinsurance Experiments for the Poor.* Microenterprise Best Practices Project, Development Alternatives Inc., Bethesda, Md.

Carrin, G., M. Desmet, and R. Basaza. 2001. "Social Health Insurance Development in Low-Income Developing Countries: New Roles for Government and Non-Profit Health Insurance Organisations." In X. Scheil-Adlung and D. D. Hoskins, eds., *Building Social Security: The Challenge for Privatization.* Geneva: International Social Security Association.

Carrin, G., R. Zeramdini, P. Musgrove, J-P. Poullier, N. Valentine, and K. Xu. 2001. *The Impact of the Degree of Risk-Sharing in Health Financing on Health System Attainment.* Report submitted to Working Group 3 of the Commission on Macroeconomics and Health, Jeffrey D. Sachs (Chairman). WHO, Geneva.

Claeson, M., C. C. Griffin, T. A. Johnston, M. McLachlan, A. Wagstaff, and A. S. Yazbeck. 2001. *Health, Nutrition, and Population Sourcebook for the Poverty Reduction Strategy Paper.* HNP Discussion Paper. Washington, D.C.: World Bank.

Criel, B., P. Van der Stuyft, and W. Van Lerberghe. 1999. "The Bwamanda Hospital Insurance Scheme: Effective for Whom? A Study of Its Impact on Hospitalisation and Utilisation Patterns." *Social Science and Medicine* 48(7): 879–911.

Dave, P. 1991. "Community and Self-Financing in Voluntary Health Programmes in India." *Health Policy and Planning* 6(1): 20–31.

DeRoeck, D., J. Knowles, T. Wittenberg, L. Raney, and P. Cordova. 1996. *Rural Health Services at Seguridad Social Campesino Facilities: Analyses of Facility and Household Surveys.* Health Financing and Sustainability Project, Technical Report No. 13. Partnerships for Health Reform Project, Abt Associates, Inc., Bethesda, Md.

Desmet, A., A. Q. Chowdhury, and K. Islam, M.D. 1999. "The Potential for Social Mobilization in Bangladesh: The Organization and Functioning of Two Health Insurance Schemes." *Social Science and Medicine* 48: 925–38.

Diop, F., A. Yazbeck, and R. Bitran. 1995. "The Impact of Alternative Cost Recovery Schemes on Access and Equity in Niger." *Health Policy and Planning* 10(3): 223–40.

Dordick G. 1997. *Something Left to Lose: Personal Relations and Survival among New York's Homeless*. Philadelphia: Temple University Press.

Dror, D., and C. Jacquier. 1999. "Microinsurance: Extending Health Insurance to the Excluded." *International Social Security Review* 52(1): 71–97.

Dror, D., A. S. Preker, and M. Jakab. 2002. "Role of Communities in Combating Social Exclusion." In D. Dror and A. S. Preker, eds., *Social Reinsurance: A New Approach to Sustainable Community Health Financing*. Washington, D.C.: World Bank/International Labour Organisation (ILO).

Duan, N., W. G. Manning Jr., C. M. Morris, and J. P. Newhouse. 1982. *A Comparison of Alternative Models for the Demand for Medical Care*. Report R-2754-HHS. The Rand Corporation, Santa Monica, Calif.

Evans, P. 1992. "The State as Problem and Solution: Predation, Embedded Autonomy, and Structural Change." In Stephan Haggard and Robert Kaufman, eds., *The Politics of Economic Adjustment: International Constraints, Distributive Conflicts, and the State*. Princeton, N.J.: Princeton University Press.

———. 1995. *Embedded Autonomy: States and Industrial Transformation*. Princeton, N.J.: Princeton University Press.

———. 1996. "Government Action, Social Capital, and Development: Reviewing the Evidence on Synergy." *World Development* 24(6): 1119–32.

Evans, R. G. 1984. *Strained Mercy*. Toronto: Butterworth.

Foster, G. 1982. "Community Development and Primary Health Care: Their Conceptual Similarities." *Medical Anthropology* 6(3): 183–95.

Granovetter, M. 1973. "The Strength of Weak Ties." *American Journal of Sociology* 78: 1360–80.

Guhan, S. 1994. "Social Security Options for Developing Countries." *International Labour Review* 33(1): 35–53.

Gumber A. 2001. *Hedging the Health of the Poor: The Case for Community Financing in India*. World Bank, HNP Discussion Paper. Washington, D.C.

Gumber, A., and V. Kulkarni. 2000. "Health Insurance for Informal Sector: Case Study of Gujarat." *Economic and Political Weekly*, 30 September, 3607–13.

Gwatkin, D. 2001. "Poverty and Inequalities in Health within Developing Countries: Filling the Information Gap." In D. Leon and G. Walt, eds., *Poverty, Inequality, and Health: An International Perspective*. Oxford: Oxford University Press.

Harding, A., and A. S. Preker. 2001. *A Framework for Understanding Organizational Reforms in the Hospital Sector*. World Bank, HNP Discussion Paper. Washington, D.C.

Hsiao, W. C. 2001. *Unmet Health Needs of Two Billion: Is Community Financing a Solution?* Report submitted to Working Group 3 of the Commission on Macroeconomics and Health, Jeffrey D. Sachs (Chairman). WHO, Geneva.

ILO (International Labour Organisation). 2000a. *Mutuelles de santé en Afrique: Charactéristiques et mise en place. Manuel de formateurs.* Programme Stratégies et Technique contre l'Exclusion sociale et la Pauvreté, Département de Sécurité Sociale (STEP). Geneva.

———. 2000b. *World Labour Report: Income Security and Social Protection in a Changing World.* Geneva.

———. 2001. "Mutuelles de santé et associations de microentrepreneurs—Guide." *Programme Stratégies et Technique contre l'Exclusion Sociale et la Pauvreté,* Département de Sécurité Sociale (STEP), Small Enterprise Development Programme (SEED). Geneva.

Jakab, M., and C. Krishnan. 2001. *Community Involvement in Health Care Financing: A Survey of the Literature on the Impact, Strengths, and Weaknesses.* Report submitted to Working Group 3 of the Commission on Macroeconomics and Health, Jeffrey D. Sachs (Chairman). WHO, Geneva.

Jakab, M., A. S. Preker, C. Krishnan, P. Schneider, F. Diop, J. Jütting, A. Gumber, K. Ranson, and S. Supakankunti. 2001. *Social Inclusion and Financial Protection through Community Financing: Initial Results from Five Household Surveys.* Report submitted to Working Group 3 of the Commission on Macroeconomics and Health, Jeffrey D. Sachs (Chairman). WHO, Geneva.

Jütting, J. 2000. *Do Mutual Health Insurance Schemes Improve the Access to Health Care? Preliminary Results from a Household Survey in Rural Senegal.* Paper presented at the International Conference on Health Systems Financing in Low-Income African and Asian Countries, November 30-December 1, Centre d'Etudes et de Recherches sur le Développement International (CERDI), Clermont-Ferrand, France.

———. 2001. *The Impact of Health Insurance on the Access to Health Care and Financial Protection in Rural Areas of Senegal.* World Bank, HNP Discussion Paper. Washington, D.C.

Litvack, J. I., and C. I. Bodart. 1992. "User Fees Plus Quality Equals Improved Access to Health Care: Results of a Field Experiment in Cameroon." *Social Science and Medicine* 37(3): 369–83.

Manning, W. G., J. P. Newhouse, N. Duan, E. B. Keeler, A. Leibowitz, and M. S. Marquis. 1987. "Health Insurance and the Demand for Medical Care: Evidence from a Randomized Experiment." *American Economic Review* 77(3): 251–77.

McPake, B., K. Hanson, and A. Mills. 1993. "Community Financing of Health Care in Africa: An Evaluation of the Bamako Initiative." *Social Science and Medicine* 3(11): 1383–95.

Midgley, J., and M. B. Tracey. 1996. *Challenges to Social Security: An International Exploration.* Westport, Conn.: Auburn House.

Musau, S. 1999. *Community-Based Health Insurance: Experiences and Lessons Learned from East and Southern Africa.* Technical Report 34. Partnerships for Health Reform Project, Abt Associates Inc., Bethesda, Md.

Musgrave, R. A., and P. B. Musgrave. 1984. *Public Finance in Theory and Practice.* New York: McGraw-Hill.

Narayan, D. 1999. "Bonds and Bridges: Social Capital and Poverty." Policy Research Working Paper 2167. World Bank, Poverty Reduction and Economic Management Network, Washington, D.C.

Navarro, V. A. 1984. "Critique of the Ideological and Political Position of the Brandt Report and the Alma Ata Declaration." *International Journal of Health Services* 2(14): 159–72.

North, D. C. 1990. *Institutions, Institutional Change, and Economic Performance.* New York: Cambridge University Press.

Otero, M., and E. Rhyne, eds. 1994. *The New World of Microenterprise Finance: Building Healthy Financial Institutions for the Poor.* West Hartford, Conn.: Kumarian Press.

Peters, D., A., G. Yazbeck, N. V. Ramana, and R. Sharma. 2001. *India—Raising the Sights: Better Health Systems for India's Poor.* Washington, D.C.: World Bank.

Platteau, J. P. 1994. "Behind the Market Stage Where Real Societies Exist" (parts 1 and 2). *Journal of Development Studies* 30: 533–77 and 753–817.

Pradhan, M., and N. Prescott. 2000. *Social Risk Management for Medical Care in Indonesia.* Paper presented at the International Conference on Health Systems Financing in Low-Income African and Asian Countries, November 30–December 1, CERDI, Clermont-Ferrand, France.

Preker, A. S. 1998. "The Introduction of Universal Access to Health Care in the OECD: Lessons for Developing Countries." In S. Nitayarumphong and A. Mills, eds., *Achieving Universal Coverage of Health Care.* Bangkok: Ministry of Public Health.

Preker A. S., H. Harding, and N. Girishankar. 2001. "Private Participation in Supporting the Social Contract in Health: New Insights from Institutional Economics." In A. Ron and X. Scheil-Adlung, eds., *Recent Health Policy Innovations in Social Security,* International Social Security Series, vol. 5. London: Transaction Publishers.

Preker, A. S., J. Langenbrunner, and M. Jakab. 2002. "Development Challenges in Health Care Financing," In D. Dror and A. S. Preker, eds., *Social Reinsurance: A New Approach to Sustainable Community Health Financing.* Washington, D.C.: World Bank/ILO.

Preker A. S., J Langenbrunner, and E Suzuki. 2001. *The Global Expenditure Gap: Securing Financial Protection and Access to Health Care for the Poor.* Report submitted to Working Group 3 of the Commission on Macroeconomics and Health, Jeffrey D. Sachs (Chairman). WHO, Geneva.

Preker, A. S., J Langenbrunner, M. Jakab, and C. Baeza. 2001. *Resource Allocation and Purchasing (RAP) Arrangements That Benefit the Poor and Excluded Groups.* World Bank, HNP Discussion Paper. Washington, D.C.

Preker A. S., G. Carrrin, D. Dror, M. Jakab, W. Hiao, and D. Arhin-Tenkorang. 2002a. "Effectiveness of Community Health Financing in Meeting the Cost of Illness." *Bulletin of the World Health Organization* 8(2): 143–50.

———, eds. 2002b. Chapter 4, "Alternative Ways of Financing Health in the Informal Sector." In Jeffrey D. Sachs, Alan Tait, and Kwesi Botchwey (Chairmen), *Report of Working Group 3 of the Commission on Macroeconomics and Health.* Geneva: WHO.

Ranson, K. 2001. *The Impact of SEWA's Medical Insurance Fund on Hospital Utilization and Expenditure in India.* World Bank, HNP Discussion Paper. Washington, D.C.

Saltman R. B., and O. Ferroussier-Davis. 2000. "The Concept of Stewardship in Health Policy." *Bulletin of the World Health Organization* 78(6): 732–39.

Schieber G., and A. Maeda. 1997. "A Curmudgeon's Guide to Health Care Financing in Developing Countries." In G. Schieber, ed., *Innovations in Health Care Financing.* Washington D.C.: World Bank. (Proceedings of a World Bank Conference, March 10–11, 1997.)

Schneider P., and F. Diop. 2001. *Synopsis of Results on the Impact of Community-Based Health Insurance (CBHI) on Financial Accessibility to Health Care in Rwanda.* World Bank, HNP Discussion Paper. Washington, D.C.

Soucat A., T. Gandaho, D. Levy-Bruhl, X. de Bethune, E. Alihonou, C. Ortiz, P. Gbedonou, P. Adovohekpe, O. Camara, J. M. Ndiaye, B. Dieng, and R. Knippenberg. 1997. "Health Seeking Behavior and Household Expenditures in Benin and Guinea: The Equity Implications of the Bamako Initiative." *International Journal of Health Planning and Management* 12(S1): 137–63.

Supakankunti, S. 1997. *Future Prospects of Voluntary Health Insurance in Thailand.* Takemi Research Paper 13. Takemi Program in International Health, Harvard School of Public Health. Harvard University, Cambridge, Mass.

———. 2001. *Determinants for Demand for Health Card in Thailand.* World Bank, HNP Discussion Paper. Washington, D.C.

van Doorslaer E., A. Wagstaff, and F. Rutten, eds. 1993. *Equity in the Finance and Delivery of Health Care: An International Perspective.* Oxford: Oxford Medical Publications.

Van Ginneken, W. 1999. "Social Security for the Informal Sector: New Challenges for the Developing Countries." *International Social Security Review* 52(1): 49–69.

Vogel, R. J. 1990. *Health Insurance in Sub-Saharan Africa.* Working Paper Series 476. World Bank, African Technical Department, Washington, D.C.

Wagstaff, A. N., N. Watanabe, and E. van Doorslaer. 2001. *Impoverishment, Insurance, and Health Care Payments.* World Bank, HNP Discussion Paper. Washington, D.C.

Woolcock, M., 1998. "Social Capital and Economic Development: Toward a Theoretical Synthesis and Policy Framework." *Theory and Society* 27: 151–208.

Woolcock, M., and D. Narayan. 2000. "Social Capital: Implications for Development Theory, Research, and Policy." *World Bank Research Observer* 15(2): 225–49.

World Bank. 1993. *World Development Report 1993: Investing in Health.* New York: Oxford University Press.

———. 1995. *World Development Report: Workers in an Integrating World.* Washington D.C.

———. 1997. *Sector Strategy for HNP.* Washington, D.C.

WHO (World Health Organization). 2000. *World Health Report 2000: Health Systems—Measuring Performance.* Geneva.

Yip, W., and P. Berman. 2001. "Targeted Health Insurance in a Low-Income Country and Its Impact on Access and Equity in Access: Egypt's School Health Insurance." *Health Economics* 10(2): 207–20.

Zeller, M., and M. Sharma. 2000. "Many Borrow, More Save, and All Insure: Implications for Food and Microfinance Policy." *Food Policy* 25(2): 143–67.

Ziemek, S., and J. Jütting. 2000. *Mutual Insurance Schemes and Social Protection.* STEP Research Group on Civil Society and Social Economy. Geneva: ILO.

CHAPTER 2

Review of the Strengths and Weaknesses of Community Financing

Melitta Jakab and Chitra Krishnan

Abstract: The chapter reviews 45 published and unpublished reports on community financing completed between 1990 and 2001. The main objective of the study was to explore performance measures reported in the literature regarding community financing. The study concluded that the reviewed literature is rich in describing scheme design and implementation. At the same time, evidence on the performance of community-financing schemes is limited.

The study focused on reporting measures on three indicators in particular:

- *Resource mobilization capacity.* Community-financing mechanisms mobilize significant resources for health care. However, there is a large variation in the resource mobilization capacity of various schemes. This review did not find systematic estimates about how much community-financing contributes to health revenues at the local or national level.

- *Social inclusion.* Community financing is effective in reaching a large number of low-income populations who would otherwise have no financial protection against the cost of illness. There is large variation in the size of various schemes. At the same time, there are no estimates about the total population covered through community financing. There are indications that the poorest and socially excluded groups are not automatically reached by community-financing initiatives.

- *Financial protection.* Community-based health-financing schemes are systematically reported to reduce the out-of-pocket spending of their members while increasing their utilization of health care services.

Community-based health-financing (CF) mechanisms play an increasingly important role in the health system of many low- and middle-income countries. The expectation is that CF mechanisms reach population groups that government and market-based health-financing arrangements do not. Populations with low income, who obtain their subsistence in the informal sector (urban and rural), and socially excluded groups (excluded because of cultural factors, physical or mental disability, or other chronic illness) are often not able to take advantage of government or market-based health-financing arrangements. Thus CF has been attracting widespread attention for its potential to provide vulnerable population groups with increased financial protection and access to health care.

With increasing interest in CF in academic, development, and policy circles, the relevant literature has also been growing. In the past decade, there has been an exponential growth in the number of conceptual works, country case studies, comparative papers, and empirical papers describing and analyzing various aspects of community-based health financing.

Despite the diverse nature of the literature, the papers reviewed for this study address many similar questions. What is community financing? How should this phenomenon that has been discussed under many different terms be described? What explains the growing enthusiasm for community financing? Are these initiatives successful in raising resources for health care, reducing the financial burden of those seeking care, and increasing access to health care? If so, what allows these schemes to succeed where the more entrenched institutions of governments and markets have failed?

This chapter provides a comprehensive review of CF literature dating from between 1990 and 2001. The chapter seeks to answer three specific questions: What is community-based health financing and what are its main modalities? How do community-financing schemes perform as health-financing instruments in terms of mobilizing resources—including the poor's—and providing financial protection by removing financial barriers to access? What are the key structural determinants that explain the performance of community financing?

In addition to addressing these specific questions, we hope to determine the focus of studies completed to date; integrate common findings; identify knowledge gaps; and present key contested issues requiring further research.

The chapter is structured as follows. In the first section, it discusses the methodology of the review. Next, it discusses the definition and possible modalities of CF. In the third section, it reviews the performance of CF with regard to resource mobilization capacity, social inclusion, and financial protection. Finally, it discusses the performance determinants of CF with regard to key technical design features and management, organizational, and institutional characteristics. Then it presents the conclusions.

METHODS

Forty-five papers were reviewed for this study. Broad selection criteria were applied: studies were included in the review if their main objective was to discuss health-financing arrangements in which the community was actively involved in some form. The selected papers included articles published in peer-reviewed journals, reports published in formal publication series of international organizations (such as the World Health Organization and the International Labour Organization), internal unpublished documents of international organizations and academic institutions, and conference proceedings. Table 2.1 presents the breakdown of the reviewed studies according to publication type.

Of these 45 papers, 6 were conceptual in nature, 8 were large-scale comparative papers (analyzing 5 or more community financing schemes), and the remaining 31 were case studies. The regional breakdown of the case studies is fairly even between Africa and Asia (15 and 11, respectively), but there are only 4 on Latin America (see table 2.2). This breakdown reflects selection bias: literature available only in Spanish was not included in the review.

TABLE 2.1   Summary Statistics of the Literature Reviewed, by Publication Type

	Peer-reviewed journal articles	Published reports	Internal documents of international organizations or academic institutions	Conference proceedings
Number of studies	20	16	5	4

The analytical approach applied to the 45 papers (see figure 2.1) followed the framework proposed by Preker and others (2001). Health care financing through community-based involvement can be seen as having three independent objectives: (1) it provides the financial resources to promote better health and to diagnose, prevent, and treat known illness; (2) it provides an opportunity to protect individuals and households against direct financial cost of illness when channeled through risk-sharing mechanisms; and (3) it gives the poor a voice and makes them active participants in breaking out of the social exclusion in which they are often trapped. These three objectives can be influenced through the design of CF schemes in terms of technical characteristics of revenue collection, pooling, and purchasing; and management, organizational, and institutional characteristics.

To approximate the three objectives of CF as proposed above, the review defined the following research questions that can be answered from available studies:

What is the potential of CF schemes to mobilize resources in a sustainable manner?

- What is the contribution of community financing to the resources available for local health systems?

- What is the share of community financing in total health revenues (of a district, state, country)?

- How does community financing compare to other resource mobilization instruments in terms of per capita amount of resources mobilized?

Is CF inclusive of the poor?

- Do community-financing schemes reach the poor? What is the socioeconomic composition of schemes?

How effective are CF schemes in preventing impoverishment due to the cost of illness?

- Do CF scheme members have better access to health care than nonmembers?

- Does CF eliminate the financial barriers to health care?

Of the 45 studies, 31 were included in the review of performance. Table 2.3 presents the list of variables we used as selection criteria for the performance section and the number of studies that reported the selected performance variable. Of the 45 studies, 26 provided some information to assess resource-generation capacity of CF, 13 provided information on social inclusion, and 20 provided useful information to assess financial protection. Appendix 2A presents the detailed list of the 45 reviewed studies and the kind of performance variables they report.

TABLE 2.2   Summary of Literature Reviewed on Community-Based Health Financing Schemes, Based on Nature of Study and by Region

Conceptual studies

1. Dror, D., and C. Jacquier. 1999. "Micro-Insurance: Extending Health Insurance to the Excluded."

2. Brown, W., and C. Churchill. 2000. *Insurance Provision in Low-Income Communities: Part II—Initial Lessons from Micro-insurance Experiments for the Poor.*

3. Ziemek, S., and J. Jütting. 2000. *Mutual Insurance Schemes and Social Protection.*

4. Criel, B. 2000. *Local Health Insurance Systems in Developing Countries: A Policy Research Paper.*

5. Ekman, B. 2001. *Community-Based Health Insurance Schemes in Developing Countries: Theory and Empirical Experiences.*

6. Hsiao, W. C. 2001. *Unmet Needs of Two Billion: Is Community Financing a Solution?*

Large-scale comparative studies (> 5 schemes)

7. Dave, P. 1991. "Community and Self-Financing in Voluntary Health Programmes in India."

8. McPake, B., K. Hanson, and A. Mills. 1993. "Community Financing of Health Care in Africa: An Evaluation of the Bamako Initiative."

9. Gilson, L. 1997. "The Lessons of User Fee Experience in Africa."

10. Atim, C. 1998. *Contribution of Mutual Health Organizations to Financing, Delivery, and Access to Health Care: Synthesis of Research in Nine Western and Central-African Countries.*

11. Bennett, S., A. Creese, and R. Monasch. 1998. *Health Insurance Schemes for People Outside Formal Sector Employment.*

12. Musau, S. 1999. *Community-Based Health Insurance: Experiences and Lessons Learned from East and Southern Africa.*

13. CLAISS. 1999. "Synthesis of Micro-Insurance and Other Forms of Extending Social Protection in Health in Latin America and the Caribbean."

14. Narula, I. S., and others. 2000. *Community Health Financing Mechanisms and Sustainability: A Comparative Analysis of 10 Asian Countries.*

Case studies—Africa

15. Arhin, D. C. 1994. "The Health Card Insurance Scheme in Burundi: A Social Asset or a Non-Viable Venture?"

16. Diop, F., R. Bitran, and M. Makinen. 1994. *Evaluation of the Impact of Pilot Tests for Cost Recovery on Primary Health Care in Niger.*

17. Arhin, D.C. 1995. *Rural Health Insurance: A Viable Alternative to User Fees.*

18. Diop F., A. Yazbeck, and R. Bitran 1995. "The Impact of Alternative Cost Recovery Schemes on Access and Equity in Niger."

19. Ogunbekun, I., and others. 1996. "Costs and Financing of Improvements in the Quality of Maternal Health Services through the Bamako Initiative in Nigeria."

20. Roenen, C., and B. Criel 1997. *The Kanage Community Financed Scheme: What Can Be Learned from the Failure?*

21. Soucat, A., T. Gandaho, and others. 1997. "Health Seeking Behavior and Household Expenditures in Benin and Guinea: The Equity Implications of the Bamako Initiative."

22. Soucat, A., D. Levy-Bruhl, and others. 1997. "Local Cost Sharing in Bamako Initiative Systems in Benin and Guinea: Assuring the Financial Viability of Primary Health Care."

(continued)

TABLE 2.2   Continued

Case studies—Africa (continued)

23. Atim, C. 1999. "Social Movements and Health Insurance: A Critical Evaluation of Voluntary, Nonprofit Insurance Schemes with Case Studies from Ghana and Cameroon."

24. Criel, B., P. van der Stuyft, and W. van Lerberghe. 1999. "The Bwamanda Hospital Insurance Scheme: Effective for Whom? A Study of Its Impact on Hospitalization Utilization Patterns."

25. Atim, C., and M. Sock. 2000. *An External Evaluation of the Nkoranza Community Financing Health Insurance Scheme, Ghana.*

26. Jütting, J. 2000. *Do Mutual Health Insurance Schemes Improve the Access to Health Care? Preliminary Results from a Household Survey in Rural Senegal.*

27. Schneider, P., F. Diop, and S. Bucyana. 2000. *Development and Implementation of Prepayment Schemes in Rwanda.*

28. Gilson, L., and others. 2000. "The Equity Impacts of Community Financing Activities in Three African Countries."

29. Okumara, J., and T. Umena. 2001. "Impact of Bamako Type Revolving Drug Fund on Drug Use in Vietnam."

Case studies—Asia

30. Hsiao, W. C. 1995. "The Chinese Health Care System: Lessons for Other Nations."

31. Ron, A., and A. Kupferman. 1996. *A Community Health Insurance Scheme in the Philippines: Extension of a Community-Based Integrated Project.*

32. Liu, Y., and others. 1996. "Is Community Financing Necessary and Feasible for Rural China?"

33. Supakankunti, S. 1997. *Future Prospects of Voluntary Health Insurance in Thailand.*

34. Supakankunti, S. 1998. *Comparative Analysis of Various Community Cost Sharing Implemented in Myanmar.*

35. Carrin, G., and others. 1999. "The Reform of the Rural Cooperative Medical System in the People's Republic of China: Interim Experience in 14 Pilot Counties."

36. Desmet, A., A. Q. Chowdhury, and K. Islam. 1999. "The Potential for Social Mobilization in Bangladesh: The Organization and Functioning of Two Health Insurance Schemes."

37. Chen, N., A. Ma, and Y. Guan. 2000. "Study and Experience of a Risk-Based Cooperative Medical System in China: Experience in Weifang of Shandong Province."

38. Gumber, A., and V. Kulkarni. 2000. "Health Insurance for Informal Sector: Case Study of Gujarat."

39. Xing-yuan, G., and F. Xue-shan. 2000. "Study on Health Financing in Rural China."

40. Preker, A. S. 2001. "Philippines Mission Report."

Case studies—Latin America and the Caribbean

41. Toonen, J. 1995. *Community Financing for Health Care: A Case Study from Bolivia.*

42. DeRoeck, D., and others. 1996. *Rural Health Services at Seguridad Social Campesino Facilities: Analyses of Facility and Household Surveys.*

43. Fiedler, J. L., and R. Godoy. 1999. *An Assessment of the Community Drug Funds of Honduras.*

44. Fiedler, J. L., and J. B. Wight. 2000. "Financing Health Care at the Local Level: The Community Drug Funds of Honduras."

Case studies—mixed regions

45. Ron, A. 1999. "NGOs in Community Health Insurance Schemes: Examples from Guatemala and Philippines."

FIGURE 2.1 Analytical Framework

Ultimate performance indicators

Health	Preventing impoverishment	Social inclusion

Intermediate performance indicators

- Level of mobilized resources
- Sustainability of resource mobilization

- Level of health care utilization
- Financial access and barriers
- Successful risk management

- Equity
- Efficiency
- Quality

Community financing schemes

Core technical design characteristics

Revenue-collection mechanisms
- Level of prepayment compared with direct out-of-pocket spending
- Extent to which contributions are compulsory compared with voluntary
- Degree of progressivity of contributions
- Subsidies to cover the poor

Arrangements for pooling of revenues and sharing of risks
- Size of the pool
- Number of pools
- Redistribution from rich to poor; from health to sick; and from gainfully employed to inactive

Resource allocation or purchasing arrangements
- Demand (for whom to buy)
- Supply (what to buy, in which form, and what to exclude)
- Prices and incentive regime (at what price and how to pay)

Management characteristics

Staff
- Leadership
- Capacity (management skills)

Culture
- Management style (top down or consensual)
- Structure (flat or hierarchical)

Access to information
- Financial, resources, health information, behavior

Organizational characteristics

Organizational forms
- Economies of scale and scope
- Contractual relationships

Organizational incentive regime
- Decision rights, market exposure, financial responsibility, accountability, social functions

Organizational integration/fragmentation
- Horizontal, vertical

Institutional characteristics

Stewardship (government oversight, coordination, regulation, monitoring, etc.)

Governance (public-private mix in ownership)

Rules on revenue transfers and risk pooling

Market structure (factor market and product market)

Source: Preker and others (2001).

TABLE 2.3   Selection Criteria to Assess the Performance of Community-Based Health Financing

Performance variable of interest	Number of studies reporting selected performance variable[a]
Resource mobilization capacity	
Contribution of CF to the resources of local health systems (providers)	26
Share of CF in total health revenues (of district, state, country)	1
Per capita amount of resources mobilized through CF	2[b]
W/ control relative to other health-financing instruments	2
Social inclusion	
Socioeconomic composition of reviewed schemes	13
Financial protection	
Utilization rate of scheme members w/ control	16
OOP payment of CF members w/ control	9

a. Studies that offered conclusions about various performance criteria but did not present supporting evidence in the study were not included in this count.

b. Dave (1991) provides total expenditures and covered populations for 12 schemes and thus the per capita amount could be calculated based on these figures. However, the author does not present them in this format.

A number of studies offered conclusions on resource mobilization, social inclusion, and financial protection based on the experience of authors or review of other studies and schemes but did not provide actual evidence in support of their conclusions. We excluded these studies from the analysis. We also dropped studies that reported performance figures for the scheme or schemes they analyzed but did not present controls that would enable us to make unbiased conclusions.

The direct and indirect determinants of financial protection, health, and social inclusion are complex. To assess these determinants, this chapter reviewed four characteristics of community-financing arrangements:

- Technical design characteristics

- Management characteristics

- Organizational characteristics

- Institutional characteristics.

Nearly all the studies reviewed provided some insight into these characteristics. The literature is particularly rich in describing the function, design, and implementation of CF arrangements.

WHAT IS COMMUNITY-BASED HEALTH FINANCING?

The term *community-based health financing* has evolved into an umbrella term that covers a wide spectrum of health-financing instruments (Hsiao 2001; Dror and Jacquier 1999). Microinsurance, community health funds, mutual health organizations, rural health insurance, revolving drug funds, and community involvement in user fee management have all been loosely referred to as community-based health financing.

The rationale of referring to these diverse financing instruments under the same heading is that they exhibit a number of similarities that effectively distinguish them from other resource mobilization instruments such as general taxation, social insurance, and out-of-pocket payments. At the same time, there are important distinctions among them in terms of their core characteristics, organizational structure, management, and institutional environment. These differences make these arrangements dissimilar enough that comparisons are impossible without some kind of typology. In this section, we present definitions and categorizations from the 45 reviewed papers and establish a typology that we will use throughout the analytical part of the chapter.

A number of studies offered an explicit definition for the type of community financing they investigated (Atim 1998; Ziemek and Jütting 2000; Hsiao 2001; Dror and Jacquier 1999; Musau 1999; McPake, Hanson, and Mills 1993). Box 2.1 presents these definitions. Regardless of the terminology used, the definitions converge on several points. In particular, the role of the community, the nature of the beneficiary group, and the social values underlying the design of the schemes stand out as key descriptors of the investigated health-financing arrangements. Each of these common characteristics will be reviewed in turn.

The first important common feature of the definitions is reference to the predominant role of *community* in mobilizing, pooling, allocating, and managing or supervising (or both) health care resources (Atim 1998; Ziemek and Jütting 2000; Hsiao 2001; Musau 1999; McPake, Hanson, and Mills 1993). The *Oxford English Dictionary* defines community as the quality of (a) "joint or common ownership, tenure or liability"; (b) "common character"; (c) "social fellowship"; (d) "life in association with others"; (e) "common or equal rights or rank"; and (f) "people organized into common political, municipal or social unity." Thus *community*—according to this definition—is a broader concept than that commonly used to refer to a geographic entity defined for political and administrative purposes.

Various forms of CF reflect most of the concepts in the above definition. Members of many CF schemes are bound together not only by geographic proximity but also by shared professional and cultural identity. A narrow geographic definition would exclude many CF schemes whose members are not geographically linked but instead belong to the same craft, profession, or religion or share some other kind of affiliation that facilitates their cooperation for financial protection. This is particularly reflected in the tradition of mutual health organizations in francophone Africa or microfinance organizations that provide health insurance to their borrowers.

The predominance of community action does not mean that CF mechanisms do not rely on government, donor, or other external support. On the contrary, reviewers of successful community initiatives often point to the role of government and donor support—both financial and nonfinancial—as a key determinant of sustainability (Carrin and others 1999; Criel, van der Stuyft,

---

BOX 2.1   DEFINITIONS OF COMMUNITY HEALTH FINANCING

Mutual Health Organizations (MHO): "A voluntary, nonprofit insurance scheme, formed on the basis of an ethic of mutual aid, solidarity, and the collective pooling of health risks, in which the members participate effectively in its management and functioning. . . . [T]hey are nonprofit, autonomous organizations based on solidarity between, and democratic accountability to, their members whose objective is to improve their members' access to good quality health care through their own financial contributions and by means of any of a range of financing mechanisms that mainly involve insurance, but that may also include simple prepayments, savings and soft loans, third-party subscription payments, and so on" (Atim 1998, p. 2).

"*Mutual insurance schemes* can be broadly defined as systems based on voluntary engagement and the principles of solidarity and reciprocity. Members usually have to meet certain obligations, e.g., payment of premiums, and are bound together by a common objective and a strong local affiliation. Many times, these schemes evolve out of traditional systems or form as a response to the low coverage provided by formal systems" (Ziemek and Jütting 2000, p. 2).

"*Community financing* can be broadly defined as any scheme that has three features: community control, voluntary, and prepayment for health care by the community members. This definition would exclude financing schemes such as regional compulsory social insurance plans and community-managed user fee programs" (Hsiao 2001, p. 4).

Microinsurance is "voluntary group self-help schemes for social health insurance. . . . The underpinning of microinsurance is that excluded populations have not been covered under the existing health insurance schemes because of two concurrent forces. The first is that . . . insurers have done little to include these population segments. The second factor has been that excluded people have forgone claiming access because of their disempowerment within society. Microinsurance proposes to change both factors" (Dror and Jacquier 1999, p. 78).

"The term *community-based health insurance* is used in this study to refer to any nonprofit health financing scheme. It covers any not-for-profit insurance scheme that is aimed primarily at the informal sector and formed on the basis of an ethic of mutual aid and the collective pooling of health risks, and in which the members participate in its management" (Musau 1999, p. 5).

"[T]he term *community financing* [means] a system comprising consumer payment (either as a user fee, some form of prepayment mechanism, or other charge) for health services at community level, the proceeds from which are retained within the health sector and managed at local level. . . . In addition it is sometimes argued that community financing is a form of community participation which ensures that communities are not just passive recipients of services" (McPake, Hanson, and Mills 1993, p. 1384).

and van Lerberghe 1999; Supakankunti 1997; Atim 1998). However, the community has a predominant role in designing the rules of the game, managing and supervising the schemes in raising resources, pooling them, and allocating them.

The second common feature of the definitions is the description of the *beneficiary group*. Typically, it is expected that community financing will attract those with no access to financial protection and no access to other health care financing arrangements. In other words, those who are not employed in the formal sector and thus are not eligible to be part of social insurance schemes; those who cannot take advantage of general tax-financed health services because of geographic access barriers, unavailability of needed care and drugs, or both; and those who cannot pay for market-based private health care.

These population groups include the poor with no means of subsistence, those engaged in economic activity in the informal sector and in agriculture; and those who are socially excluded because of ethnicity, religion, mental and physical disability, or other illness (Musau 1999; Dror and Jacquier 1999; Atim 1998; Atim and Sock 2000; Gumber and Kulkarni 2000).

Finally, the third common feature of the definitions is reference to the *social values and principles* underlying the design of community-based financing. This includes the principles of voluntary participation, built-in solidarity mechanisms, and reciprocity. In many societies, these principles originate from the poor's traditional self-help mechanisms, which embrace not only health (or primarily not health) but also many other risks with potentially devastating financial implications (Atim 1999; Musau 1999; DeRoeck and others 1996).

Based on the above, we adopted a broad definition of community financing that reflects all three of these common characteristics. For the purpose of this review, we included studies of health-financing arrangements characterized by the following:

- The community (geographic, religious, professional, ethnic) is actively engaged in mobilizing, pooling, and allocating resources for health care.

- The beneficiaries of the scheme have predominantly low income, earning a subsistence from the informal sector (rural and urban), or are socially excluded.

- The schemes are based on voluntary engagement of the community (although not necessarily of the individual community members).

- The structure of resource mobilization and benefits reflect principles of solidarity.

- The primary purpose of the schemes is not commercial (that is, not-for-profit).

The advantage of this broad definition is that it is inclusive of many different health-financing arrangements with these common characteristics. Further, it effectively distinguishes community-based health financing from other resource mobilization instruments, including out-of-pocket payments, voluntary private insurance, social insurance, and general taxation.

At the same time, the disadvantage of this definition is that it does not address the problem of "apples and oranges." In other words, this definition does not facilitate comparability across the schemes. Health-financing arrangements that meet the above definition can still differ significantly from each other in terms of objectives, structure, management, organization, and institutional characteristics. For example, community-level revolving drug funds in Honduras would qualify as CF, and so would the hospital-based prepayment–risk-sharing scheme of Bwamanda (DRC) and the individual savings account for pregnant women in Indonesia. Yet these various arrangements have different capacities to mobilize resources, to provide financial protection, and to include the poor.

We aimed to address this problem by grouping community-financing schemes. The possibilities for creating a typology are endless, and this is reflected in the reviewed papers. Four of the 45 papers reviewed propose a typology, and each proposes different ways of grouping CF. The common characteristics in the proposed typologies are that they combine the technical health-financing characteristics of the schemes with descriptors of the organizational structure that governs the operation of the schemes.

- Bennett, Creese, and Monasch (1998) separate the schemes based on the nature of the health risks they cover and ownership. The authors distinguish between high-cost, low-frequency events (type 1) and low-cost, high-frequency events (type 2). Additionally, schemes are also presented by ownership arrangements, distinguishing them by health facility, community, cooperative or mutual, nongovernmental organization (NGO), government, or joint ownership.

- Atim (1998) reviews the experience of mutual health organizations in West and Central Africa and separates schemes based on their ownership (traditional clan or social network, social movement or association, provider and community comanaged, community) and their geographic and socioprofessional criteria (rural, urban, and profession, enterprise, or trade union-based).

- Criel, van der Stuyft, and van Lerberghe (1999) distinguish between two poles of voluntary health insurance systems: the mutualistic, or participatory, model, and the provider-driven, or technocratic, model. Their starting point is the risk categorization offered by Bennett, Creese, and Monasch, and they arrive at these two typologies by adding three additional characteristics: size of target population, degree of overlap between the scheme and the existing providers, and intermediary institutions between the source of funding and the destination of the funds.

- Hsiao (2001) distinguishes among five types of CF initiatives: direct demand-side subsidies channeled to individuals (for example, Thai health card), cooperative health care, community-based third-party insurance, provider-sponsored insurance, and producer or consumer cooperative. The categorization takes into account not only whether community involvement is present but also the strength of community involvement.

From our review of three dozen case studies, four commonly encountered and well identifiable modalities emerged that proved useful for our analytical purpose. The first modality groups schemes in which the resource mobilization instrument is out-of-pocket payments but the community is actively involved in fee design, collection, allocation, and management. We refer to this modality as "community cost-sharing" to distinguish it from cost-sharing arrangements in which the community is not involved in any aspect of health financing. The second modality is the community-based prepayment scheme or mutual health organization. The third one is provider-based community health insurance. We label the final category community-based prepayment scheme linked to government or social insurance system. Table 2.4 summarizes these four types of schemes based on their core design features and management, organizational, and institutional characteristics.

Community cost-sharing. In these types of arrangements, the community participates in mobilizing resources for health care through user fees. The health-financing instrument in this case is out-of-pocket payments, but the community is involved in setting user fee levels, allocating the collected resources, developing and managing exemption criteria, and general management and oversight. The community may also be involved in management of at least the first level of health care, the health centers, through participatory structures. The most important characteristics distinguishing this type of financing arrangement from the other three modalities is the lack of prepayment and risk sharing. The Bamako Initiative is a good illustration of this kind of health-financing mechanism.

Community prepayment or mutual health organizations. These schemes are characterized by voluntary membership, prepayment of usually a one-time annual fee, and risk sharing. Some of these schemes cover catastrophic benefits (including hospital care and drug expenditures); others do not. The community is strongly involved in designing and managing the scheme. Schemes are typically not-for-profit. Examples include the Grameen Health Plan in Bangladesh and the Boboye District Scheme in Niger.

Provider-based health insurance. These schemes often revolve around single provider units such as a town or city or regional hospital. They are characterized by voluntary membership, prepayment of usually a one-time annual fee, risk sharing, and coverage of catastrophic risks. They are frequently started by the providers themselves or through donor support. The involvement of the community is often more supervisory than strategic. Examples include the Bwamanda Hospital Insurance Scheme in the Democratic Republic of the Congo and the Nkoranza Community Health-financing Scheme in Ghana.

Government or social insurance-supported community-driven scheme. These community-based health-financing schemes are attached to formal social insurance arrangements or government-run programs. The community actively participates in running the scheme, but the government (Thailand) or the social insurance system (Ecuador) contributes a significant amount of the financing. These schemes are not always voluntary (Burundi), and some have referred to this category as district or regional health insurance. Often such financing initiatives are initiated by the government and not the community. One example of this type of scheme is Ecuador's Seguro Social Campesino.

Table 2.5 presents the list of reviewed papers grouped by these modalities. The comparative studies review several types of schemes of varying modalities.

TABLE 2.4   Often Encountered Forms of Community Financing

	Community involvement in user fee collection	Community prepayment scheme or mutual health organization	Provider-based community health insurance	Community-driven prepayment scheme attached to social insurance or government-run system
Example	❑ Bamako Initiative in Benin and Guinea	❑ Grameen in Bangladesh ❑ Mutual health organizations in Thiès, Senegal ❑ CMS in China	❑ Bwamanda in Democratic Republic of Congo ❑ Nkoranza in Ghana	❑ Seguro Social Campesino, Ecuador ❑ Thai Health Card Scheme ❑ Indonesia ASKES
Technical design characteristics	❑ Point-of-service payment ❑ No risk sharing ❑ Preventive care subsidized by curative care	❑ Prepayment ❑ Risk sharing ❑ Typically primary care; also some drug and sometimes hospital care	❑ Prepayment ❑ Risk sharing ❑ Hospital care	❑ Prepayment ❑ Risk sharing ❑ Primary and hospital care
Management characteristics	❑ Community involvement in setting fees and exemptions schedules and allocation of collected resources	❑ Strong community involvement in management and strategy ❑ Community not necessarily defined in geographic sense but also by professional associations	❑ Community involvement is more informational and supervisory than managerial	❑ Community involvement in decisionmaking
Organizational characteristics	❑ No formal organizational form but informal links with health centers	❑ Separated financing and provision ❑ Varying degree of linkages between schemes and providers ranging from third-party payment to durable institutionalized relationships	❑ Integrated financing and provision ❑ Often poor linkages with primary care if not included	❑ Durable organizational structures ❑ Linkages with social security and government entities
Institutional characteristics	❑ Government commitment to Bamako ❑ Donor support	❑ Often started and supported by donor and government initiatives	❑ Often donor initiated and donor supported	❑ Very strong government involvement (financial, supervisory)

TABLE 2.5   Summary of Case Studies by Modalities

Modality 1: Community involvement in user fee collection

1. McPake, B., K. Hanson, and A. Mills. 1993. "Community Financing of Health Care in Africa: An Evaluation of the Bamako Initiative."

2. Ogunbekun, I., and others. 1996. "Costs and Financing of Improvements in the Quality of Maternal Health Services through the Bamako Initiative in Nigeria."

3. Soucat, A., T. Gandaho, and others. 1997. "Health Seeking Behavior and Household Expenditures in Benin and Guinea: The Equity Implications of the Bamako Initiative."

4. Soucat A., D. Levy-Bruhl, and others. 1997. "Local Cost Sharing in Bamako Initiative Systems in Benin and Guinea: Assuring the Financial Viability of Primary Health Care."

5. Gilson, L. 1997. "The Lessons of User Fee Experience in Africa."

6. Supakankunti, S. 1998. *Comparative Analysis of Various Community Cost Sharing Implemented in Myanmar.*

7. Fiedler, J.L., and R. Godoy. 1999. *An Assessment of the Community Drug Funds of Honduras.*

8. Fiedler, J. L., and J. B. Wight. 2000. "Financing Health Care at the Local Level: The Community Drug Funds of Honduras."

9. Gilson, L., and others. 2000. "The Equity Impacts of Community Financing Activities in Three African Countries."

10. Okumara, J., and T. Umena. 2001. "Impact of Bamako Type Revolving Drug Fund on Drug Use in Vietnam."

Modality 2: Community prepayment or mutual health organizations

11. Arhin, D. C. 1995. *Rural Health Insurance: A Viable Alternative to User Fees.*

12. Toonen, J. 1995. *Community Financing for Health Care: A Case Study from Bolivia.*

13. Hsiao, W. C. 1995. "The Chinese Health Care System: Lessons for Other Nations."

14. Ron, A., and A. Kupferman. 1996. *A Community Health Insurance Scheme in the Philippines: Extension of a Community-Based Integrated Project.*

15. Liu, Y., and others. 1996. "Is Community Financing Necessary and Feasible for Rural China?"

16. Desmet, A., A. Q. Chowdhury, and K. Islam. 1999. "The Potential for Social Mobilization in Bangladesh: The Organization and Functioning of Two Health Insurance Schemes."

17. Ron, A. 1999. "NGOs in Community Health Insurance Schemes: Examples from Guatemala and Philippines."

18. Gumber, A., and V. Kulkarni. 2000. "Health Insurance for Informal Sector: Case Study of Gujarat."

19. Carrin, G., and others. 1999. "The Reform of the Rural Cooperative Medical System in the People's Republic of China: Interim Experience in 14 Pilot Counties."

20. Chen, N., A. Ma, and Y. Guan. 2000. "Study and Experience of a Risk-Based Cooperative Medical System in China: Experience in Weifang of Shandong Province."

21. Xing-yuan, G., and F. Xue-shan. 2000. "Study on Health Financing in Rural China."

22. Jütting, J. 2000. *Do Mutual Health Insurance Schemes Improve the Access to Health Care? Preliminary Results from a Household Survey in Rural Senegal.*

23. Schneider, P., F. Diop, and S. Bucyana. 2000. *Development and Implementation of Prepayment Schemes in Rwanda.*

24. Preker, A. S. 2001. "Philippines Mission Report."

(continued)

TABLE 2.5   Continued

Modality 3: Provider-based community health insurance

25. Roenen, C., and B. Criel. 1997. *The Kanage Community Financed Scheme: What Can Be Learned from the Failure?*

26. Criel, B., P. van der Stuyft, and W. van Lerberghe. 1999. "The Bwamanda Hospital Insurance Scheme: Effective for Whom? A Study of Its Impact on Hospitalization Utilization Patterns."

27. Atim, C., and M. Sock. 2000. *An External Evaluation of the Nkoranza Community Financing Health Insurance Scheme, Ghana.*

Modality 4: Community-driven prepayment scheme attached to social insurance or government-run system

28. Arhin, D. C. 1994. "The Health Card Insurance Scheme in Burundi: A Social Asset or a Non-Viable Venture?"

29. DeRoeck, D., and others. 1996. *Rural Health Services at Seguridad Social Campesino Facilities: Analyses of Facility and Household Surveys.*

30. Supakankunti, S. 1997. *Future Prospects of Voluntary Health Insurance in Thailand.*

Studies that address multiple modalities

31. Dave, P. 1991. "Community and Self-Financing in Voluntary Health Programmes in India."

32. Diop, F., R. Bitran, and M. Makinen. 1994. *Evaluation of the Impact of Pilot Tests for Cost Recovery on Primary Health Care in Niger.*

33. Diop F., A. Yazbeck, and R. Bitran 1995. "The Impact of Alternative Cost Recovery Schemes on Access and Equity in Niger."

34. Atim, C. 1998. *Contribution of Mutual Health Organizations to Financing, Delivery, and Access to Health Care: Synthesis of Research in Nine Western and Central-African Countries.*

35. Bennett, S., A. Creese, and R. Monasch. 1998. *Health Insurance Schemes for People Outside Formal Sector Employment.*

36. Musau, S. 1999. *Community-Based Health Insurance: Experiences and Lessons Learned from East and Southern Africa.*

37. Atim, C. 1999. "Social Movements and Health Insurance: A Critical Evaluation of Voluntary, Nonprofit Insurance Schemes with Case Studies from Ghana and Cameroon."

38. CLAISS. 1999. "Synthesis of Micro-Insurance and Other Forms of Extending Social Protection in Health in Latin America and the Caribbean."

39. Narula, I. S., and others. 2000. *Community Health Financing Mechanisms and Sustainability: A Comparative Analysis of 10 Asian Countries.*

40. Hsiao, W. C. 2001. *Unmet Needs of Two Billion: Is Community Financing a Solution?*

Conceptual papers that did not address any specific schemes classified under the modalities

41. Dror, D., and C. Jacquier. 1999. "Micro-Insurance: Extending Health Insurance to the Excluded."

42. Brown, W., and C. Churchill. 2000. *Insurance Provision in Low-Income Communities: Part II—Initial Lessons from Micro-insurance Experiments for the Poor.*

43. Ziemek, S., and J. Jütting. 2000. *Mutual Insurance Schemes and Social Protection.*

44. Criel, B. 2000. *Local Health Insurance Systems in Developing Countries: A Policy Research Paper.*

45. Ekman, B. 2001. *Community-Based Health Insurance Schemes in Developing Countries: Theory and Empirical Experiences.*

PERFORMANCE OF COMMUNITY-BASED HEALTH FINANCING

This section synthesizes the conclusions and evidence presented in the 45 reviewed studies regarding the performance of community-financing arrangements. Although there are several interesting performance aspects, this review focuses specifically on three questions.

Question 1: What is the potential of community-based health-financing schemes as sustainable health care financing mechanisms? Which modality of community financing performs better in terms of resource mobilization?

Question 2: How inclusive of the poor are CF schemes? Which modality is more inclusive? Do the rich participate in pooling arrangements?

Question 3: How effective are CF schemes in providing financial protection for their members? Which modality of community financing performs better to provide financial protection?

Summary findings for resource mobilization capacity

- Community-financing arrangements contribute significantly to the resources available for local health care systems, whether for primary care, drugs, or hospital care.

- It appears that the involvement of the community—in various forms—results in access to more household resources than would otherwise be available for health care.

- At the same time, there is large variation in the share of CF in the total resources of local health systems.

- There continues to be a need for more rigorous evaluation of the resource generation capacity of community-based schemes.

Summary findings for social inclusion

- Community-based health financing is effective in reaching a large number of low-income populations who would otherwise have no financial protection against the cost of illness.

- The poorest and socially excluded groups are not automatically included in CF initiatives.

- High-income groups are frequently underrepresented relative to the entire population, undermining redistribution of resources from the rich to the poor.

Summary findings for financial protection

- Generally, community-based health-financing schemes (modalities 2–4) are reported to reduce the out-of-pocket spending of their members while increasing their utilization of health care services.

Resource Mobilization Capacity

The most striking conclusion from the review of the literature is that *there is little systematic evidence that would allow assessment of the overall resource generation capacity of various CF initiatives.* It is also difficult, at this point, to assess how the various modalities fare when compared with each other as well as when compared with other health-financing instruments. None of the reviewed studies reported the amount of resources raised through community-financing arrangements as a share of the country's total health revenues. In a few cases, there are estimates about the per capita expenditures of the schemes. However, in the absence of concurrent estimates about the proportion of the population covered, extrapolation to a national level was not possible.

This lack of evidence is not surprising. In most cases, community-financing arrangements are not registered. For example, 60 percent of 50 reviewed CF schemes in West and Central Africa were not registered with authorities (Atim 1998). Thus centrally maintained data do not exist. Surveys of a nationally representative nature do not ask questions based on which extrapolation would be statistically appropriate.

In the absence of systematic assessments, the following findings aim to provide a synthesis of authors' conclusions and an approximation of sustainability of resource mobilization through community financing.

Community-financing arrangements contribute significantly to the resources available for local health care systems, be it primary care, drugs, or hospital care. Twenty-six studies report the contribution of community-financing schemes to the operational revenues of local providers. A few examples are shown in box 2.2. The most striking finding is the large variation in the capacity of CF schemes to contribute to the operational expenditures of local providers. Some schemes achieve full financing of the recurrent costs of their local health center, even some drug and referral expenditures. Others, particularly hospital-based schemes (modality 3), have a modest contribution to the resources of the facility and external contributions are required.

This large variation in the resource-generation ability holds not only across countries but also within countries. For example, Dave (1991) compares the experience of 12 community-financing schemes in India. The Sewagram scheme, for example, was found to generate enough revenues through membership fees to cover 96 percent of all community-based health care costs, including salaries, drug costs, and mobile costs. On the other hand, the RAHA scheme covered only between 10 percent and 20 percent of the total community costs. The author attributes the difference to the subscription policies: at Sewagram at least 75 percent of the households had to enroll in the scheme before services were reimbursed. This increased the risk-pooling and resource mobilization ability of the scheme. On the other hand, at RAHA, subscription occurred on an individual basis.

It appears that the involvement of the community—in various forms—results in access to more household resources than would be otherwise available for health care. Most of the evidence in this regard originates from the analysis of the Bamako Initiative.

BOX 2.2   Contribution of CF Schemes to Operational Revenues

Community cost sharing/total local operating costs

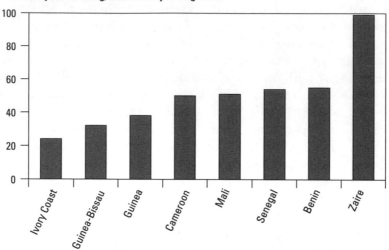

This graph is based on data from a study conducted by Soucat, Gandaho, Levy-Bruhl, and others on cost sharing in Benin and Guinea. The level of cost recovery from user fees in the health centers of those countries varies from 24 percent to 99 percent of the total local operating costs. This excludes the salaries generally paid by the government.

Source: Soucat, Gandaho, Levy-Bruhl, and others (1997).

Percent of recurrent costs from prepayment

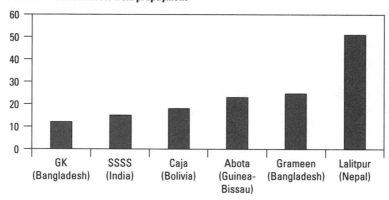

Based on data from Bennett, Creese, and Monasch, this graph shows the cost recovery from prepayment of six modality 2 schemes. The range is from 12 percent to 51 percent of recurrent expenditure. This shows that for these schemes the resources collected do not cover the full recurrent costs, thereby necessitating other sources of funding: out-of-pocket payments, donor, and government subsidy.

Source: Bennett, Creese, and Monasch (1998).

(continued)

BOX 2.2   Continued

Percent of health facility operation costs financed by scheme

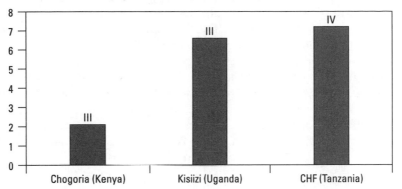

Based on data from Musau, the graph shows the cost-recovery level of three schemes: Chogoria, Kisiizi (modality 3 schemes), and Community Health Fund of Tanzania (modality 4). The contribution of the schemes to the financing of the health facility ranges from 2.1 percent to 7.2 percent. Compared to Chogoria, the higher resource mobilization capacity of Kisiizi is attributed to lower premiums, which attracts more members. The CHF scheme is highly subsidized by the government from funds provided under a World Bank project. *Source:* Musau (1999).

The Bamako Initiative is categorized in our typology as modality 1: the community is involved in setting the level of user fees, designing and managing exemption schemes, and allocating the collected funds. (See box 2.3 for a more detailed description of the Bamako Initiative.) The financing instrument still lacks risk-pooling and prepayment elements a priori. However, the involvement of the community appears to alleviate the collection difficulties providers have experienced with user-fee mechanisms and the regressivity associated with out-of-pocket payments. In particular, community involvement can lead to better allocation of collected resources to services and drugs that community members value and want (McPake, Hanson, and Mills 1993; Diop, Yazbeck, and Bitran 1995; Soucat 1997).

A few highlights:

• Soucat, Gandaho, and others (1997) analyzed the impact of the Bamako Initiative in Benin and Guinea. They showed that direct household expenditure (through user fees) contributed to 25 percent of the health centers' local operating costs in Benin and 40 percent in Guinea. The revenue was used to cover drug costs, outreach, local maintenance, and replacing supplies, and preventive care was subsidized more than curative care, thereby promoting utilization. In another study Soucat, Levy-Bruhl, and others (1997) found that in Benin, about

---

BOX 2.3   THE BAMAKO INITIATIVE

The Bamako Initiative (BI) was launched in 1987 by a group of African ministers of health in Bamako, Mali, in a meeting sponsored by WHO and UNICEF.
The BI was a response to the rapid deterioration of access experienced in several health systems during the 1980s. Deterioration in access was partially
attributed to the imposition of user fees on public facilities. In contrast, the BI
model emphasizes that revenue should be raised and controlled at the local
level through community-based activities that are national in scope. Community participation is seen as a mechanism to build accountability to the users of
health care in that the revenues are used in ways that address the persistent
quality weaknesses of primary care (Gilson 1997). By late 1994, the BI had been
implemented in 33 countries, of which 28 were in sub-Saharan Africa. The
other 5 were in Cambodia, Myanmar, Peru, Vietnam, and Yemen.

---

half of the local operating costs was covered by the government, 23 percent by
donors, and 28 percent by a surplus generated by community financing. In
Guinea, 44 percent of the operating costs were covered by the government, 26
percent by donors, and 30 percent by community financing, with a lower average surplus than in Benin.

- Pilot studies conducted in Niger compared three resource mobilization methods:
newly introduced user fees, prepayment scheme plus user fees, and the control district where health services remained "free" (Diop, Yazbeck, and Bitran 1995). Revenues from fees were managed by local providers and by local health committees
organized by the population. Revenues were pooled at the district level and used
mainly to purchase drugs. The study found that both intervention districts showed
substantial increases in revenue collection compared with the control district. It also
revealed that the revenue generation per capita under the prepayment method was
two times higher than under the user-fee method. The authors add that the sustainability of these financing mechanisms critically depends on cost-containment.

There is little evidence from the analysis of other modalities to determine how
well modalities 2, 3, and 4 fare relative to each other in mobilizing resources for
health care.

While some of the literature is enthusiastic about the contribution of CF to
health care resources, others are less optimistic about the sustainable resource-
generation capacity of these arrangements. In the studies in which the schemes'
contribution was low in the total financing of providers, authors tended to be
pessimistic about sustainable resource generation through CF arrangements. (Bennett, Creese, and Monasch 1998; Atim 1998; Musau 1999; Arhin 1994; Roenen and
Criel 1997; CLAISS 1999). The key factor that undermines the revenue-raising
potential of community financing is their predominantly poor contributing population. Whether in rural or in urban areas, community-based health-financing
schemes reach the poorest half of the population. If most members of community-

financing schemes are poor, redistribution within the community takes place within a much limited overall resource pool (Hsiao 2001; Jütting 2000; Atim 1998; Bennett, Creese, and Monasch 1998).

- Bennett, Creese, and Monasch (1998) recognize that prepaid premiums are important resource-generating instruments, but the authors conclude that "there is little evidence that voluntary prepayment schemes for those outside the formal sector can be 'self-financing' for anything other than the short term." They show that for most schemes the resources collected from the combination of prepayment and user fees does not cover the recurrent costs of the scheme, and thus external funding is required. See table 2.6 for their findings.

- In six Central and West African countries, Atim (1998) concludes that mutual health organizations (MHOs) "have had little impact on the finances of health facilities." For instance, in the Thiès region of Senegal, 30 percent of the admissions into St. Jean de Die are MHO members, and yet MHO resources account for less than 2.5 percent of hospital revenues. Atim notes, however, that these findings are not surprising, given the recent growth in the MHO phenomenon in the region. He concludes that the potential of MHOs to mobilize resources is much greater than current figures on contribution revenues would suggest.

- Similar experiences are reported from five schemes in East Africa. Two hospital-based prepayment schemes in Uganda and Kenya contributed 8 percent and 2 percent, respectively, to the operational expenditures of their hospitals. Similar results were observed in Tanzania with regard to dispensaries: 5.4 percent of the participating dispensaries' income came from the prepayment scheme (Musau 1999).

- A study of the National Health Card Insurance Scheme (CAM) in Burundi revealed that the revenue generated from "premiums was insufficient to fund even the recurrent costs of outpatient drugs consumed by participating households" (Arhin 1994).

- In the review of Latin American community-financing schemes, 9 out of 10 schemes were found to need large external contributions to ensure future sustainability (CLAISS 1999).

- Roenen and Criel (1997) reported that the sum of the premiums generated in the Kanage Community Financed Scheme covered only a fraction of what members spent on care. The scheme was largely financed by the revenues of the Murunda hospital to which the scheme was affiliated.

Social Inclusion

In this section, we explore whether CF schemes are effective in reaching the poor and socially excluded groups. To address this question, we looked at the socioeconomic composition of CF scheme membership. In particular, we were interested in whether CF arrangements reach the poor and whether higher income groups participate in pooling and income redistribution arrangements.

TABLE 2.6 Cost Recovery from Prepaid Premiums

No.	Scheme	Country	Cost recovery from prepayment Last date available
42	SWRC	India	10 percent of recurrent expenditure
25	RAHA	India	10–20 percent off community costs & 100 percent referral costs[a]
24	SSSS	India	15 percent of recurrent expenditure[b]
18	Caja-Tiwanaku	Bolivia	18 percent of recurrent expenditure[c]
31	Abota	Guinea Bissau	23 percent of recurrent expenditure[d]
64	Bajada	Philippines	30 percent of recurrent expenditure
58	CAM	Burundi	34 percent of outpatient drug costs[e]
17	GK	Bangladesh	12 percent of recurrent expenditure[f]
14	Grameen	Bangladesh	24.7 percent of recurrent expenditure[g]
41	BRAC	Bangladesh	50 percent of recurrent expenditure
62	Health Card	Thailand	50 percent[h]
67	Bwamanda	former Zaire	65–70 percent recurrent, excluding personal allowances
79	SWHI	Thailand	50–60 percent[i]
59	Lalitpur	Nepal	51 percent of recurrent expenditure[j]
21	Kisiizi	Uganda	72 percent of recurrent expenditure[k]
46	KSSS	India	88 percent of recurrent expenditure
60	Boboye	Niger	89 percent of drug and management costs[l]
26	Sewagram	India	96 percent of community health program costs
32	Medicare II	Philippines	100 percent of recurrent expenditure[m]
33	PHACOM	Madagascar	100 percent of drug costs[n]
61	UMASIDA	Tanzania	100 percent of costs
2	ORT	Philippines	100 percent excluding professional salaries
66	Nsalasani	Congo-Brazzaville	100 percent
29	Bao Hiem Y Te	Vietnam	130 percent[o]

Source: Bennett, Creese, and Monasch (1998, p. 40)

a. Nonmember fee collections cover roughly 60 percent of community cost.

b. Copayments cover 31 percent of costs and balance is financed from fund-raising activities.

c. Without the costs associated with expatriate assistance the caja contribution would have been 48 percent of budget.

d. In a study of 18 village schemes the cost recovery ranges from 3 percent to 123 percent based on the assumption that all communities consume a given amount of drugs estimated by government.

e. There is no link between prepayment revenues collected and financing of services as revenues revert to government. A study in Muyinga Province showed that the revenue from premiums was sufficient to fund approximately 34 percent of drug costs.

f. The remaining was covered by user fees (24 percent), subsidies from GK commercial ventures (14 percent), and international solidarity (50 percent).

g. The remaining was covered by user fees (41.3 percent members and nonmembers) and a long-term loan from Grameen Bank (34 percent).

h. The scheme is currently half-financed by government budget and half by cardholders; this is a relatively recent reform, and previous estimates show recovery of approximately 35 percent of recurrent costs.

i. Balance from cross-subsidy from richer households.

j. Cost recovery from prepayment ranges from 30 percent to 56.6 percent.

k. Average cost recovery for the hospital as a whole is 48 percent.

l. 149 percent of drug costs only.

m. Fund utilization is relatively low, ranging from 38 to 78 percent of total collections. Only in 1992 after a large drop of membership disbursement exceeded collection in Unisan, Quezon, pilot scheme.

n. Drugs are bought with membership fees but often only last three months of the year.

o. The 130 percent includes a cross-subsidy from formal sector workers to informal sector workers.

Of the 13 studies that report evidence regarding the socioeconomic composition of CF members, the findings appear to be consistent. *Community-based health-financing schemes extend coverage to a large number of people who would otherwise not have financial protection. However, there seems to be some doubt whether the poorest are included in the benefits of community-based health financing.* Where data are available, the most frequently cited reason for not being included in a community-financing scheme is lack of affordability. Distance to scheme hospital is also reported as affecting the decision to enroll in the scheme in several cases. These findings do not show systematic variation with the modality of the reviewed scheme. Table 2.7 summarizes these findings.

TABLE 2.7   Summary of Findings (1): Who Is Covered by CF Arrangements?

	Scheme reaches the poor	Poorest of the poor are not covered	Ability to pay is the main reason for not being covered	Rich do not participate	Distance gradient to scheme provider
Modality 1					
Diop, Yazbeck, and Bitran (1995), Niger	✔				
McPake, Hanson, and Mills (1993), Burundi	✔	✔	✔		
Gilson and others (2000), Benin, Kenya, Zambia	✔				
Modality 2					
Desmet, Chowdhury, and Islam (1999), Bangladesh	✔		✔	✔	✔
Jütting (2000), Senegal	✔	✔	✔		
Diop, Yazbeck, and Bitran (1995), Niger	✔				
Liu and others (1996), China	✔				
Carrin and others (1999), China	✔				
Modality 3					
Criel, van der Stuyft, and van Lerberghe (1999), Dem. Rep. of Congo	✔	✔		✔	
Atim and Sock (2000), Ghana	✔	✔	✔		✔
Modality 4					
Arhin (1994), Burundi	✔	✔	✔		
DeRoeck and others (1996), Ecuador	✔			✔	✔
Supakankunti (1997), Thailand	✔		✔		
Total number of studies confirming selected finding	**13**	**5**	**6**	**3**	**3**

Findings for modality 2 schemes: Community health fund or mutual health organization:

- The Gonosasthya Kendra (GK) in Bangladesh is effective in reaching the poor. Of the households classified as destitute in the area, 80 percent are covered by the scheme—46 percent of the poor, 20 percent of the middle class, and 10 percent of the rich, amounting to an overall subscription rate of 27.5 percent. The reason among the destitute and the poor for not subscribing, even after 15 years of operation of the scheme, is the level of the premium and copayments associated with it. The distribution of the scheme's membership by income group is as follows: 33.5 percent are classified as destitute and poor, 57.5 percent as middle income, and 9 percent as rich. In terms of equity, this suggests that pooling and income redistribution does take place but predominantly between the middle income and the poor (Desmet, Chowdhury, and Islam 1999).

- Subscription rates to the scheme demonstrate a distance gradient to the GK hospital: subscription rates between the two lowest socioeconomic groups were 90 percent for the villages near the hospital and 35 percent for the distant villages. Lack of transportation to the GK hospital was the second most-cited reason among the destitute and the poor for not subscribing to the scheme (Desmet, Chowdhury, and Islam 1999).

- The Grameen Bank (GB) health scheme is operated by the microfinance organization in Bangladesh. The GB scheme covered 57.8 percent of the poor in the areas while only 1.8 percent of the nonpoor families signed up for the scheme. This suggests that the scheme effectively enlisted the membership of the local poor. At the same time, solidarity and income redistribution is undermined as the rich do not take part in the pooling arrangement (Desmet, Chowdhury, and Islam 1999).

- In Rwanda, the pilot prepayment scheme increased the utilization rate of members as compared with nonmembers despite a copayment charge.
  - Consultation rates of nonmembers = 0.2 per capita in all five districts.
  - Consultation rates of members = 1.3 per member in Byumba, 1.87 in Kabgayi, and 1.76 in Kabutare.
  - Comparing utilization rates pre- and post-intervention, members' consultation rates were three to six times higher than reported before implementation of the prepayment scheme.

- Similar findings are reported for Senegal's Thiès district. Analyzing the membership characteristics of four mutual health organizations, Jütting (2000) reports that the average income of members is three times that of nonmembers. He concludes that the poorer people do not participate in MHOs because they do not have the financial resources to pay the regular premium. At the same time, Jütting suggests that this finding does not mean that MHOs increase inequality for the population. Based on the national poverty line, most of the scheme members qualify as poor. Thus on average it can be concluded that these mutual health organizations have helped poor rural populations cope with health risks, even though they have not been able to include the very poorest.

Findings for modality 3 schemes: Provider-based community health insurance:

- In the Bwamanda hospital prepayment scheme in the Democratic Republic of the Congo, the very low- (less than US$20/month) and high-income (greater than US$200/month) groups were less represented among scheme members than in the nonmember population. Of the member population, 14.9 percent was from very low-income HHs versus 18.7 percent among nonmembers; 5.9 percent of the member population was from high-income HHs versus 10.5 percent among nonmembers (Criel, van der Stuyft, and van Lerberghe 1999).

- In the Nkoranza scheme in Ghana, being "hard core poor" (defined as those falling below one-third of average income) is one of the reasons for not joining prepayment schemes. Eight percent of the Nkoranza town and 17 percent of the whole district are identified as hard core poor. The reason most often stated for not being a part of the scheme was "financial" and the fact that the registration period coincided with a low financial situation. One focus group also cited distance from the hospital as a reason for being uninsured (Atim and Sock 2000).

Findings for modality 4 schemes: Community financing supported by government, social insurance, or both:

- Under the Thai health card scheme in Khon Kaen province, health cardholders have significantly lower income than those without a health card. This suggests a pro-poor targeting of the health card program. Separating cardholders into new cardholders, renewed cardholders, and dropouts, Supakankunti (1997) reports that dropouts have the lowest income, suggesting that the health card scheme may pose affordability problems to the lowest income population groups in addition to adverse selection due to lower levels of reported chronic illness in this group.

- Comparing revolving drugs funds and the prepaid health card scheme in Burundi, 25 percent of the households were reported to be part of the prepayment scheme. Socioeconomic status and membership in the prepayment scheme were positively correlated. The poor were more likely to pay through user charges than purchase a prepayment plan. The low subscription rate in the prepayment scheme was associated with difficulty in coming up with one-time large payments in cash-constrained situations and the poor quality of services at government facilities. These factors limited ability, as well as willingness to pay (McPake, Hanson, and Mills 1993). Arhin's findings corroborate that the primary reason for not purchasing a prepayment plan was financial affordability. She reports that in Burundi 27 percent of survey respondents did not purchase the health card because they could not afford it (Arhin 1994).

Financial Protection

In this section, we explore whether CF schemes are effective in providing protection from the impoverishing effects of catastrophic health care events. At this point, only imperfect measures are available to approximate this question. Specifically, we looked for the following indicators to assess whether community-financing schemes reduce the financial burden of seeking care. What is the level of out-of-pocket payments of members relative to nonmembers? What is the utilization of CF scheme members relative to nonmembers?

Analyzing utilization and out-of-pocket expenditure patterns together allows us to take into account forgone use due to the high cost of seeking health care. Assessing financial protection based only on point-of-service spending information does not allow delayed or forgone care due to high costs to be factored in.

Twenty studies present evidence regarding the financial protection impact of the CF schemes they reviewed. In 13 studies, scheme members are more likely to use health care services than nonmembers, and 2 report no difference between members and nonmembers. One study compared user fees with prepayment schemes (Diop, Yazbeck, and Bitran 1995) and found a slight decrease in the use of health care for the user-fee modality compared with the prepayment scheme of CF. In 9 of these, members pay less out-of-pocket. These findings do not appear to systematically vary with the modality of the scheme. We summarize these findings in table 2.8.

Findings for modality 1 schemes:

- Soucat and others (1997) have reported the increased utilization of health services after the introduction of the Bamako Initiative in Benin and Guinea. The authors attribute this development to the availability of drugs and improved quality of services brought about by community involvement. The poor in Guinea had fewer alternative sources of care compared with what they could find in the illegal drug market in Benin, which led Guinea's poor to opt out of seeking care. This study emphasized that improvements in quality, access to care, availability of drugs, and community involvement play an important role in increasing utilization of schemes that rely on user fees as the predominant health-financing mechanisms.

Findings for modality 2 schemes:

- Pilot studies conducted in Niger compared three resource-mobilization methods: newly introduced user fees, prepayment scheme plus user fees, and the control district where health services remained "free" (Diop, Yazbeck, and Bitran 1995). Revenues from fees were managed by local providers and by local health committees organized by the population. Revenues were pooled at the district level and used mainly to purchase drugs. In both intervention districts, quality improvements and availability of drugs stimulated use of health care while utilization continued to decline in the control district. The authors conclude that the "positive effects of the quality improvements cancelled out the negative effects of the introduction of use fees." A few details:

TABLE 2.8   Summary of Findings (2): Does CF Reduce the Burden of Seeking Health Care?

	Utilization of members relative to nonmembers	Level of OOPs for members relative to nonmembers
Modality 1		
Soucat and others (1997), Benin and Guinea	Higher	
Diop, Yazbeck, and Bitran (1995), Niger	Lower	Lower
McPake, Hanson, and Mills (1993), Burundi	Higher	
Gilson and others (2000), Benin, Kenya, Zambia	Higher	
Modality 2		
Desmet, Chowdhury, and Islam (1999), Bangladesh	Same	
Gumber and Kulkarni (2000), India		Lower
Arhin (1995), Ghana	Higher	
Diop, Yazbeck, and Bitran (1995), Niger	Higher	Lower
Schneider, Diop, and Bucyana (2000), Rwanda	Higher	
Jütting (2000), Senegal	Same	
Liu and others (1996), China		Lower
Carrin and others (1996), China		Lower
Xing-yuan and Xue-shan (2000), China	Higher	Lower
Chen, Ma, and Guan (2000), China		Lower
Modality 3		
Criel, van der Stuyft, and van Lerberghe (1999), Dem. Rep. of Congo	Higher	
Roenen and Criel (1997), Rwanda	Higher	
Atim (1999), Ghana	Higher	
Modality 4		
Arhin (1994), Burundi	Higher	Lower
DeRoeck and others (1996), Ecuador	Higher	Lower
Musau (1999), Tanzania	Higher	
Total number of studies confirming selected finding	**16**	**9**

Note: OOPs = out-of-pocket payments.

- People using improved services in the fee-for-service district saved 40 percent of the amount they spent on health care for an episode of illness before the intervention.
- In the prepayment district, out-of-pocket health spending declined by 48 percent, and total health spending (including the tax component) declined by 36 percent.
- The number of initial visits to the health care facility increased by about 40 percent in the prepayment district. Utilization among the poorest quartile doubled. Utilization decreased slightly in the fee-for-service district.
- Even for short travel distances, utilization in the fee-for-service district decreased from 45 percent to 37 percent and increased from 36 percent to 43 percent in the prepayment district.

- The SEWA Scheme in India improves financial protection for its members. Among the rural population, the total cost of seeking care for SEWA members was significantly less than for ESIS members and the uninsured (Rs 295 versus Rs 380 and Rs 401, respectively, for acute morbidity; Rs 451 versus Rs 644 and Rs 697, respectively, for chronic morbidity). However, the burden of seeking care on the household budget continued to be higher among SEWA members than among those insured by other mechanisms (Gumber and Kulkarni 2000).

- Arhin (1995), in assessing the viability of rural health insurance as an alternative to user fees, also found that the scheme in Ghana removed a barrier to admission and led to earlier reporting of patients and increased utilization among the insured.

- There is no convincing evidence that the two reviewed Bangladesh schemes fare strongly in terms of improving access to hospital care for the poor. Desmet, Chowdhury, and Islam (1999) report that the use of hospital services among members shows a significant income gradient. Hospital admissions per 100 persons per year amount to 2 for the destitute, 2.3 for the poor, 3.72 for the middle income, and 10.7 for the rich. Whether this is due to overuse by the higher income groups or underuse by the lower income groups needs to be tested. The Grameen Bank scheme does not include hospital care, and the lack of coverage for hospital care is the most frequently raised complaint in the implementation committee.

- Jütting (2000) finds no significant difference among the contact rates between members of three Senegal schemes and nonmembers. An interesting finding in one of the schemes is the low contact rate, which Jütting attributes to the availability of malaria medication.

- In China, various attempts to revive the Cooperative Medical System (CMS) are described in detail in Hsiao (2001). A number of studies assess the success of these experiences in terms of reducing out-of-pocket payments and increasing utilization by its members. A few examples are provided below:

  - In Shandong Province, a study was conducted to determine the level of disease-induced poverty. It was measured by calculating average medical expenditures for those diseases classified as contributing to a high economic burden based on income level and disease type. Disease-induced poverty was found to have decreased from 23 percent to 3.7 percent in Shougang County, and from 30 percent to 3 percent in Pingdu County after the introduction of CMS coverage (Chen, Ma, and Guan 2000).
  - Carrin and others (1999) assessed "ratios of insurance protection" in China's Rural Cooperative Medical System (RCMS). The authors measured the ratio of average health insurance contribution (destined for reimbursement of health care costs) per capita to average health care expenditure per capita. They found wide variation in the level of insurance protection across counties, from less than 10 percent in Lingwu and Xiaoshan Coun-

ties to more than 30 percent in Yihuang County. However, the authors also observed that "on average" health insurance contributions are not enough to offer RCMS members a reasonable health insurance benefit because out-of-pocket expenditures are still associated with seeking care.

- Another study based on household data compared out-of-pocket expenses and utilization by members and nonmembers of the Cooperative Health Care Scheme (CHCS) pilot study. The average fee per outpatient visit was 10.1 yuan for CHCS members compared with 21.7 yuan for nonmembers. At the same time, higher utilization of medical care among CHCS members was observed in the two pilot sites. Hospital admission rates were 60 percent among members, compared with 43 percent in the control group. In the township of Wuzhan, 17.3 percent of CHCS members used outpatient services compared with 7.4 percent in the control group (Xing-yuan and Xue-shan 2000).

- Liu and others (1996) compared households covered by community-financing schemes and the uninsured in China's poverty regions. They show that the cost per visit is twice as high for the uninsured as for the insured (3 yuan per visit for the uninsured as compared with 1.5 yuan for a member of a household insured under community-financing schemes). They also find that the higher average charge per outpatient visit for the uninsured can be attributed to the fact that these "schemes can exercise their bargaining power in demanding discounted prices or the providers can be paid on a partial-capitation basis" (Liu and others 1996; Hsiao 2001).

Findings for modality 3 schemes:

- Criel, van der Stuyft, and van Lerberghe (1999) looked at the utilization of hospital services associated with the Bwamanda hospital insurance scheme in the Democratic Republic of Congo. They found that hospital utilization was significantly higher among the insured population than among the uninsured. The innovative aspect of their study was assessing whether the additional utilization was justified or the result of insurance coverage in terms of moral hazard and induced demand. They concluded that the impact of insurance increased access to justified care in the case of caesarian sections and hernias. Thus the Bwamanda scheme succeeded in increasing utilization of high-priority hospital care services (strangulated hernias and C-sections).

- A distance gradient was observed in both insured and uninsured populations, suggesting that insurance can overcome the financial barriers to use but not necessarily the geographic barriers. The indirect costs of travel and hospitalization time in rural areas may outweigh the direct costs of hospitalization. When looking at specific high-priority interventions (strangulated hernias and C-sections), the distance gradient is reduced, suggesting that the insurance scheme improved equity in the district. The same impact is not observed for nonurgent care. This suggests that the impact of geographic barriers was more successfully compensated for in the case of high-priority service use than in the case of low-priority service use. In addition, these findings suggest

inelastic demand for high-priority services as well as effective resource allocation practices (Criel, van der Stuyft, and van Lerberghe 1999).

- In 1993, three-fourths of the consultants at the hospital-clinic level and half
  of the hospitalized patients were members of the Kanage cooperative scheme
  in Rwanda. Members used the hospital services 8.5 times as often as nonmembers. Although utilization of the services was high among the members,
  there was a lack of equality, which could have contributed to the failure of the
  system. The size of the premium was independent of income or distance from
  the hospital. It was not an integrated system and lacked quality care and services, which led to the failure of the scheme (Roenen and Criel 1997).

Findings for modality 4 schemes:

- The Health Card Scheme (CAM) in Burundi studied by Arhin illustrates that,
  in the month preceding the study, 27.9 percent of the households that held
  valid CAM cards had incurred out-of-pocket expenses for medical consultations, drug purchases, or both, while the corresponding figure for those
  households without valid cards was 39.9 percent. The mean expenditure per
  treatment was also lower for scheme members (Arhin 1994).

- The formal treatment rate (modern, or western, care sought outside the home)
  was more than 50 percent higher for the CAM group than for the non-CAM
  members. This high rate for the CAM group may be explained by the fact that
  some government health centers gave incomplete treatments, delaying recovery
  and requiring visits to collect the remaining drugs. It is also possible that this
  high utilization rate among CAM households was the outcome of "supplier-
  induced demand," that is, an increase in the demand and consumption of
  health care by patients as a result of the providers' actions. In addition, households participating in the CAM scheme were three times more likely to use the
  government facilities than non-CAM households (Arhin 1994).

- The Ecuador Seguridad Social Campesino (SSC) rural health facility significantly
  increased financial protection for its members: out-of-pocket expenditure for
  health care of SSC members was only one-third of that for nonmembers. Members of the SSC rural health facility were more likely to seek care for illness than
  nonmembers (80 percent versus 66 percent). Demand analysis conducted
  demonstrated that improving the quality of care and increasing the referral rates
  and availability of drugs would increase the utilization rates of SSC health services. The analysis also showed that there was no significant relationship
  between household income and distance and travel time to reach the health
  facility and the decision to seek care outside the home. Lower income households were more likely to belong to the scheme (DeRoeck and others 1996).

Discussion of Performance Results

Our review found that community-financing arrangements—regardless of the
modality—contributed a significant amount to the resources available to local

health systems. At the same time, there was a large variation in terms of the share of community financing in the local health revenues. It is also apparent that community-financing arrangements alone can rarely support hospital-level care in full, and thus other mechanisms of health financing are frequently used in conjunction with such arrangements.

It has to be noted, however, that the evidence base regarding the resource-generation capacity of community-financing schemes requires further strengthening. Currently, the total amount of resources mobilized through community-based health financing is anyone's guess. What is the share of health financing through CF arrangements in terms of total health care financing? How many resources are mobilized through CF arrangements relative to general taxation, social insurance, private insurance, and out-of-pocket payments?

In the absence of more comprehensive information and improved methodologies, it is difficult to assess the global impact and the potential of community financing as resource mobilization instruments to finance health care for the poor. Having a systematic assessment of the volume of resources raised through community financing would allow exploration of the following issues:

- Comparability with other sources of health financing would allow assessment of effectiveness, efficiency, and equity of community financing as health-financing mechanisms.

- Assessment of the impact of community financing on the amount of government funding. A critical question is whether community financing complements or displaces government funding. Does the existence of CF make governments allocate fewer resources to a region with a lot of CF initiative, or is the reverse true?

- Assessment of sustainability of CF arrangements over the long run.

More evidence can be found about CF's impact on social inclusion and financial protection. The targeting outcome of community-financing schemes is impressive although there are indications that the very poorest are not automatically included. In terms of financial protection, CF reduces financial barriers to access through increased utilization by members, as opposed to nonmembers, and reduced out-of-pocket spending. There were no studies suggesting an inverse relationship, and two studies found no difference between use by members and nonmembers.[1]

However, a number of methodological concerns warrant some caution in interpreting the reported results. The most important one is that selection into membership status is nonrandom. People with higher risk for illness and higher propensity to use health care will be more likely to purchase insurance. Thus the impact of membership on utilization and out-of-pocket payments cannot be validly discerned by looking at sample averages of members and nonmembers. Such measures are biased and magnify the impact of community financing on utilization because these individuals would also have had higher use in the absence of membership.

DETERMINANTS OF SUCCESSFUL RESOURCE MOBILIZATION, SOCIAL INCLUSION, AND FINANCIAL PROTECTION

The key determinants that contribute to successful resource mobilization, combating social exclusion, and financial protection include: (a) ability to address adverse selection, accommodate irregular revenue stream of membership, prevent fraud, and have arrangements for the poorest; (b) good management with strong community involvement; (c) organizational linkages between the scheme and providers; and (d) donor support and government funding. Table 2.9 summarizes successful and unsuccessful design features.

TABLE 2.9   Determinants Associated with Effective Revenue Collection and Financial Protection

	Design features	
	Supporting effective revenue collection and financial protection	*Undermining revenue collection and financial protection*
Technical design characteristics	❑ Addressing adverse selection through group membership ❑ Accommodating irregular income stream of members (allow in-kind contributions, flexible revenue collection periods) ❑ Sliding fee scales and exemptions for the poor make schemes more affordable	❑ Noncompliance, evasion of membership payments ❑ Adverse selection ❑ Lack of cash income ❑ No cash income at collection time
Management characteristics	❑ Community involvement in management can exert social pressure on member compliance with revenue collection rules ❑ Extent of capacity building ❑ Information support	❑ Provider capture—high salary of providers at the expense of service-quality improvement ❑ Weak supervision structures increase the chance of fraud with membership card ❑ Poor control over providers and members contributes to moral hazard and cost escalation, and undermines sustainability of the scheme
Organizational characteristics	❑ Linkages with providers to negotiate preferential rates raises attractiveness of schemes and contributes to successful membership	❑ Fragmentation between inpatient and outpatient care leads to inefficiency and waste ultimately resulting in loss of membership
Institutional characteristics	❑ Government and donor support make the schemes more sustainable and pro-poor.	

Technical Design Characteristics

Revenue Collection

Most community-financing schemes rely on a combination of revenue sources including prepayment, user charges, government subsidy, and donor assistance. For example, in the Kanage Cooperative Scheme in Rwanda, the sum of the premiums collected covered only a fraction of what members spent on care, and the scheme was largely financed by the revenues of the hospital. The share of each these sources varied widely by scheme (Roenen and Criel 1997).

Despite large variations in the composition of revenue sources, it appears that schemes can rarely raise enough resources from prepayment only. As a result, user charges are often utilized in conjunction with other resources, and most schemes rely on some form of external financing (government subsidy, donor support). For example, the CLAISS study (1999) compared 11 schemes in Latin America and found that 9 received significant external financial support.

Most prepayment schemes collect membership fees on the basis of annual premium rates, which are typically a flat rate (community rated). Annual collection is consistent with the agrarian-based structure of income-generating capacities (Diop, Yazbeck, and Bitran 1995; Roenen and Criel 1997; Atim and Sock 2000; Bennett, Creese, and Monasch 1998; Arhin 1994). Sliding scales and exemptions for the poor are rare and reported more frequently from Asia than Africa (Desmet, Chowdhury, and Islam 1999; Dave 1991). Flat rate contributions simplify the collection procedure and are less subject to manipulation. At the same time, such contribution schemes may prevent the poorest from joining.

Revenue collection appears to be more successful when the contribution scheme takes into account the nature of the membership population's revenues. Synchronizing the contribution collection period with cash-earning periods makes a difference in terms of the ability of the schemes to raise resources. Some examples include:

- In Central and West Africa, 73 percent of the 22 MHOs reviewed had already designed their contribution scheme to coincide with a more cash-endowed period (Atim 1998).

- The Kanage Cooperative Scheme in Rwanda scheduled registration in the coffee-harvesting period between June and September. Roenen and Criel (1997) suggested that this may have been too short a time period and, along with low membership levels, may have contributed to the scheme's failure.

- The Bwamanda Hospital Insurance Scheme also has a community-rated system of premium collection during the crop-selling season. The scheme offers voluntary membership to the family as a subscription unit (Criel, van der Stuyft, and van Lerberghe 1999).

- The Nkoranza community-financing scheme in Ghana was found to have a low coverage rate of 30 percent. The registration period did not coincide with the cash-earning period of the community. This was one of the main reasons behind the low enrollment (Atim 2000).

BOX 2.4   TURNING POTATOES AND LABOR INTO CASH REVENUES IN BOLIVIA

Toonen argues that allowing farmers to provide in-kind contributions either in terms of farm products or labor increases the ability of the scheme to attract members and thus resources. He presents the example of a rural prepayment plan from Bolivia in which membership dues were in the form of contributing seed potatoes to the community organization. In addition, at least one family member had to work on the community lot for production of potatoes. Some of the harvest was kept for use as seed potatoes for the following year, and the remainder was sold on the market. Proceeds were used to pay for drugs, to pay a bonus to the auxiliary nurse, and to renovate the health centers.

Source: Toonen (1995).

In-kind contributions are rarely allowed (Atim 1998; Bennett, Creese, and Monasch 1998; Musau 1999; Dave 1991). There are a few exceptions, and in all cases the authors appear enthusiastic about the potential of generating resources from in-kind contributions. For example, Preker (2001) found that in the Philippines' Pesos for Health community scheme, when people fell ill and had to visit the hospital, or for members who could not pay the premiums, they could monetarize agricultural produce such as chickens into cash in the hospital and were able to pay for health care. See also box 2.4.

Dave (1991) also found schemes in India where membership payments were accepted in the form of rice and sorghum. In-kind contributions, however, are accepted as payment for prepayment insurance scheme membership and not as an on-going payment option—RAHA scheme (rice), Sewagram (sorghum), Goalpara (community labor)—to ensure that the poor are not excluded. Schemes such as Sewagram employ a community health worker (CHW) to collect the contributions once a year, usually at harvest time; the CHW then sells the grain in the open market. From the funds generated the CHW purchases drugs, pays Sewagram for mobile support, and retains the difference as his or her salary.

Pooling

There is wide variation in the size and number of risk-pools. At the two extremes are schemes that start up with a few dozens households (such as Guatemala and ASSABA) and schemes that operate with several million members (such as Burundi and the health card scheme). From the database of 82 schemes complied by Bennett, Creese, and Monasch (1998), the following conclusions emerge about the size of community-financing schemes:

- The population covered varied between 40 households and 700 million (Niger).

- The share of eligible population in the total local population also varied from less than 1 percent to 90 percent.

- The average level of coverage of eligible population in the sample amounted to 37 percent.

In addition to small size, pooling is further undermined by adverse selection. As community-based schemes are mostly voluntary and charge a flat premium, adverse selection is often reported as a key difficulty in ensuring financial sustainability (Atim 1998; Bennett, Creese, and Monasch 1998; Arhin 1994; Ekman 2001). For example, in the Burundi Health Card Scheme the overall low membership rate (23 percent of households) was associated with community-rated premiums that discouraged low-risk individuals from purchasing CAM cards. Non-CAM members referred to higher care often purchased cards prior to the treatment or at the time of the referral to reduce their financial barrier to expensive curative care without having to participate in the risk sharing. Larger households were also more likely to be current or past cardholders (Arhin 1994).

Prepayment schemes apply several mechanisms to increase and diversify their risk pool. These include waiting time between registration and eligibility for benefits; (mandatory) group-based membership at the family or enterprise or professional association levels; and incentives to register entire families (Atim 1998; Musau 1999; Bennett, Creese, and Monasch 1998; Dave 1991; Atim and Sock 2000). For example, membership in the Chogoria Hospital Insurance Scheme in Kenya is open, but the premium structures favor group memberships. Coffee and tea cooperative societies and schools were the target groups in the community. However, coverage fell to only a group of hospital employees in 1998–99 because of an inability to attract group memberships, high premium rates for individual memberships, slow services, and insufficient benefits (Musau 1999).

Purchasing and Resource Allocation

The purchasing and resource allocation function of community-financing schemes is less extensively discussed in the literature than other aspects of their operations. Some schemes rely on third-party reimbursement to members; others pay providers directly. Often, sustainable financing is associated with the community's ability to negotiate preferential rates with providers.

Through several mechanisms, the community aims to ensure social control over the doctor-patient relationship and prevent unjustified overuse of services. There are examples of mandatory referrals to use higher level care, treatment guidelines, and various limitations and caps on utilization to prevent moral hazard and induced demand.

For example, the MHO in Senegal is community-based and covers only hospitalization. The membership fee is per person insured, although, in general, the household is a member of the mutual and participates in the decisions. If a member needs surgery, he or she has to pay 50 percent of the costs of the operation. Any excess stay at the hospital (beyond 10 to 15 days) is initially covered by the mutual, and then the member has to reimburse it. This seems to keep overutilization of services in check (Jütting 2000).

Management Characteristics

Besides getting the technical characteristics of the contribution scheme right, good management can also contribute to the success or failure of resource mobilization mechanisms. Good management is often as visible for members as the care they receive. For example, if the claims settlement process and other administrative measures prove cumbersome and lengthy, members may be less willing to join the scheme.

Perhaps the strongest agreement among the reviewed articles concerns the issue of community involvement in management of schemes as a prerequisite for success (Atim 1999; Atim and Sock 2000; Arhin 1995; Roenen and Criel 1997; Gumber and Kulkarni 2000; Carrin and others 1999; Desmet, Chowdhury, and Islam 1999). Community involvement in scheme management leads to improvements in not only revenue collection but also in cost containment, access, and quality of services. These performance measures, in turn, are prerequisites for sustaining membership levels and thus revenue flows (Hsiao 2001).

For example, Atim (1998) identifies the fact that MHOs owe their success to democratic governance, which is one of the original contributions of these schemes. MHOs represent their communities or members before the health authorities, including the providers influencing decisions of resource allocation, and ensure responsiveness of the health authorities to community concerns, which enhances the sustainability of the schemes.

The absence of community involvement in management may lead to provider capture and monopoly pricing. For example, the Kanage Cooperative Scheme described by Roenen and Criel (1997) did not have any community participation in its governance. There was a lack of adequate and relevant technical information to help in the decisionmaking process. There was no dialogue between the population and the hospital, leading to a dominant position for the health service. This may have rendered the system fragile and led to its failure.

Even when the community is involved in scheme management, representational issues might arise. Gilson and others (2000) reviewed the experience of Kenya, Zambia, and Benin. Community structures often were not seen as reflecting the views of the wider population, critical decisions often did not take into account the interest of the poorest, and the poorest were rarely involved directly in decisionmaking. The authors conclude that the voice of the poorest within the communities often is not heard or is not influential. As a result, community mechanisms by themselves may not adequately address the poor's lack of financial protection.

The problem encountered by most schemes, however, is that community-based schemes lack the management and administrative skills necessary for the successful design and operation of prepayment schemes. Such skills would include being able to calculate premium rates, determine benefits packages, market the scheme, communicate with members, negotiate with providers, keep accounting and bookkeeping records, work with computers, and monitor and evaluate the scheme (Atim 1998). See also box 2.5.

BOX 2.5   POOR MANAGEMENT IN THE NKORANZA SCHEME

The Nkoranza community-financing health insurance scheme was launched in 1992 in Ghana. The scheme is a hospital-based (modality 3) scheme. It was designed in association with Memisa, a Dutch Christian NGO. The scheme is affiliated with a private district hospital, St. Theresa's Hospital, for which the hospital bills are paid and which is paid on a fee-for-service basis. The scheme has voluntary membership based on a community-rated premium. The founding NGO offered to meet any deficits in the first three years of the scheme's operation. The scheme has a low coverage rate of 30 percent of the area's population.

Poor management of the Nkoranza scheme affected the enrollment and attractiveness of the scheme. Staff members were not aware of their formal job descriptions. There was a lack of training for staff in marketing and community participation methods, general management skills, risk-management techniques, negotiation skills, accounting and bookkeeping, computing skills, scheme-monitoring and evaluation of the scheme, and some of the hospital staff displayed negative attitudes toward the patients. The management approach was also top-down, with no supervisory body, reflecting the nonparticipatory design of the scheme.

The community was not effectively involved in the governance of the project. The community's participation was restricted to education and information campaigns. It was a hospital-based scheme, run as another department of the hospital. However, there are rules and regulations governing membership and access to services, which are revised annually and circulated within the community.

Source: Atim and Sock (2000).

Yet hiring someone with adequate skills to run and manage the scheme may cost the scheme too much. For example, in the Kanage Cooperative Scheme, the salary of the person hired to manage the scheme and register members proved too much for the scheme to bear (about US$670 a year), so the hospital took over. The scheme's total administrative costs were evaluated at 12 percent of its revenues, which may have been grossly underestimated as the rent on the leases was never included (Roenen and Criel 1997).

Organizational Characteristics

Of the organizational characteristics reviewed, linkages between schemes and providers are reported to be an important determinant of the performance of community-based schemes. Schemes that have a durable partnership arrangement or contractual arrangement with providers can negotiate preferential rates for their members. This, in turn, increases the attractiveness of the scheme to the population and contributes to sustainable membership levels.

For example, the schemes in the Thiès region of Senegal negotiated preferential rates with the nearby private St. Jean de Dieu Hospital. The hospital is run by a religious organization that is driven by altruistic objectives and has been very supportive of the activities of the Mutual Health Organizations. The negotiated rates allow the schemes to offer considerable benefits with acceptable contribution rates. This makes the schemes very attractive to the population and explains the high penetration rate among the target groups (Atim 1998).

Close ties with providers also allow the community to monitor provider behavior and exert social pressure on providers. This can lead to efficiency gains, allowing the schemes to use the resources for noticeable service improvement, which again increases the schemes' attractiveness to the population and is the cornerstone of sustainability. Conversely, inefficiencies due to weak gatekeeping, for example, may lead to moral hazard and wasted resources. In this case, membership may drop if service and quality do not improve and if the costs of the membership are higher than the perceived value of the benefits. The Nkoranza health insurance scheme is an example of this (Atim and Sock 2000).

Another level of organizational linkages is the relationship of the scheme to other schemes, in particular to the national government health system and/or social security system. In the Thai Health Card Scheme, the beneficiaries were allowed to use the health provider units under the Ministry of Public Health via the health center or community hospital and follow the referral line. Providers were compensated for the care they provided to health cardholders on a per case basis. They were also reimbursed for administrative expenses incurred by being part of the health card program (Supakankunti 1997).

Institutional Characteristics

Information is available about certain institutional characteristics of community-financing schemes, such as stewardship and regulation, ownership forms and related governance structures, and markets. However, better understanding is necessary to assess how various institutional characteristics contribute to scheme performance. This is particularly the case regarding issues of ownership in which modalities are well-formulated, but their impact on performance is less understood.

Stewardship. The role of government-level stewardship is often hypothesized as a critical determinant of sustainable health financing through community structures. Some researchers argue that government and donor support are critical for successful and sustainable community-based health financing. This can be financial support but it can also be a supportive policy environment and the provision of training and information opportunities.

In Thailand, for example, the government subsidizes half of the cost of the health card. The household contributes half the price of the insurance card during the income-earning season, while the other half is subsidized by general tax revenue through the Ministry of Public Health. The Ministry of Public Health decentralized the management and decisionmaking to the provincial level, allowing provinces to define their own policies. The premiums, however, remained the same. The health card officers helped increase access to the scheme by providing clear information to the community (Supakankunti 1997).

In some provinces of China, the Rural Cooperative Medical System is a joint effort between the government, the villages, and the rural population. Counties and townships played a vital role in the design of the scheme, which was adapted to different local situations (Carrin and others 1999).

At the same time, there are community-financing schemes that were created in response to a vacuum in government stewardship—and managed to survive. Criel, van der Stuyft, and van Lerberghe (1999) offer the example of the Bwamanda scheme in the Democratic Republic of Congo, which "succeeded in generating stable revenue for the hospital in a context where government intervention was virtually absent and where external subsidies were most uncertain."

A more systematic assessment of the various forms of government support (financial, nonfinancial) for community financing and their performance impact would make a much-needed contribution toward our understanding of what makes certain schemes work and others fail.

Ownership. There are various forms of ownership and related forms of governance: by members (that is, cooperative), by providers, by nongovernmental organizations, by microfinance organizations, and by churches. (See Bennett, Creese, and Monasch 1998 for a comprehensive discussion of ownership forms of community financing.) Each form of ownership can demonstrate successful as well as unsuccessful resource-mobilization schemes. Thus the same conclusion holds as for government regulation—linking alternative ownership forms with performance measures is a much-needed contribution to the field.

Markets. Community-financing schemes compete on the factor markets (particularly labor and supplies) with other organizations involved in financing and providing health care. Attracting physicians to remote rural areas where most community-financing schemes work is difficult. Community-financing schemes' effective demand for factors of health services production is hampered by their low ability to pay due to their predominantly poor contributing population.

In the health services markets, community-financing schemes often fill a vacuum, and thus competitive forces do not necessarily apply: community-financing schemes are often initiated in response to the complete absence of other income-protection instruments for the poor against the cost of illness. Thus their members often do not have a meaningful choice of alternative schemes or other health-financing modalities.

At the same time, competition is more likely when the scheme is involved in active purchasing of health services from providers and employs selectivity in the resource allocation process and performance rewards. This is again hampered by the geographic monopoly of providers in poor rural areas where many of the schemes operate. Further understanding of how market mechanisms apply to community-financing schemes and how they affect performance would be helpful.

In conclusion, the reviewed literature is very rich in terms of describing various technical, managerial, organizational, and institutional features of community-financing schemes. At the same time, better understanding is needed to assess how these structural characteristics contribute to scheme performance. This is particularly true where modalities are now well-formulated but their impact on performance is less understood.

CONCLUDING REMARKS

This review of 45 studies on community-based health financing has found a number of interesting observations. Perhaps the most obvious conclusion is that the literature on community-based health financing is growing exponentially. This reflects enthusiasm among policymakers and researchers alike about the potential of these schemes to mobilize resources for the health care of the poor.

Although this growing literature is varied in terms of focus, content, scope, and approach, the following observations emerge:

- The reviewed literature is very rich in describing the nature of community financing and its variants. There is plenty of information about the design of various schemes and also about the implementation process.

- Evidence regarding the performance of community financing is building up. In particular, there is rather convincing evidence that community involvement in resource mobilization increases access to health care for those covered by these programs while reducing the financial burden of those seeking health care.

- At the same time, the need persists for further evidence about the performance of community-based health-financing arrangements along various measures. Most striking is the lack of knowledge about the number of people covered globally, the extent of their coverage, and the volume of resources mobilized. In the absence of these indicators, assessment of the potential of community financing at a global scale is difficult.

- There are a number of definitions and typologies presented in the literature, and this chapter is guilty in adding an additional one. It would be an important step, however, to arrive at a common definition so that individual studies and presented schemes could be compared more easily.

- Accepting that community financing comes in many shapes and forms, a key unanswered question is, What form of community financing is more effective in terms of mobilizing resources for the health of the poor and providing financial protection against the cost of illness?

See page 114 for acknowledgments, notes, and references.

APPENDIX 2A. PERFORMANCE VARIABLES REPORTED IN THE REVIEWED STUDIES

In this section, we list the reviewed 45 studies, grouped according to the modality of the scheme or schemes it reviews (table 2.10). Sections 1 through 4 are the four modalities, Section 5 summarizes studies that address multiple modalities and were large comparative papers, and Section 6 lists the conceptual papers. The performance variables include resource generation, social inclusion, and financial protection.

TABLE 2.10   Performance Variables Reported in the Reviewed Studies

Modality 1: Community cost sharing	Countries reviewed	Resource generation	Social inclusion	Financial protection	Others
1. McPake, B., K. Hanson, and A. Mills. 1993. "Community Financing of Health Care in Africa: An Evaluation of the Bamako Initiative."	Burundi Guinea Kenya Uganda	✔	✔	✔	
2. Ogunbekun, I., and others. 1996. "Costs and Financing of Improvements in the Quality of Maternal Health Services through the Bamako Initiative in Nigeria."	Nigeria	✗	✗	✗	
3. Soucat, A., T. Gandaho, and others. 1997. "Health Seeking Behavior and Household Expenditures in Benin and Guinea: The Equity Implications of the Bamako Initiative."	Benin Guinea	✔	✗	✔	
4. Soucat, A., D. Levy-Bruhl, and others. 1997. "Local Cost Sharing in Bamako Initiative Systems in Benin and Guinea: Assuring the Financial Viability of Primary Health Care."	Benin Guinea	✔	✗	✗	
5. Gilson, L. 1997. "The Lessons of User Fee Experience in Africa."	Africa	✔	✗	✗	Efficiency Equity Sustainability
6. Supakankunti, S. 1998. "Comparative Analysis of Various Community Cost Sharing Implemented in Myanmar."	Myanmar	✗	✗	✗	

(continued)

TABLE 2.10   Continued

Modality 1: Community cost sharing	Countries reviewed	Resource generation	Social inclusion	Financial protection	Others
7. Fiedler, J. L., and R. Godoy. 1999. *An Assessment of the Community Drug Funds of Honduras.*	Honduras	✗	✗	✗	
8. Fiedler, J. L., and J. B. Wight. 2000. "Financing Health Care at the Local Level: The Community Drug Funds of Honduras."	Honduras	✗	✗	✗	Quality
9. Gilson, L., and others. 2000. "The Equity Impacts of Community Financing Activities in Three African Countries."	Benin Kenya Zambia	✔	✔	✔	
10. Okumara, J., and T. Umena. 2001. "Impact of Bamako Type Revolving Drug Fund on Drug Use in Vietnam."	Vietnam	✗	✗	✗	

Modality 2: Community prepayment or mutual health organizations	Countries reviewed	Resource generation	Social inclusion	Financial protection	Others
11. Arhin, D.C. 1995. *Rural Health Insurance: A Viable Alternative to User Fees.*	Ghana Guinea-Bissau Burundi	✔	✗	✔	
12. Toonen, J. 1995. *Community Financing for Health Care: A Case Study from Bolivia.*	Bolivia	✔	✗	✗	
13. Hsiao, W.C. 1995. "The Chinese Health Care System: Lessons for Other Nations."	China	✗	✗	✗	
14. Ron, A., and A. Kupferman. 1996. *A Community Health Insurance Scheme in the Philippines: Extension of a Community-Based Integrated Project.*	Philippines	✗	✗	✗	
15. Liu, Y., and others. 1996. "Is Community Financing Necessary and Feasible for Rural China?"	China	✔	✔	✔	
16. Desmet, A., A. Q. Chowdhury, and K. Islam. 1999. "The Potential for Social Mobilization in Bangladesh: The Organization and Functioning of Two Health Insurance Schemes."	Bangladesh	✔	✔	✔	

(continued)

TABLE 2.10   Continued

Modality 2: Community prepayment or mutual health organizations	Countries reviewed	Resource generation	Social inclusion	Financial protection	Others
17. Ron, A. 1999. "NGOs in Community Health Insurance Schemes: Examples from Guatemala and Philippines."	Guatemala Philippines	✗	✗	✗	
18. Carrin, G., and others. 1999. "The Reform of the Rural Cooperative Medical System in the People's Republic of China: Interim Experience in 14 Pilot Counties."	China	✔	✔	✔	
19. Chen, N., A. Ma, and Y. Guan. 2000. "Study and Experience of a Risk-based Cooperative Medical System in China: Experience in Weifang of Shandong Province."	China	✗	✗	✔	
20. Xing-yuan, G., and F. Xue-shan. 2000. "Study on Health Financing in Rural China."	China	✗	✗	✔	Drug use behavior
21. Gumber, A., and V. Kulkarni. 2000. "Health Insurance for Informal Sector: Case Study of Gujarat."	India	✗	✗	✔	
22. Jütting, J. 2000. "Do Mutual Health Insurance Schemes Improve the Access to Health Care? Preliminary Results from a Household Survey in Rural Senegal."	Senegal	✗	✔	✔	
23. Schneider, P., F. Diop, and S. Bucyana. 2000. *Development and Implementation of Prepayment Schemes in Rwanda.*	Rwanda	✔	✗	✔	Quality
24. Preker, A. 2001. "Philippines Mission Report."	Philippines	✗	✗	✗	

Modality 3: Provider-based community health insurance	Countries reviewed	Resource generation	Social inclusion	Financial protection	Others
25. Roenen, C., and B. Criel 1997. *The Kanage Community Financed Scheme: What Can Be Learned from the Failure?*	China Rwanda Sub-Saharan Africa	✔	✗	✔	Effectiveness Efficiency

(continued)

TABLE 2.10   Continued

Modality 3: Provider-based community health insurance	Countries reviewed	Resource generation	Social inclusion	Financial protection	Others
26. Criel, B., P. van der Stuyft, and W. van Lerberghe. 1999. "The Bwamanda Hospital Insurance Scheme: Effective for Whom? A Study of Its Impact on Hospitalization Utilization Patterns."	Democratic Republic of Congo	✔	✔	✔	Efficiency
27. Atim, C., and M. Sock. 2000. *An External Evaluation of the Nkoranza Community Financing Health Insurance Scheme, Ghana.*	Ghana	✗	✔	✔	

Modality 4: Community-driven prepayment scheme attached to social insurance or government-run system	Countries reviewed	Resource generation	Social inclusion	Financial protection	Others
28. Arhin, D. 1994. "The Health Card Insurance Scheme in Burundi: A Social Asset or a Non-Viable Venture?"	Burundi	✔	✔	✔	Benefit to women
29. DeRoeck, D., and others. 1996. *Rural Health Services at Seguridad Social Campesino Facilities: Analyses of Facility and Household Surveys.*	Ecuador	✔	✔	✔	Cost and demand analysis
30. Supakankunti, S. 1997. *Future Prospects of Voluntary Health Insurance in Thailand.*	Thailand	✔	✔	✗	Quality of care

Studies that address multiple modalities	Countries reviewed	Resource generation	Social inclusion	Financial protection	Others
31. Dave, P. 1991. "Community and Self-Financing in Voluntary Health Programmes in India."	India	✔	✗	✗	
32. Diop, F., R. Bitran, and M. Makinen. 1994. *Evaluation of the Impact of Pilot Tests for Cost Recovery on Primary Health Care in Niger.*	Niger	✔	✔	✔	Quality
33. Diop F., A. Yazbeck, and R. Bitran. 1995. "The Impact of Alternative Cost Recovery Schemes on Access and Equity in Niger."	Niger	✔	✔	✔	Quality

(continued)

TABLE 2.10   Continued

Studies that address multiple modalities	*Countries reviewed*	*Resource generation*	*Social inclusion*	*Financial protection*	*Others*
34. Atim, C. 1998. *Contribution of Mutual Health Organizations to Financing, Delivery, and Access to Health Care. Synthesis of Research in Nine West and Central-African Countries.*	Benin Burkina- Faso Cameroon Côte d'Ivoire Ghana Mali Nigeria Senegal Togo	✔	✗	✗	Efficiency Quality Sustainability

35. Bennett, S., A. Creese, and R. Monasch. 1998. *Health Insurance Schemes for People Outside Formal Sector Employment.*	Bangladesh
	Burundi
	Cameroon
	China
	Dem. Rep.
	  of Congo
	Ecuador
	Guatemala
	Guinea-Bissau
	India
	Indonesia
	Kenya
	Madagascar
	Mali
	Mexico
	Nepal
	Nigeria
	Papua New
	  Guinea
	Philippines
	Tanzania
	Thailand
	Vietnam
		✔	✗	✗	Efficiency

36. Musau, S. 1999. *Community-Based Health Insurance: Experiences and Lessons Learned from East and Southern Africa.*	Kenya Tanzania Uganda	✔	✗	✔	Efficiency Quality Sustainability
37. Atim, C. 1999. "Social Movements and Health Insurance: A Critical Evaluation of Voluntary, Nonprofit Insurance Schemes with Case Studies from Ghana and Cameroon."	Cameroon Ghana	✔	✗	✗	Efficiency

(continued)

TABLE 2.10   Continued

Studies that address multiple modalities	Countries reviewed	Resource generation	Social inclusion	Financial protection	Others
38. CLAISS. 1999. "Synthesis of Micro-Insurance and Other Forms of Extending Social Protection in Health in Latin America and the Caribbean."	Argentina Bolivia Colombia Dominican Republic Ecuador Guatemala Honduras Nicaragua Peru Uruguay	✔	✗	✗	Equity Financial Sustainability Quality
39. Hsiao, W. C. 2001. *Unmet Needs of Two Billion: Is Community Financing a Solution?*	China Indonesia	✔	✗		
40. Narula, I. S. and others. 2000. *Community Health Financing Mechanisms and Sustainability: A Comparative Analysis of 10 Asian Countries.*	Cambodia China Indonesia Lao PDR Mongolia Myanmar Papua New Guinea Philippines Thailand Vietnam	✔	✗	✗	Quality Financial Sustainability

Conceptual papers that did not address any schemes classified under the modalities	Countries reviewed	Resource generation	Social inclusion	Financial protection	Others
41. Dror, D., and C. Jacquier. 1999. "Micro-Insurance: Extending Health Insurance to the Excluded."		✗	✗	✗	
42. Brown, W., and C. Churchill. 2000. *Insurance Provision in Low-Income Communities: Part II—Initial Lessons from Micro-insurance Experiments for the Poor.*		✗	✗	✗	
43. Ziemek, S., and J. Jütting. 2000. *Mutual Insurance Schemes and Social Protection.*		✗	✗	✗	

(continued)

TABLE 2.10   Continued

Conceptual papers that did not address any schemes classified under the modalities	Countries reviewed	Resource generation	Social inclusion	Financial protection	Others
44. Criel, B. 2000. *Local Health Insurance Systems in Developing Countries: A Policy Research Paper.*		✗	✗	✗	
45. Ekman, B. 2001. *Community-Based Health Insurance Schemes in Developing Countries: Theory and Empirical Experiences.*		✗	✗	✗	

APPENDIX 2B. CORE CHARACTERISTICS OF COMMUNITY FINANCING SCHEMES FROM THE REVIEW OF LITERATURE

In this section, we list 21 schemes reviewed in the literature grouped by their modality (table 2.11). The design characteristics of the schemes are detailed: technical design characteristics, management characteristics, organizational characteristics, and institutional characteristics.

TABLE 2.11   Core Characteristics of Community Financing Schemes, from the Review of Literature

Modality 1: *Community cost sharing*

Authors (year)	Soucat and others (1997)
Name of the scheme	Bamako Initiative in Benin and Guinea
Technical design characteristics	
Revenue collection mechanisms	• User fee • Voluntary
Pooling and risk-sharing arrangements	
Purchasing and resource allocation	• Curative care covered in revitalized health centers • Reduced prices or free care for the poor provided based on a case-by-case basis interview and visual inspection • Highly utilized by children, and low SES exclusion only due to financial reasons • Low price for preventive care due to cross-subsidization of long-term curative care
Management characteristics	
Staff	• Large proportion of operating costs covered through user fee funds • Funds retained at health center level and managed locally
Culture	
Access to information	
Organizational characteristics	
Organizational forms	
Incentive regime	
Linkages	
Institutional characteristics	
Stewardship	• Community involved in monitoring and budgeting, increases accountability and autonomy
Governance	• Community sense of ownership
Insurance markets	
Factor and product markets	

(continued)

TABLE 2.11   Continued

Modality 2: Community prepayment scheme or mutual health organization

Authors (year)	Gumber and Kulkarni (2000)	Desmet, Chowdhury, and Islam (1999)	Desmet, Chowdhury, and Islam (1999)
Name of the scheme	Self Employed Women's Association (SEWA), India	Grameen Health program, Bangladesh	Gonosasthya Kendra, Bangladesh
Technical design characteristics			
Revenue collection mechanisms	• Voluntary membership for families • Women beneficiaries • Fixed premium, which is low as assets of the NGO assist the running of the scheme	• Prepayment with a form of scaling in fee structure • Members are beneficiaries of the Grameen Bank cooperative	• Sliding scale fee structure of premiums and copayments • Voluntary per household based on signing of contract
Pooling and risk-sharing arrangements			
Purchasing and resource allocation			
Management characteristics			
Staff	• Preference for management at the panchayat level • Easy and quick settlement of claims by administrative staff		
Culture		• Top-down approach of management	• Power struggle in management scaling down of the interaction with the community to family and individual
Access to information			
Organizational characteristics			
Organizational forms			
Incentive regime			
Linkages			
Institutional characteristics			
Stewardship		• No active subscriber involvement	• No active subscriber involvement
Governance			
Insurance markets			
Factor and product markets			

(continued)

TABLE 2.11   Continued

Modality 2: Community prepayment scheme or mutual health organization (continued)

Authors (year)	Jütting (2000)	ATIM (1999)	Arhin (1994)
Name of the scheme	**Mutual Health Organization (MHO), Senegal**	**Mutuelle Famille Babouantou de Yaoundé, Cameroon**	**Abota Village Health Insurance Scheme, Guinea-Bissau**
Technical design characteristics			
Revenue collection mechanisms	• Fee per member insured • Generally household is a member • 50 percent of costs to be paid in case of surgery to check overutilization, any excess stay in the hospital of more than 10–15 days initially paid by the mutual and eventually reimbursed by the member	• Individual or family membership—high premiums • Members of same ethnic group	• Revenue collection varies from village to village, from individual to household basis, in-kind contribution in the form of agricultural produce accepted • Prepayment contributions collection time varied from once to twice a year
Pooling and risk-sharing arrangements		• 3 months probationary period to check for adverse selection • Family registration incentives to check for adverse selection	• Social cohesion responsible for reducing adverse selection and moral hazard
Purchasing and resource allocation	• Covers only hospitalization	• Association pays a lump sum to member in the event of hospitalization for a specified time, surgery for at least 15 days • Cannot claim benefits more than once a year • As check on moral hazard, scheme pays fixed amount per person per year	• If Abota scheme member, referred patients to the public health facilities exempt from consultation fees

(continued)

TABLE 2.11   Continued

Modality 2: Community prepayment scheme or mutual health organization (continued)

**Management
characteristics**

Staff		• Mutual aid organization draws on voluntary labor of its members for management and other tasks • No full-time paid staff • No external grants in the income • Potentially good management staff— skilled in their own workplaces, and stiff sanctions exist for dereliction of duty	• Decreasing capacity of government health workers to train and supervise village health workers • Abota funds misappropriated by village health workers or staff of the Ministry of Health • Drug shortages • Village health workers attend refresher training courses
Culture	• Household participates in the decisionmaking	• Community participation in meetings and elections of management • Social control to check fraud, moral hazard, etc.	

Access to information

**Organizational
characteristics**

Organizational forms

Incentive regime

Linkages	• Contract with nonprofit St. Jean de Dieu hospital provides a reduction of up to 50 percent for treatment		• Supplier of drugs is the Central Medical Store in the capital to government health centers and sectoral hospitals • Government obligated to train and supervise village health workers, supply essential drugs • Support also provided by NGOs such as GVC and WHO/UNICEF evaluation teams

(continued)

TABLE 2.11   Continued

Modality 2: Community prepayment scheme or mutual health organization (continued)

Institutional characteristics		
Stewardship	• No enforcement of essential drug list policy or generic drugs for refunds	• Government involvement apart from management by both traditional and political leaders through the village committees • Individual communities develop financing system based on local appropriateness • However, no control of community in purchasing of inputs
Governance	• Social solidarity is prominent • Democratic accountability, participation and a sense of ownership is strong	• Has the characteristics of a social institution • Community involvement beyond mobilization of local material and labor resources
Insurance markets		
Factor and product markets		
Authors (year)	**Musau (1999)**	**Musau (1999)**	**Schneider, Diop, and Bucyana (2000)**
Name of the scheme	**Mburahati Health Trust Fund, Tanzania**	**Atiman Insurance Scheme, Tanzania**	**Community-Based Health Insurance—Prepayment Schemes, Rwanda**
Technical design characteristics			
Revenue collection mechanisms	• Two types of payments: registration fees to cover operational costs related to start-up of scheme and regular contributions (daily) in cash or in-kind for daily income earners • Membership based on a nuclear family, flat fee per day per person	• Monthly premiums paid directly to the Parish Office • Family or individual membership • Voluntary membership	• Annual premium per family • Copayment is paid per episode of care • In the pilot project, two districts had voluntary subscription and one subscription was through health solidarity fund

(continued)

TABLE 2.11   Continued

Modality 2: Community prepayment scheme or mutual health organization (continued)

Pooling and risk-sharing arrangements	• To prevent moral hazard, there is social control as the group is small • There is a 3-month probation period, and the whole family must enroll in scheme to prevent adverse selection	• Schemes practice a short probation or waiting period for a month, in practice varies and adverse selection exists • Moral hazard risk is minimized by social control	• One-month waiting period • On a health center level, risk is shared within the community; on a hospital level, the risk is shared on a district level
Purchasing and resource allocation	• Includes outpatient care in designated dispensary, and covers 10 percent of costs of hospitalization in public hospital • No MCH services included • Family photograph in dispensary is required to prevent fraud, and the patient signs for treatment received	• Includes outpatient care at local church dispensary, no limit to cost • Primary care available at St. Camillus Dispensary • Members have an ID card with photograph to minimize fraud	• Covers basic health center package of services, drugs, and ambulance referral to district hospital • Subsidization of premiums by employers and religious authorities • Prepayment schemes reimburse health centers by capitation payment • District hospital reimbursed by district federation on a per episode basis from the schemes' monthly disbursement

Management characteristics

Staff	• Manual recordkeeping by different officials of the scheme • All members receive training from the SSMECA regarding need for social protection and characteristics of mutual health insurance schemes • On-the-job training related to administration and management received • Health care provider also receives training regarding administration requirements and adherence to established procedures prior to medical treatment	• Manual records kept in church office, incomplete after theft • Weak management of the dispensary resulted in irregularities in leadership and accountability of the dispensary over prescription of drugs, and poor quality care • No fraud check systems in place • Scheme's leaders, staff, and health care provider have no training on management of health insurance	• Provided regular training before and after launch of the prepayment scheme on scheme modalities, accounting tools, administration, organizational and financial issues, etc. • In order to strengthen financial and organizational management capacities on the provider side, members prepay for care, and schemes pay a capitation rate instead of fee-for-service payment

(continued)

TABLE 2.11 Continued

Modality 2: Community prepayment scheme or mutual health organization (continued)

Culture	• Operates through an elected Health Committee composed of a chairperson, secretary, and treasurer, and monthly meetings and annual general meeting		• Staff receives regular feedback on service utilization, financial standing, and membership status • Contractual relationship with the partners of scheme lends democratization in Rwanda
Access to information			• Population informed about introduction of prepayment schemes via radio spots, newspaper articles, and community and church meetings

Organizational characteristics

Organizational forms			
Incentive regime			
Linkages	• With public hospital • Technical assistance from the SSMECA (Strengthening Small and Micro Enterprise and their Cooperatives/Association) • Contract with the Harlem Agape Dispensary to provide health care • The Medical Department of the Catholic Secretariat of the Tanzania Episcopal Church assists the group in checking the treatment forms on a regular basis	• With local church dispensary that reports to the diocese medical director and the medical board • Linkages with the Christian Mutual Association in Belgium to develop control measures such as treatment guidelines and official agreement between scheme and dispensary	

(continued)

TABLE 2.11 Continued

Modality 2: *Community prepayment scheme or mutual health organization (continued)*

Institutional characteristics

Stewardship	<ul><li>The Scheme Management Committee is elected by members</li><li>There are formal links with the local government; Kinondoni district cooperative officer provides training on aspects related to cooperative management</li></ul>	<ul><li>The Parish Office and Scheme Executive Committee manage the scheme</li><li>Consultations with MOH, and ILO's SSMECA STEP project</li><li>Some sort of subsidy reliance exists</li></ul>	<ul><li>Two districts chose for the schemes to be managed by providers and population, while one chose to be managed directly by the population</li></ul>
Governance	<ul><li>Members run the scheme, active involvement in the design and implementation of scheme</li></ul>	<ul><li>Community participation, members attend general meeting and elect their representatives in the Executive Committee</li></ul>	

Insurance markets

Factor and product markets

Modality 3: *Provider-based community health insurance*

Authors (year)	Atim and Sock (2000)	Roenen and Criel (1997)	Criel, van der Stuyft, and van Lerberghe (1999)
Name of the scheme	**Nkoranza Community Health Financing Scheme, Ghana**	**Kanage Cooperative Scheme, Rwanda**	**Bwamanda Hospital Insurance Scheme, Democratic Republic of Congo**

Technical design characteristics

Revenue collection mechanisms	<ul><li>Community-rated premiums</li><li>Collected Dec.–Jan.</li><li>Voluntary membership</li><li>Entire families covered</li></ul>	<ul><li>Community-rated premiums</li><li>Collected June–Sept.</li></ul>	<ul><li>Voluntary scheme</li><li>Community-rated premiums</li><li>Collected during the crop-selling season</li></ul>
Pooling and risk-sharing arrangements	<ul><li>Scheme insists at the time of admission of patient, that whole family be registered</li><li>Medical officer determines access to benefits to prevent moral hazard</li></ul>	<ul><li>Inverse relationship— poor ends up financing the services offered to the more affluent members of the cooperative</li></ul>	<ul><li>Family is the subscription unit</li></ul>

(continued)

TABLE 2.11   Continued

Modality 3: *Provider-based community health insurance (continued)*

Purchasing and resource allocation		• No good surveillance system leading to fraudulent use of services	• 20 percent copayment in case of hospital admission, which helps reduce adverse selection
Management characteristics			
Staff	• Lack of training in community participation skills, negotiation skills, accounting and book-keeping, computing skills, monitoring and evaluation of scheme	• One staff initially managed enrollment, but hospital took over due to high costs	
Culture	• Top-down approach of management	• No community involvement	
Access to information			
Organizational characteristics			
Organizational forms	• Contract with St. Theresa's Hospital, admission costs are covered		
Incentive regime	• Scheme pays the hospital on a fee-for-service basis	• Subsidized by Murunda Hospital	
Linkages	• With private district hospital—St. Theresa's Hospital	• Linked to the Murunda Hospital	• Linked to hospital as health care provider
Institutional characteristics			
Stewardship	• Hospital based	• Hospital based	
Governance	• No community involvement	• Hospital played a dominant role, no community participation	• Managed by the District Health Team
Insurance markets			
Factor and product markets			

(continued)

TABLE 2.11 Continued

Modality 3: Provider-based community health insurance (continued)

Authors (year)	Musau (1999)	Musau (1999)
Name of the scheme	**Kisiizi Hospital Health Society, Uganda**	**Chogoria Hospital Insurance Scheme, Kenya**
Technical design characteristics		
Revenue collection mechanisms	• Premium rates depend on family size and time period for which premiums are paid • The scheme is for those who can afford it, access for the poor is not considered	• Fixed premiums based on individual or family enrollment and benefits included • All members should also belong to the Kenya National Hospital Insurance Fund (NHIF) • Voluntary membership to scheme
Pooling and risk-sharing arrangements	• To prevent moral hazard, copayments are charged for out- and in-patient services • At least 60 percent of the group has to be enrolled for the scheme to work and prevent adverse selection • There is also a waiting period before coverage commences to stop people from joining scheme when they have just fallen sick	• To prevent moral hazard, out-patient visits have a copayment • There is a two-week waiting period, exclusion of preexisting conditions, and discount for those who join as a group to prevent adverse selection
Purchasing and resource allocation	• Includes out-patient care and in-patient care in general ward bed, and has no annual limit • Member ID cards are used to prevent fraud	• Includes outpatient and inpatient care subject to annual limits • To prevent fraud and abuse, there is a member ID card with photograph
Management characteristics		
Staff	• Manual data management with no regular reports kept in scheme office • Good internal control over use of hospital services, and external audit to prevent fraud • Some hospital staff have a negative attitude toward scheme members • Not enough staff members • Delay in processing claims so that they can collect drugs from pharmacy • Hospital has a computerized financial accounting system	• Computerized data management with monthly reports kept in the scheme office • Good internal controls over use of service and external audit along with monthly reports on utilization help prevent fraud and abuse of scheme
Culture		
Access to information	• Scheme conducts education meetings to help prospective members understand the scheme	

(continued)

TABLE 2.11 Continued

Modality 3: Provider-based community health insurance (continued)

Organizational characteristics		
Organizational forms		
Incentive regime		
Linkages	• No separation between the scheme and the hospital, and the scheme is part of the hospital and hence no contractual agreement exists	• With the Chogoria Hospital under the Presbyterian Church of East Africa • Current members are all employees of the hospital
Institutional characteristics		
Stewardship	• The Kisiizi Hospital Committee Consultative group manages along with the community members • Scheme recognized and supported by the MOH and the Ugandan Community-Based Health Financing Association • The scheme falls under the Community-Based Health Care program of the hospital	• The Hospital Committee manages the scheme • Technical assistance from the MOH and USAID funded Kenya Health Care Financing Project
Governance	• Community participation in design and implementation of scheme, and management of scheme	• No community participation
Insurance markets		
Factor and product markets		

Modality 4: Community-driven prepayment scheme attached to social insurance or government-run system

Authors (year)	**Xing-yuan and Xue-shan (2000)**	**Supakankunti (1997)**	**Carrin and others (1999)**
Name of the scheme	**Cooperative Health Care Scheme (CHCS), China**	**Thai Health Card Scheme, Thailand**	**Rural Cooperative Medical System (RCMS), China**
Technical design characteristics			
Revenue collection mechanisms	• Funded by peasants and government	• Voluntary prepaid scheme • Half the price of the insurance card is paid by the household during the cycle, depending on seasonal fluctuations, and the other half is subsidized by general tax revenue through the MOPH	• Voluntary • One-time registration, contributions collected once a year • Subsidy by government

(continued)

TABLE 2.11 Continued

Modality 4: Community-driven prepayment scheme attached to social insurance or government-run system (continued)

Pooling and risk-sharing arrangements		• Problem of adverse selection and over-utilization of services	• All funds pooled into one account except in 8 townships where risk sharing was limited due to separate accounts for farmers and workers
Purchasing and resource allocation	• Provides curative and preventive care	• 80 percent of the funds from the health card is allocated to compensate providers, and 20 percent for administrative costs	• Provides hospital care at the township and county level
Management characteristics			
Staff	• Effective as most of the funds were spent on health care and only 6–7 percent on management		• Technical support provided by a Central Technical Team, comprising representatives from the MOH, medical universities, and WHO
Culture		• Decentralized by the MOPH to the provincial level to define their own policies	
Access to information		• Health card officers effective in providing clear information to the community	
Organizational characteristics			
Organizational forms			
Incentive regime			
Linkages		• Beneficiaries used health provider units under the MOPH via health center or community hospital and referral line	
Institutional characteristics			
Stewardship			• Joint financial effort by the government, villages, and the rural population
Governance			• Counties and townships played a vital role in the design of the scheme adapted locally

(continued)

TABLE 2.11 Continued

Modality 4: Community-driven prepayment scheme attached to social insurance or government-run system *(continued)*

Insurance markets

Factor and product markets

Authors (year)	DeRoeck and others (1996)	Arhin (1994)	Musau (1999)
Name of the scheme	Seguridad Social Campesino (SSC), Ecuador	La Carte d'Assurance Maladie (CAM), Burundi	Community Health Fund (CHF), Tanzania
Technical design characteristics			
Revenue collection mechanisms	• Urban payroll tax and subsidies from government's general budget and investment income pay for the rural population enrolled in the scheme • SSC members contribute a small monthly fee that makes up less than 5 percent of the program's budget • Voluntary membership for whole family • Scheme study found user fees being charged largely for drugs, even to members	• CAM card purchased by household entitles two adults and all children younger than 18 to free health care at all public health facilities • Fixed price (community-rated premium) • Valid for one year and purchased at any time	• Voluntary participation except for civil servants employed by the Ministry of Local Government • Pricing of benefits package based on out-patient department health services
Pooling and risk-sharing arrangements	• From urban workers to the rural poor	• Adverse selection of households was a major problem due to larger households being more likely to purchase card • Moral hazard also a huge problem	• There is adverse selection in the scheme • Fixed premiums do not recognize the ability of the community to pay • There is a mechanism for the very poor to be exempt from paying for participation in the scheme • However, mandatory user-fee program together with CHF, has eliminated inappropriate use of services
Purchasing and resource allocation	• Provides medical and dental outpatient services, maternity, pre- and postnatal care, outreach activities, health education, and follow-up home visits	• If no card, user charges determined by health worker • Names of members written on card, thus preventing fraudulent use	• Includes outpatient care and has no limit • Member ID cards are used to prevent fraud

(continued)

TABLE 2.11   Continued

Modality 4: Community-driven prepayment scheme attached to social insurance or government-run system (continued)

**Management
characteristics**

Staff	• Shortages of drugs and fulltime medical staff led to the 50 percent decrease in utilization of clinics • Medical staff stresses the need for frequent in-service training; training in specialized in-patient care appropriate to urban area problems is often provided	• Shortage of drugs is a problem • Health worker discriminated against CAM holders in favor of cash payers • Few female medical technicians (poor ante-natal care)	• Manual recordkeeping at facilities and district headquarters, and computer spreadsheets at headquarters • Friendly staff • Good drug availability
Culture	• Top-down management from central office to regional community clinics	• Revenue retained by local committees that have financial responsibilities, although in practice only a small fraction used for health	• Top-down approach from MOH to DMO to CHF Ward Committee and community

Access to information

**Organizational
characteristics**

Organizational forms

Incentive regime

Linkages	• Provides primary health care outpatient services through a network of 549 small health clinics in remote rural areas and coastal and mountain regions	• Health worker salaries and drugs funded by government	• No contract between the CHF and service providers • Public health facilities and health centers and dispensaries participate in the CHF

**Institutional
characteristics**

Stewardship	• Administered through the government division of Instituto Ecuadoriano Seguro Social (IESS), including procurement of medicines, hiring employees, management, budget	• National health insurance scheme implemented by government	• The management is by the District CHF Board, Ward Health Committee, and facility staff • Initiated by the MOH government initiative, and receives full recognition

(continued)

TABLE 2.11   Continued

Modality 4: Community-driven prepayment scheme attached to social insurance or government-run system (continued)

Governance	• Community participation in the management of the fund and running of the public health facilities
Insurance markets	
Factor and product markets	

Acknowledgments: The authors of this chapter are grateful to the World Health Organization (WHO) for having provided an opportunity to contribute to the work of the Commission on Macroeconomics and Health and to the World Bank for having published the material in this chapter as an HNP Discussion Paper.

Many individuals from various organizations helped us compile an extensive list of published and unpublished studies for this review. We are grateful to all who helped us with this exciting investigative work. We would particularly like to thank Chris Atim (Abt Associates) for his insightful comments and suggestions. We are grateful to Christian Baeza (International Labour Organisation) who shared with us ILO's extensive experience and research results. Andrew Creese (WHO) and Sara Bennett (Abt Associates) greatly helped our work by making available the database of their research on health insurance in the informal sector.

NOTE

1. There may be some bias in the above conclusion as a result of "publication bias." It could be that research that found no difference on performance is less likely to be published. In addition, successful schemes are more likely than failed ones to make their way into studies.

REFERENCES

Arhin, D. C. 1994. "The Health Card Insurance Scheme in Burundi: A Social Asset or a Non-Viable Venture?" *Social Science and Medicine* 39(6): 861–70.

———. 1995. *Rural Health Insurance: A Viable Alternative to User Fees.* London School of Hygiene and Tropical Medicine, Discussion Paper. London.

Atim, C. 1998. *Contribution of Mutual Health Organizations to Financing, Delivery, and Access to Health Care: Synthesis of Research in Nine West and Central African Countries.* Technical Report 18. Partnerships for Health Reform Project, Abt Associates Inc., Bethesda, Md.

———. 1999. "Social Movements and Health Insurance: A Critical Evaluation of Voluntary, Non-Profit Insurance Schemes with Case Studies from Ghana and Cameroon." *Social Science and Medicine* 48(7): 881–96.

Atim, C., and M. Sock. 2000. *An External Evaluation of the Nkoranza Community Financing Health Insurance Scheme, Ghana.* Technical Report No. 50. Partnerships for Health Reform Project, Abt Associates Inc., Bethesda, Md.

Bennett S., A. Creese, and R. Monasch. 1998. *Health Insurance Schemes for People Outside Formal Sector Employment.* ARA Paper 16. World Health Organization (WHO), Geneva.

Brown, W., and C. Churchill. 2000. *Insurance Provision in Low-Income Communities: Part II—Initial Lessons from Microinsurance Experiments for the Poor.* Microenterprise Best Practices Project, Development Alternatives Inc., Bethesda, Md.

Carrin, G., R. Aviva, H. Yang, H. Wang, T. Zhang, L. Zhang, S. Zhang, Y. Ye, J. Chen, Q. Jiang, Z. Zhang, J. Yu, and L. Xi. 1999. "The Reform of the Rural Cooperative Medical System in the People's Republic of China: Interim Experience in 14 Pilot Counties." *Social Science and Medicine* 48: 961–72.

Chen, N., A. Ma, and Y. Guan. 2000. "Study and Experience of a Risk-Based Cooperative Medical System in China: Experience in Weifang of Shandong Province." Paper presented at the International Conference on Health Systems Financing in Low-Income African and Asian Countries, November 30–December 1, Centre d`Etudes et de Recherches sur le Développement International (CERDI), Clermont-Ferrand, France.

CLAISS (Latin American Center for Health Systems Research). 1999. "Synthesis of Micro-Insurance and Other Forms of Extending Social Protection in Health in Latin America and the Caribbean." Under the supervision and guidance of the ILO and PAHO counterparts, for the ILO-PAHO initiative of extending social protection in health in Latin America. Paper presented to the Mexico City tripartite meeting of ILO with the collaboration of PAHO, Mexico City.

Criel, B. 2000. *Local Health Insurance Systems in Developing Countries: A Policy Research Paper.* Departement Volksgezondheid, Instituut voor Tropische Geneeskunde, Antwerp.

Criel, B., P. Van der Stuyft, and W. Van Lerberghe. 1999. "The Bwamanda Hospital Insurance Scheme: Effective for Whom? A Study of Its Impact on Hospitalisation and Utilisation Patterns." *Social Science and Medicine* 48(7): 879–911.

Dave, P. 1991. "Community and Self-Financing in Voluntary Health Programmes in India." *Health Policy and Planning* 6(1): 20–31.

DeRoeck, D., J. Knowles, T. Wittenberg, L. Raney, and P. Cordova. 1996. *Rural Health Services at Seguridad Social Campesino Facilities: Analyses of Facility and Household Surveys.* Health Financing and Sustainability Project, Technical Report 13. Partnerships for Health Reform Project, Abt Associates Inc., Bethesda, Md.

Desmet, A., A. Q. Chowdhury, and K. Islam, M.D. 1999. "The Potential for Social Mobilization in Bangladesh: The Organization and Functioning of Two Health Insurance Schemes." *Social Science and Medicine* 48: 925–38.

Diop, F., R. Bitran, and M. Makinen. 1994. *Evaluation of the Impact of Pilot Tests for Cost Recovery on Primary Health Care in Niger.* Technical Report 16. Health Financing and Sustainability Project, Abt Associates Inc., Bethesda, Md.

Diop, F., A. Yazbeck, and R. Bitran. 1995. "The Impact of Alternative Cost Recovery Schemes on Access and Equity in Niger." *Health Policy and Planning* 10(3): 223–40.

Dror, D., and C. Jacquier. 1999. "Microinsurance: Extending Health Insurance to the Excluded." *International Social Security Review* 52(1): 71–97.

Ekman, B. 2001. *Community-Based Health Insurance Schemes in Developing Countries: Theory and Empirical Experiences.* Lund University Center for Health Economics (LUCHE), Department of Economics. Lund University.

Fiedler, J. L., and R. Godoy. 1999. *An Assessment of the Community Drug Funds of Honduras.* Technical Report No. 39. Partnerships for Health Reform, Abt Associates, Inc., Bethesda, Md.

Fiedler, J. L., and J. B. Wight. 2000. "Financing Health Care at the Local Level: The Community Drug Funds of Honduras." *International Journal of Health Planning and Management* 15: 319–40.

Gilson, L. 1997. "The Lessons of User Fee Experience in Africa." *Health Policy and Planning* 12(4): 273–85.

Gilson, L., D. Kalyalya, F. Kuchler, S. Lake, H. Oranga, and M. Ouendo. 2000. "The Equity Impacts of Community Financing Activities in Three African Countries." *International Journal of Health Planning and Management* 15: 291–317.

Gumber, A., and V. Kulkarni. 2000. "Health Insurance for Informal Sector: Case Study of Gujarat." *Economic and Political Weekly*, September 30, 3607–13.

Hsiao, W. C. 1995. "The Chinese Health Care System: Lessons for Other Nations." *Social Science and Medicine* 41(8): 1047–55.

———. 2001. *Unmet Health Needs of Two Billion: Is Community Financing a Solution?* World Bank, HNP Dicussion Paper. Washington, D.C.

Jütting, J. 2000. *Do Mutual Health Insurance Schemes Improve the Access to Health Care? Preliminary Results from a Household Survey in Rural Senegal.* Paper presented at the International Conference on Health Systems Financing in Low-Income African and Asian Countries, November 30–December 1, CERDI, Clermont-Ferrand, France.

Liu, Y., S. Hu, W. Fu, and W. C. Hsiao. 1996. "Is Community Financing Necessary and Feasible for Rural China?" *Health Policy* 38: 155–71.

McPake, B., K. Hanson, and A. Mills. 1993. "Community Financing of Health Care in Africa: An Evaluation of the Bamako Initiative." *Social Science and Medicine* 3(11): 1383–95.

Musau, S. 1999. *Community-Based Health Insurance: Experiences and Lessons Learned from East and Southern Africa.* Technical Report 34. Partnerships for Health Reform Project, Abt Associates, Inc., Bethesda, Md.

Narula, I. S., J. T. G. Tan, R. Knippenberg, and N. Jahanshahi. 2000. *Community Health Financing Mechanisms and Sustainability: A Comparative Analysis of 10 Asian Countries.* Paper presented at the International Conference on Health Systems Financing in Low-Income African and Asian Countries, November 30–December 1, CERDI, Clermont-Ferrand, France.

Ogunbekun, I., O. Adeyi, A. Wouters, and R. H. Morrow. 1996. "Costs and Financing of Improvements in the Quality of Maternal Health Services through the Bamako Initiative in Nigeria." *Health Policy and Planning* 11(4): 369–84.

Okumara, J., and T. Umena. 2001. "Impact of Bamako Type Revolving Drug Fund on Drug Use in Vietnam." Http://www.who.int/dap-icium/posters/3D3_TXTF.html.

Preker, A. S. 2001. "Philippines Mission Report." Internal document. The World Bank.

Preker, A. S., G. Carrin, D. Dror, and M. Jakab. 2001. *Health Care Financing for Rural and Low-income Populations: The Role of Communities in Resource Mobilization and Risk Sharing.* A draft background report submitted to the Commission on Macroeconomics and Health. WHO, Geneva.

Roenen, C., and B. Criel. 1997. *The Kanage Community Financed Scheme: What Can Be Learned from the Failure?* Antwerp: Institute of Tropical Medicine.

Ron, A. 1999. "NGOs in Community Health Insurance Schemes: Examples from Guatemala and Philippines." *Social Science and Medicine* 48: 939–50.

Ron, A., and A. Kupferman. 1996. *A Community Health Insurance Scheme in the Philippines: Extension of a Community-Based Integrated Project.* Geneva: WHO; London: International Cooperation–World ORT Union.

Schneider, P., F. Diop, and S. Bucyana. 2000. *Development and Implementation of Prepayment Schemes in Rwanda.* Technical Report 45. Partnerships for Health Reform Project, Abt Associates Inc., Bethesda, Md.

Soucat A., T. Gandaho, D. Levy-Bruhl, X. de Bethune, E. Alihonou, C. Ortiz, P. Gbedonou, P. Adovohekpe, O. Camara, J. M. Ndiaye, B. Dieng, and R. Knippenberg. 1997. "Health Seeking Behavior and Household Expenditures in Benin and Guinea: The Equity Implications of the Bamako Initiative." *International Journal of Health Planning and Management* 12(S1): 137–63.

Soucat, A., D. Levy-Bruhl, P. Gbedonou, K. Drame, J. P. Lamarque, S. Diallo, and R. Osseni. 1997. "Local Cost Sharing in Bamako Initiative Systems in Benin and Guinea: Assuring the Financial Viability of Primary Health Care." *International Journal of Health Planning and Management* 12(S1): 109–35.

Supakankunti, S. 1997. *Future Prospects of Voluntary Health Insurance in Thailand.* Takemi Research Paper 13. Takemi Program in International Health, Harvard School of Public Health. Harvard University, Cambridge, Mass.

Supakankunti, S. 1998. *Comparative Analysis of Various Community Cost Sharing Implemented in Myanmar.* Paper presented to the Workshop of Community Cost Sharing in Myanmar, November 26–28.

Toonen, J. 1995. *Community Financing for Health Care: A Case Study from Bolivia.* Bulletin 337. Royal Tropical Institute, Amsterdam.

Xing-yuan, G., and F. Xue-shan. 2000. "Study on Health Financing in Rural China." Paper presented at the International Conference on Health Systems Financing in Low-Income African and Asian Countries, November 30–December 1, CERDI, Clermont-Ferrand, France.

Ziemek, S., and J. Jütting. 2000. *Mutual Insurance Schemes and Social Protection.* Bonn: Center for Development Research (ZEF) Bonn.

CHAPTER 3

Experience of Community Health Financing in the Asian Region

William C. Hsiao

Abstract: One of the most urgent and vexing problems around the world is how to finance and provide health care for the more than two billion peasants and ghetto dwellers in low- and middle-income countries. The first part of this chapter develops a conceptual framework for community financing and uses it to clarify and classify the variety of community-financing schemes. This section of the chapter discusses the impact of community-financing schemes on outcomes and compares them to several scheme outcomes in African countries. The second part of the chapter uses the conceptual framework developed above to explain why some community-financing schemes in Asia have been successful and why some have failed. The review points to a number of measures governments could take to strengthen such community financing. Those measures include subsidizing the premiums of the poor, providing technical assistance to improve scheme management capacity, and forging links with formal health care networks. Satisfaction with a particular scheme was often related to the nature of direct community involvement in its design and management. A critical factor was the matching willingness and ability of individuals to pay, with the expectation of benefits to be received at some later time. The review also highlights several areas of government actions that appear to have a negative impact on the function of community-financing schemes. Top-down interference with scheme design and management appear to have a particularly negative impact on their functioning and sustainability.

Amost urgent and vexing problem around the world is how to finance and provide health care for the more than two billion peasants and ghetto dwellers in low- and middle-income countries.[1] Most of them are poor. Today, these two billion people do not have adequate health care to meet their basic needs (World Bank 2001). Most countries try to serve this population by operating public clinics in rural areas, but getting qualified practitioners to staff the clinics is often difficult. Practitioners frequently evade or refuse assignment there or do not attend the clinics regularly; when they are there, they often provide poor customer service. In addition, the facilities lack drugs and supplies. Thus when people become ill, they turn first to home remedies. Unsuccessful self-treatment frequently leads to big bills for extensive use of outpatient services by traditional healers, private practitioners, and pharmacists. When serious illness strikes, the poor flood into, and overcrowd, the public and charity hospitals. In numerous countries, the patients have to pay for inpatient hospital services, and many of them have to bankrupt their families to pay for the services or forgo the treatment and die. Studies found higher proportions of women and children forgoing medical treatment. Studies also consistently found that poor households use a very large part of their income for health care, even when the government theoretically provides free, or nearly free, services.[2] Studies in several countries, including China, found that large medical expenditure (for example, inpatient hospital services and costly outpatient drugs) is the major cause of poverty (Liu 2001). These facts raise at least three serious questions.

First: Is a nation spending a reasonable amount for its health? Many countries do not spend enough for the health care of their rural residents and urban poor. Can the governments spend more? It depends. Most low-income nations have a tax base that is too narrow and a tax collection system that is too ineffective to yield large sums of general revenue. The result is inadequate public funding for basic health care for the rural and ghetto households.[3] Other well-known financing modalities are unfeasible or undesirable. Social and private insurance are unviable. User fees are inequitable and create high barriers for the poor who need access to health care. (Whether foreign sources and domestic governments can allocate additional funds to support the health care of this population is being addressed in another chapter.)

Second: Does a nation have the capacity to transform money into effective services for the rural and poor population? In many countries where the government funds and provides free, or nearly free, services for rural residents and the poor, the target population is not utilizing those public health services. These households use their meager income to pay for services and drugs from the private sector. Why? Detailed country studies have consistently found a disturbing fact. In most low-income countries, although governments fund public provision of primary care at the village and township (subdistrict) levels,[4] they cannot manage and monitor these publicly funded services at the grassroots level. Whatever the amount of funds spent, it does not produce the services people want and value, though facilities are built and staffed (Bitran 1995; Gilson 1995; Zere, McIntyre, and Addison 2001). As a result, when people become ill, they pay to see the private practitioners and buy drugs themselves. (The findings of these studies are also summarized in another chapter on efficiency.)

Third: Can these services be organized so they will be used more efficiently and effectively? Out-of-pocket payments to private providers have some serious drawbacks. For one, there is no risk pooling. Patients also have to pay whatever private practitioners and drug peddlers charge. At the village level, the prices can be high since the population size is not likely to be able to support competing providers. At the subdistrict (township) level, the competition is also limited because of population size. In addition, the health service market suffers from well-documented market failures that can result in price gouging, poor quality of medical care, and induced demand for drugs sold at a high profit.[5] If households are willing to prepay the amount that they now pay out of pocket into an organized financing scheme, *collective gains* can be obtained. The organized fund could pool risks, improve quality and expand the delivery of health care, using the same amount of money.

Combinations of the above three problems lead to unmet health needs around the world. The different combinations that cause the problem must be identified since they need different policy remedies. For many very low-income countries in Africa, the causes of their unmet health needs are clear: underfunding as well as the inability of their health systems to transform their money into effective health care for rural and poor populations. China, Egypt, India, and Kenya spend reasonable amounts, but their health systems cannot transform the money into effective services for rural and poor populations. In contrast, Sri Lanka, spending a modest amount, has produced enviable results in health status and risk protection. As a result, we have some confidence that additional public spending by Sri Lanka could yield significant gains, but we cannot say that about India.

Throughout the world, community financing has been used to mobilize resources to fund and deliver health care for rural and ghetto communities. Some types of community-financing schemes have been successful in addressing all of the three issues discussed above, while others are primarily income-generating schemes for providers (for example, the Community Health Fund in Tanzania).

In recent years, *community financing* has become a term used loosely by health-financing specialists to label any financing scheme that may involve some community contribution or participation. Schemes range from the Drug Revolving Funds, which rely on user fees to fund a continuous availability of drugs, to government-managed prepayment schemes that require a community's residents to contribute to funding for public facilities, to hospital-sponsored and -managed insurance schemes that principally cover only that hospital's services. These schemes are very different in nature and purpose, in population covered, in benefit structure, in the extent of risk pooling, and in management.[6] Labeling any scheme that involves the community as a community-based health financing (CF) scheme has confused health policy leaders about which types of schemes are viable and how CF can alleviate the health needs of two billion people. It also impairs researchers in their investigations of the key common characteristics of community financing that explain the success or failure of such a scheme so that countries around the world can have a generalized concept of CF to assess when they can take the individual successful cases of it to scale.

This chapter has two parts. The first develops a conceptual framework for community financing and uses it to clarify and classify different types of schemes. The framework is intended to clarify the ambiguity, variations, and perplexity of community-financing schemes to gain some insight into the characteristics that make community financing a success or failure. To do that, we have to ask, Success or failure in what? This chapter offers two criteria: the potential community financing has to cover a significant percentage of the target population and mobilize resources and the value CF adds to the outcomes that matter to a society. We evaluate the schemes' impact on outcomes and compare them to several schemes in Africa. The comparative analysis provides some insight into which characteristics matter the most for establishing and sustaining community financing and what benefits schemes bring. The second part of the chapter uses the conceptual framework to explain several community-financing schemes in Asia and reasons for their success or failure.

WHAT IS COMMUNITY FINANCING?

Community-based health funds have existed for centuries. The earliest ones were largely sponsored by local religious organizations such as churches and synagogues. In the last century, community cooperatives, local mutual aid societies, and local funeral funds have sponsored and managed local health funds. The initiation of a nationwide community-based and -managed program in China—the Cooperative Medical System (CMS)—in the late 1950s captured the world's attention with the potential of community-based efforts to mobilize resources and provide cost-effective health care for the rural population. Other well-known, successful community-based financing and provision programs include the Thai Health Card Scheme and Indonesia's Dana Sehat. Each scheme covers millions of rural people for primary care and some secondary hospital services. Other local schemes such as Grameen Health Program, Dhaka Community Hospital Insurance Program, and the Self-Employed Women's Association (SEWA) have been successfully established and cover thousands of low-income households.

Several major studies have reviewed and summarized the numerous community-financing schemes around the world. Stinson (1982) was the first to compile an inventory and brief description of close to 200 financing schemes. Bennett, Creese, and Monasch (1998) analyzed the risk-pooling characteristics of more than 80 schemes globally. Most recently, Atim (1998) conducted a study of 22 mutual health organizations in Africa. These three comprehensive studies covered schemes ranging from local prepaid user fee plans and church-sponsored, traditional, third-party insurance schemes to universal compulsory social insurance for target populations. The schemes' wide variations make it almost impossible to understand what constitutes a community-financing scheme much less grasp what made these schemes successful.

Community financing can be broadly defined as any scheme that has three features: community[7] control, voluntary membership, and prepayment for health care by the community members.[8] This definition would exclude financing schemes such as regional compulsory social insurance plans and community-managed user fee programs. However, the definition here is still too vague for analytical purposes when we try to understand what makes a community-financing scheme a success or failure.

Two analytical definitions of community financing can be derived from our strategic framework in mobilizing domestic resources for health outlined in chapter 1 of the Report of Working Group 3, Commission on Macroeconomics and

Health. Our framework argued that community financing is one of several financing modalities to raise funds. *Then one way to differentiate community-financing schemes is by examining their capability to mobilize resources and population coverage.* Our framework also suggests another way to differentiate CFs. Financing is an instrument used to achieve societal goals. We are ultimately interested in a financing scheme's impacts on the outcomes of a health system. Therefore, *another way to differentiate CFs is by the final outcomes they produce.* We explain in greater detail about the two approaches in classifying and studying CFs below.

Classify and Analyze Community-Financing Schemes by Their Potential to Mobilize Fiscal Resources and Attract a Large Percent of Target Population to Enroll

A CF scheme's ability to raise funds from households depends on their ability to pay. A scheme's capacity to raise funds from community businesses depends on the number of rural enterprises and cooperatives. Poverty households have to be heavily subsidized, and poor households also require some subsidizing.

What would motivate households that have some ability to prepay to do so? Their willingness to prepay must be the primary determinant. Economic and social factors influence their willingness to prepay (Hsiao 1995, Bennett, Creese, and Monasch 1998). From the economic perspective, the expected economic and quality gains have to be equal or greater than the prepayment. Social norms and close relationships, however, may shape people's preference for prepayment that involves elements of income transfer. The economic and social considerations are discussed below. The chapter then discusses which specific gains members are likely to value. In examining a CF scheme's ability to produce economic and quality gains, we argue that it is dependent on the management's motivation. Management's motivation and competence are manifest in certain organizational and incentive characteristics known to improve efficiency and quality of health care. We identify and discuss them in detail.

Major Determinants of Community Members' Willingness to Prepay

Economic theory suggests that households' willingness to prepay depends on their belief that by doing so they will gain economically or in health care or both. In other words, the expected benefit has to be greater than the cost. That could happen in three ways. First, the existing facilities could produce the patient-valued services more efficiently (including reducing corruption) so that the prepayment would buy more than it presently does. Second, the prepayment could purchase something new that is valued by the household, such as risk protection. Third, the government could provide a direct and visible subsidy to motivate community members to join a CF. For example, when the government matches every dollar the community member prepays, members can easily see the economic gain. Other forms of subsidy can be the discounting of the price CF members pay for services or drugs or both.

As for the social characteristics of a community that may influence households' willingness to prepay, we hypothesize that social capital could influence people's preference to prepay. Prepayment implicitly involves risk pooling and cross-subsidizing between the healthy and the less healthy, and between the rich and the poor. Young and healthy people will not enroll if they have to prepay a similar amount as the elderly and less healthy people. But sociologists have long argued that social capital is an important determinant of people's willingness to cooperate with each other. This theory has been supported by several empirical economic and political studies (Putnam 1993; Liu 2001; Narayan and Pritchett 1997).

We hypothesize that the degree of mutual concern that community members have for each other (social cohesion and solidarity) could have a significant influence on their willingness to prepay, even when an individual household is uncertain that the expected benefit will be greater than the amount to be pre-paid. In economic terms, it means social cohesion and mutual concern shape people's preference for prepayment. We hypothesize that *the greater the social capital, the more people are willing to prepay.*

In a simple diagram, we can illustrate the interactions between economic gains and social capital and that their sum has to reach a threshold—the prepayment required. We show that a CF scheme can be successful even when the prepayment amount is greater than the expected economic or health gain because of the social capital. This hypothesis is illustrated in figure 3.1. While community A can produce the same level of economic and quality gains as community B, A has less social capital; the sum of the two for A did not exceed the prepayment amount required. Consequently, community A did not establish a CF scheme. Community B, with its

---

FIGURE 3.1   Feasibility of Establishing Community Financing and the Amount the Average Person Is Willing to Pay as a Function of Expected Gains and Social Capital

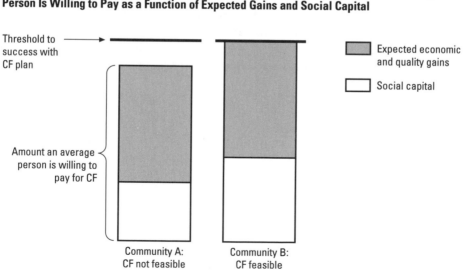

greater social capital, was able to establish a scheme. Our hypothesis may explain why some CF schemes have been successful while others have failed since they vary in their ability to produce gains, and communities have varied social capital.

Supported by the Chinese government and UNICEF, we have been conducting social experiments in 10 poor rural counties in eight different provinces in China, testing whether social capital affects rural households' willingness to prepay. Liu (2001) developed several measurements of social capital, including the degree of mutual assistance a household has given and the participation in civic activities in the villages. His preliminary regression analysis found a statistically significant association between these social capital variables and people's willingness to pay and their actual enrollment in CF schemes.

What Gains May Be Valued by Community Members?

Numerous studies have examined the reasons why rural population have voluntarily enrolled and stayed enrolled in different schemes. Market surveys have also been conducted in China and in Indonesia to glean what kind of health care and risk pooling people prefer to prepay and how much they are willing to prepay. Overall, these studies found that people most often mentioned the following items among the top three products they valued most: availability of close-by and affordable[9] primary care and drugs; some protection against high financial risks such as hospital charges; neat and clean facilities particularly outhouses or bathrooms; reasonably competent practitioners; and good customer service. Various studies conducted in Africa, Asia, and Latin America also had similar findings. We summarize the products valued by community members in table 3.1.

When Would a CF Scheme Give Priority to Producing Economic Gains and Improving Quality of Services for the Patients?

Though we can understand what products community members value highly, the producers may still not have supplied them, particularly under public provision. Under what circumstances would CF schemes be motivated to produce the economic and quality gains valued by the community members? Management control is one critical determinant. Household interview surveys consistently found community members' key concern was whether their funds would be used exclusively

---

TABLE 3.1   How Community Members Valued Service Availability, Quality, Risk Protection, and Costs

Availability of affordable services			Quality of services (competence, cleanliness, and custom service)			Extent of risk protection	Costs	
Preventive	Primary care and drugs	Hospital	Preventive	Primary care and drugs	Hospital		Travel	Charges at time of use
High	High	Modest	Modest	High	High	Modest	High	High

for their benefit. Corruption is a major worry together with excessive spending on staff compensation and services that have less value to the patients. Consequently, to be willing to pay, people must trust and have confidence in the organization that manages the fund. In most low-income countries, the government has not earned the trust and confidence of the people at the village and township levels (Gilson and others 1994; Hsiao 1995). When this is the case, nongovernmental organizations (NGOs) that have the people's confidence must manage the fund. Other managers could include local agricultural cooperatives, churches and mosques, funeral funds, or a newly formed community organization. This aspect—*people's confidence and trust in the organization managing the fund*—is a precondition for a scheme's success.

We believe that in general, governments are less capable than the local community in managing the services for the patients' benefit at the village and subdistrict levels. The reasons are straightforward. Governments face financial and human resource constraints in managing thousands of clinics at village and township levels. But CF scheme members have a self-interest in seeing that their prepayment is used wisely and efficiently for services they value. When the local community has significant control over the scheme, members can have a greater voice in deciding how the funds should be spent. Members can manage the efficiency and quality of services much more effectively because they can readily monitor the staff's regular attendance at the clinic and the availability of drugs and supplies. They can directly experience a practitioner's technical competency and the service quality and can observe daily the cleanliness of the health facilities. Therefore we can expect greater economic and quality gains as community control and management increases. This relationship is illustrated in figure 3.2.

The curve in figure 3.2 represents the hypothetical relationship between the gains and community control. Their relationship is nonlinear because we assume the community members have limited education, management knowhow, and knowledge of medical affairs. At some point, the gains reach an asymptotic point because of the community's limited ability to manage. Thus the best combination of control and management may be a combination of community, government, and health professionals.

Experience from local community-controlled schemes and household interview surveys conducted in China and Indonesia support our hypothesis. As described in the second part of this chapter, one large Chinese survey conducted in five provinces found that more than two-thirds of the community residents want significant control over the CF schemes before they will enroll. In examining the CF experience, we have consistently found that agricultural and lumber cooperatives managed schemes in Indonesia. Community-managed Dana Sehat and CMS have increased the availability and access of health care at the village and subdistrict levels. Moreover, the Indonesian experience also illustrates the limited managerial capability of the community members. The most successful Dana Sehat plans were the ones in which villages grouped themselves by subdistrict. The board members were chosen by community members, but full-time qualified managers were hired to manage the plan at the subdistrict level.

FIGURE 3.2   Plausible Relationship between Locus of Control and Economic and Quality Gains

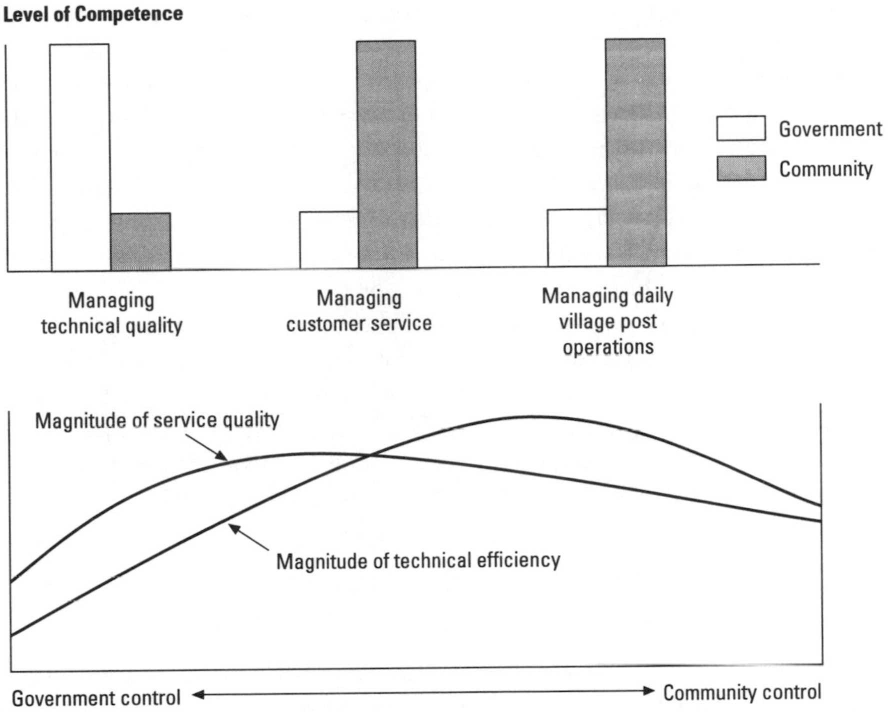

What Operational Characteristics of a CF Scheme Represent Managerial Efforts to Improve Efficiency and Quality?

Four key factors emerged in our examination of which organizational and management characteristics and incentives structures are more likely to yield efficiency and quality gains valued by community members. First, market surveys in China and Indonesia and household interview surveys consistently found that availability and proximity of reasonably competent practitioners matter the most to community members. They have a paramount concern about the distance they have to travel for basic primary care and drugs. They also highly value home visits by health practitioners such as midwives. Second, studies found that economic gains can be produced by organizational arrangements such as integrating financing and provision of preventive and primary care at the village level,[10] using an essential drug list, centralizing the bulk purchase of drugs, and having an organized drug distribution network (Carrin and Vereecke 1992; Saurborne, Nougtara, and Latimer 1994). Quality gains can be obtained through organizational arrangements such as establishing a formal referral system, regular monitoring of clinical performance of practitioners at lower level facilities by higher level facilities, and cleanliness and hygiene at the clinic, particularly in the bathrooms. Efficiency and quality gains can also be obtained by using patient and provider incentives such as imposing a copayment on drugs to reduce moral hazard, allowing patients some choice to create competition, paying practitioners separately for health education and prevention to improve self-care and prevention, and paying salary plus bonus to practitioners to improve working hours and custom services (McPake, Hanson, and Mills 1992).

Using the factors gathered from various CF experiences and marketing studies, we can classify and examine a CF by the local community's relative control and managerial power over it and its organizational, managerial, and incentive characteristics. These are important because they may indicate the relative gains that a CF can produce, gains valued by those who have to prepay. Once we can examine the magnitude of the gains and the kind of gains a CF can produce, we can infer what a CF's likelihood of success is in raising funds from the community and the size of the population likely to enroll. In table 3.2, we summarize the major characteristics of CFs that enable them to produce significant economic and quality gains. It is important to stress that most of the cost reductions produced by CFs came from purchasing drugs in bulk and using them more appropriately (Carrin and Vereeke 1992; Saurborne, Nougtara, and Latimer 1994).

When Households Are Willing to Prepay: Lessons from Specific Community-Financing Schemes in Asia

By closely examining the CF schemes mentioned in this chapter, we determined that there are several types, based on the key factors that can explain the success or failure of the various schemes. We summarize them here.

Direct government subsidy to individuals. The Thai Health Card represents this generic model. Its success seems to come from four factors: (1) patients have to pay high user fees unless they enroll, (2) the government directly and visibly matches the premium paid by the enrollee, (3) patients have free choice of public providers, and (4) most people can readily calculate that the benefits would exceed the premium they pay. This model should not even be included as a community-financing scheme since it has little grassroots community involvement.

Cooperative health care. China's CMS and Dana Sehat represent this generic model. Financing and provision are integrated at the village and subdistrict levels. The original success of CMS was largely due to its extremely efficient and low-cost health care delivery system, which brought clear benefits to the enrollees and was also compulsory. Its major weakness was in public control and management. The local officials in many communities abused their power and misused CMS funds for their own gain. When the compulsory feature was removed after agriculture reform in the early 1980s, only the uncorrupted CMSs (between 50 and 60 percent of them) had any chance of surviving on a voluntary basis. The CMSs that continued, despite the government's effort to abolish them in the mid-1980s, can be divided into two groups. The first were those found in better-off communities with enough middle-class rural households to be able to give some subsidy. The second

TABLE 3.2 A Typology of Selected Characteristics of Community-Financing Schemes

Name	Control	Operational Features							
		Organization					Incentives		
	Degree of community control	Integration of financing and provision at village level	Organized referral system, monitoring by continuous education by upper level	Organized purchase and use of drugs	Contracting hospitals	Allow choice and competition	Subsidy	Copayment to reduce overuse of services and drugs	Salaried practitioners
Thai Health Card									
Tanzania Community Health Fund									
CMS—*Jiangsu County*									
CMS—*14 Counties*									
CMS—*10 Counties*									
CMS—*Tibet*									
Dana Sehat									
	Increased efficiency	Increased quality		Increased efficiency and quality	Increased efficiency	Increased efficiency	Greater participation	Increased efficiency and quality	Increased efficiency

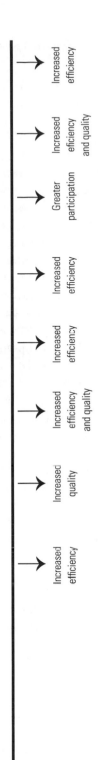

were those found in poorer communities that had local government leaders who were enthusiastic about continuing with the scheme and were able to mobilize subsidies from either local government or rural enterprises. In addition, the CMSs in these poorer communities had to account to the enrollees for use of the fund and were able to integrate financing and provision at village and township levels to produce efficient, quality health care. The experience of Dana Sehat was similar to that of CMS. Dana Sehat's slow expansion can be explained by two factors. First, the government gives no subsidy, and the poor and near-poor households could not pay. Dana Sehat succeeded largely in areas where a religious charity or rural industries such as a lumber cooperative were able to provide some subsidy. Second, a village is too small a unit to support an entire scheme and to provide management know-how and risk pooling.

Community-sponsored third-party insurance. A social experiment designed and operated by the Rand Corp. was conducted in China. The experiment aimed to assess how many people were willing to join a voluntary community-based health insurance plan, what premiums the Chinese peasants were willing to pay without a government subsidy, and the price elasticity of demand. The Rand experiment set the premiums at 1.5 percent of average income. The system was designed as an insurance plan, and the insured paid a significant copayment or coinsurance when they sought health care from village, township, and county health facilities. They could visit county hospitals only in an emergency or with the approval of the township health center. More than 90 percent of households in the test areas voluntarily joined the program, and 95 percent reenrolled after the first year. Administrative costs were kept low (8 percent of total reimbursements).

Provider-sponsored prepayment plan. The Dhaka Community Hospital (DCH) Plan represents this generic model. The DCH system operates a health insurance scheme at its clinics, known as the Health Card Program. There are five types of health cards. The Family Health Card, intended for rural households, costs 40 taka per month (about US$1) for an initial enrollment and 20 taka for renewal, covering up to 12 members per household, including servants living there. This plan entitles the whole household to consult the clinic doctor at any time and to monthly home visits by DCH-trained health workers. Patients with the health card do not pay additional fees for consulting a doctor but have to buy medicines outside the clinic. The School Children Card, free to schoolchildren living near the health clinics, offers children free physical examinations and health education. The Worker Health Card, for workers in enterprises near the clinics, costs 2 taka per month per worker. Premiums are paid by the companies or the owners' associations. The benefit package includes free consultation but no monthly home visits by health workers. The Sports Card, for professional sports players, is intended mainly to publicize the clinics. No premium is charged for enrollment, and medical consultations are free. Poor families in the communities received a special Destitute Card at no cost, which allows members of poor households to visit the clinic at 5 taka per visit. The community committees decide which families in the village qualify as "poor" and should receive Destitute Cards.

Consumer or producer cooperatives. The Grameen Bank (GB) represents this generic model. GB is internationally known for its successful group-based credit program and as a provider of credit to the rural poor, particularly women, who own less than a half acre of land or whose assets do not exceed the value of one acre of land. Grameen has 2.3 million members and, through its 1,167 branches, covers almost half of the villages in the country. GB established the Grameen Health Program (GHP) to provide basic health care services to its members as well as nonmembers living in the same operational area and to provide insurance to cover the cost of basic care. The GHP functions as an insurer as well as a health care provider. The GHP's prepaid health insurance program is open to everyone covered by a GB branch regardless of whether they are GB members. The insurance scheme utilizes the organization structure of the GB credit program.

At the GB branch operational level, which normally has 2,500 GB families and 3,500 non-GB families, GHP organizes health centers to provide outpatient services, routine pathological tests, and basic drugs. Each center is staffed with a doctor, who also acts as the center director, a paramedic, a lab technician, and an office manager. Some centers have subcenters, usually staffed by one paramedic and two health workers (Grameen Bank 1995). The number of Grameen health centers gradually expanded from 5 in 1993 to 10 in 1997. The families enrolled in the insurance increased from 13,000 in 1994 to 25,935 in 1996. About 85 percent of the subscribers are GB members. This ratio has not changed much over the years.

In summary, we can classify community-financing schemes into five types:

- *Direct Subsidy to Individual*
  Thai Health Card
  Tanzania Community Health Fund

- *Cooperative Health Care*
  High-income communities: Jiangsu Province
  Middle-income communities: 14-county (WHO)
  Low-income communities: 30-county study
                                  10-county experiment
                                  Tibet

- *Community-Based Third-Party Insurance*
  Rand Experiment in Sichuan Province
  Dana Sehat

- *Provider-Sponsored Insurance*
  Dkaha Community Hospital
  Gonoshasthaya
  Bwamanda

- *Producer or Consumer Cooperative*
  Grameen

General Findings

The general findings can be summed up as follows:

- Rural households and urban poor households are willing to prepay a portion of their health services. The amount they are willing to prepay depends on economic and social factors. The economic factors include the household's ability to pay, the size of out-of-pocket payments they have to make if not enrolled in a CF scheme, direct subsidy given, and who controls the funds and delivery of basic primary care services. The social factor includes the sense of kinship and mutual concern for each other in a community (social capital).

- The poor and near poor need simple and direct government or donor subsidies to make the economic gains very visible to motivate them to prepay. The subsidy could be as low as half the prepayment amount to be paid by the people. Poverty households need almost full subsidy.

- The revealed preference seems to show that people prefer to have both primary care and insurance and are willing to make a tradeoff. Among the CF schemes in Asia, people most wanted coverage of primary care and drugs. This is logical because people want to have a direct payoff. Understanding and appreciation for risk pooling is rudimentary.[11] Furthermore, greater coverage of primary care reduces adverse selection by including individuals who have no serious health problems, but they may drop out once they learn their prepayment has little immediate direct payoff.

- In most communities, a CF scheme must have its members' trust and confidence. This means the community must have reasonable control over the scheme and the services delivered at the village level.

- CMS and many Dana Sehat plans have demonstrated that they can produce measurable economic gains and improvements in service quality.

- The government or an established NGO must initiate the scheme and conduct training.

- Community-sponsored third-party insurance schemes have seldom succeeded in covering a significant percentage of the target population.

- Some nations rely on community cooperatives and have found that consumer cooperatives have done better than producer cooperatives in looking out for the patients' interests.[12]

Classify and Assess Community-Financing Schemes by Outcomes

Another approach in analyzing and assessing CF schemes is by their impacts on the health system outcomes. Outcome data by community have seldom been collected. A few studies have found measurable improvements in health out-

FIGURE 3.3   The Trade-Offs between Health Gains and Risk Protection by Type of Service Funded

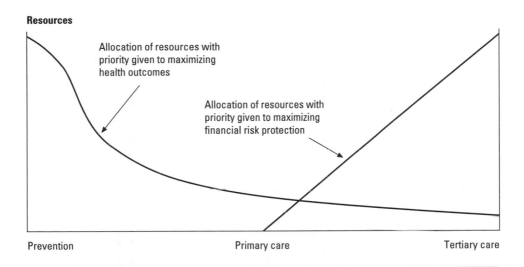

come and financial risk protection after the introduction of certain types of CF at the regional or national level. The Chinese experience is a good example. In the absence of reliable data, we can examine the health services that are provided under a scheme and infer the potential impacts on health and risk pooling. The relationship between covered health services and health outcomes and risk pooling are shown in figure 3.3. It also illustrates the trade-offs when resources are very limited. The most painful trade-off is between improvement of health status and prevention of impoverishment.

The CF schemes can be compared by their likely impacts on health status and risk pooling. Table 3.3 summarizes the outcomes by which the schemes should be assessed; the use of this framework is illustrated with several selected CF schemes.

A SUMMARY OF THE VALUE ADDED BY TYPES OF COMMUNITY-FINANCING SCHEMES

For low-income countries, CF schemes have only modest ability to increase the total amount of funds for health care. The reason is straightforward. The target population consists of largely poor and low-income households whose ability to pay is modest. The major value added by such schemes is their organization of what households and government are already spending directly and their use of the funds to buy more and better services.

Properly structured CF schemes can significantly improve efficiency, reduce the cost of health care, improve quality and health outcomes, and pool risks.

TABLE 3.3 Assessment of Potential Value Added by Selected Types of Community-Financing Schemes

Name of CF	Potential to mobilize funds	Equity in financing	Increase efficiency and reduce cost	Improve access	Improve quality	Greater risk pooling
Thai Health Card						
CMS						
Dana Sehat						

Equity · Consumer satisfaction · Better health outcomes · Financial risk protection

Community-financing schemes could improve preventive services and reduce the incidence of disease. They could also improve people's access to health care and the quality of services, thus improving their health status. The schemes could improve risk pooling and reduce health-induced impoverishment as well.

CF schemes can be grouped by their basic purposes:

- Mobilizing additional funds for government facilities and improving access—*prepaid user fees* (for example, Community Health Funds in Tanzania, Health Card in Thailand)

- Mobilizing funds from rural population and urban poor and improving access, efficiency, and quality of care with modest risk pooling—*cooperative healthcare* (for example, CMS, Dana Sehat, Grameen Kalyan, Boboye, Abota)

- Assuring more stable funding for providers—*provider sponsored insurance* (for example, Dhaka Hospital, Nkoranza, Bwamanda).

We summarize the five types of CF schemes and their potential impact on the final outcomes of a health system. Table 3.4 gives our evaluation, based on studies of a limited number of schemes.

A REVIEW OF SELECTED ASIAN COMMUNITY-FINANCING SCHEMES

Community financing is an ambiguous term that has been used loosely over the years to describe some level of community involvement in financing health care. Community involvement alone, however, cannot be used as the single dimensional factor for all the various schemes, including copayment for government services, prepayment schemes for hospital services, financing schemes for immunization, private insurance schemes, and even revolving drug funds.

Community financing can be broadly defined as any scheme that has two features: a community base[13] and prepayment into an identifiable fund by the community members[14] that entitles them to some health benefits. This definition would exclude some financing schemes such as regional social insurance plans and community-managed user fee programs. Using this definition, we selected several well-known national and local financing schemes for analysis. These case studies may shed light on why some schemes have succeeded and others have failed.

National Schemes

China's Cooperative Medical System

In China, about 800 million people live in rural areas, most of them engaged in farming. Most of them were living on bare subsistence before the 1979 agricultural reform. The average disposable income per person was roughly equivalent to US$115 in 1985, ranging from under US$25 per capita for the poorest households to US$175 (1,390 yuan) for those in the highest income quartile.

TABLE 3.4 Potential Value Added by Types of Community-Financing Schemes

Type of CF	Who controls use of fund	Potential pop. to be covered and raise fund	Equity in financing	Increase efficiency and reduce cost	Improve access	Improve quality	Greater risk pooling
Prepay user fees	Government	Low	Low	None	Low	Low	Low
	Individual households	Modest	Low	None	Modest	Low	Low
Cooperative healthcare	Local community and special purpose NGO	High	Low	High	High	High	Modest unless government subsidy
Community-based third party insurance	Community	Cover higher income families	Low	Low	High for those insured	Low	High
Provider-sponsored insurance	Hospitals	Cover higher income families	Low	Low	High for those insured	Low	High
Provider or consumer cooperative	Cooperatives	Cover member	Low	High	High	High	Medium

Beginning in the late 1950s, health care for China's rural population was organized and financed through the Cooperative Medical System (CMS), an integrated part of the overall system of collective agriculture production and social services.

Health care for the rural population was organized into a three-tier structure. Village health stations served an average of 500 to 1,000 residents; township health centers served 15,000 to 20,000 people; and county hospitals served a catchment area of 200,000 to 300,000 people. Village stations were staffed by part-time village doctors whose training consisted of three to six months' basic medical education after junior middle school. Their role was to provide basic preventive care (for example, immunization, prenatal consultation) and simple curative services (treating common illnesses and injuries). Most township health centers were owned and operated by the town government. An average facility had 7 to 10 beds and 10 staff members, led by a physician with a three-year medical school education after senior middle school. County hospitals, serving as medical referral centers for rural residents, were owned and operated by the county government and staffed by physicians with four to five years of medical school training. The typical county hospital had 135 beds and 186 staff members, of whom 8 percent had bachelor of medicine degrees. County hospitals had at least the five basic specialty services—obstetrics-gynecology, pediatrics, internal medicine, general surgery, and radiology. Under this system, village health stations, township health centers, and county hospitals were integrated within the three-tier system by a vertical administrative system. County hospitals and township health centers provided regular technical assistance and supervision to the lower level organizations.

At CMS's peak, 90 percent of the rural population was covered by its schemes. Health services, financed through CMS, relied on prepayment plans. Most of the villages funded CMS from three sources:

- *Compulsory prepayment by residents.* Depending on the benefit structure of the plan and the local community's economic status, 0.5 to 2 percent of a peasant family's annual income (4 to 8 yuan) was to be paid into the fund as premiums.

- *Village contributions.* Each village contributed a certain portion of its income from collective agricultural production or rural enterprises to a welfare fund, and a portion of this fund was used to finance health care.

- *Government subsidies.* Subsidies from higher level governments funded the compensation of health workers and capital investments.

China achieved remarkable health improvements for its rural population before 1985. CMS was characterized by its collective financing, prepayment, and organization of health services through the three-tier system. This community financing and organization model of health care was believed by many observers to have contributed in a significant way to China's success in accomplishing its "first health care revolution," by providing preventive and primary care to almost every Chinese and reducing infant mortality from about 200 per 1,000 live births (1949) to 47 per 1,000 live births (1973–75), increasing life expectancy from 35 years to about 65.

In the early 1980s, when China's rural reforms decollectivized Chinese agricultural production, most CMS schemes collapsed. Most villages had to dissolve their CMSs after the main source of financing, the welfare fund, supported by collective farming income, disappeared. An ideological shift prompted some high government officials to declare that the remaining CMS programs should be abolished. Thus most communities that still had CMSs were forced to disband their systems by the mid-1980s, much to the dismay of local people. Last but not least, patronage, corruption, and poor management contributed to the downfall of CMS. CMS, though based in local communities, was controlled and managed by local officials who were not held accountable to the people. Some of these officials abused their power for selfish ends. As a result, people lost confidence in the government-run CMS program and refused to make financial contributions once the system became voluntary in the early 1980s.

The health status of the rural population in China has deteriorated. This deterioration has been closely related to the collapse of CMS. For example, a World Bank study found that China's earlier progress in improving child health appears, in the aggregate, to have come to a stop, despite rapid economic growth since the early 1980s. The analysis found that mortality of children under five years of age (under-5) declined steadily until the early 1980s and then began a slight upward drift. Experiences from other countries suggest that the under-5 mortality rate need not reach a plateau, as China's has done. This indicates that China's performance has deteriorated not only in absolute terms but also relative to other countries. The China Network–Harvard study of 30 poor counties confirmed the World Bank's study. China's poverty areas have experienced steady economic growth since the beginning of economic reform, in 1980; per capita gross domestic product, or GDP, (in real terms) increased from US$56 in the late 1970s to US$88 in the late 1980s. However, the median infant mortality rate in the surveyed counties increased from about 50 per 1,000 live births to 72 per 1,000 live births during the same period of time.

Preventive services provided under CMS, financed out of central government and local welfare funds, were essentially free. Now, the vast majority of the rural population obtain their health services on a fee-for-service (FFS) basis instead of the previous prepaid basis.

CMS Schemes that Survived: A Natural Experiment

Despite the government's policy of abolishing CMS and the absence of central and provincial government support, some CMSs survived. That these were now voluntary schemes underscored the fact that they survived principally because peasants in those communities had chosen to continue the schemes. However, these natural experiments have several biases. The peasants were already familiar with CMS; they knew the scheme and its possible benefits and drawbacks. It is important to bear in mind that this level of awareness makes the experiment unrepresentative.

How Many CMSs Survived?

A survey of five poor provinces in China, conducted in 1993 in preparation for the World Bank's loan for the Rural Health Workers Development Project, found that among the five provinces, one relatively poor province, Shanxi, had the greatest coverage—close to two-thirds of the villages maintained some form of community financing (see table 3.5). But in another very poor province, Guizhou, few villages had community financing (0.8 percent). In these poor provinces, the schemes were financed largely by household contributions, and benefits covered only primary care services because the very poor households could make only small contributions.

The *Study of Thirty Poor Counties* was conducted in 1993–95 by a network of Chinese universities and Harvard University. The study found that 16.5 percent of the villages surveyed still maintained some type of community-based health-financing scheme, covering 11.6 percent of the sampled population (see table 3.6). About two-thirds of the schemes covered only primary care services at the village level; a third covered comprehensive services, ranging from primary care to inpatient services. The benefit structures all incorporated coinsurance and often set high copayment rates for inpatient services. The study found that the most prevalent type of community fund management was by village committee or by the village and township jointly (see table 3.7).

TABLE 3.5   Prevalence and Benefits of Community Health Financing in 5 Provinces, 1991 (percent)

Province	Number of villages with community financing	Percent of villages with community financing	Percent of schemes with comprehensive coverage	Percent of schemes with primary care services only
Fujian	512	6.3	25	75
Guizhou	160	0.8	6	94
Hebei	3,992	13.1	42	58
Henan	1,590	6.2	7	93
Shanxi	4,727	65.6	15	85
Total	10,981	12.2	24	76

Note: Data from the *Study of Thirty Poor Counties* indicate that almost 80 percent of the category "services and drugs coverage" is comprehensive coverage. Therefore, for the purposes of this table, the *Five Province Survey* data were recategorized, with services and drugs plans counted as comprehensive coverage and the remaining categories (services only, drugs only, other) counted as primary care services coverage only.

Source: World Bank (1993).

TABLE 3.6   Prevalence and Benefits of Community Health Financing in 30 Poor Counties, 1993

Type of benefits	Number of villages covered	Percentage of villages covered	Percentage of population covered
Comprehensive	29	5.1	4.4
Primary care services only	59	11.4	7.2
Total	88	16.5	11.6

Note: Comprehensive benefits refers to schemes that reimburse 30–100 percent of hospitalization charges for township and county-level hospitals and 50–100 percent of outpatient fees. Primary care services refers to coverage of fees (or discounted prices) for most village-level services with fees at the township and county levels paid out-of-pocket by patients.

Source: China Network and Harvard School of Public Health (1996).

TABLE 3.7   Management of Community Health Financing in 30 Poor Counties, 1993 (percent)

	Type of benefits	
Form of management	Comprehensive	Primary care services only
Township government	17.2	3.4
Township health center	20.7	6.8
Village and township jointly	20.7	10.2
Village committee	34.5	47.5
Village and township doctors	6.9	32.1

Source: China Network and Harvard School of Public Health (1996).

A summary of results:

Overall, about 13 percent of the rural villages continued with CMS. More affluent areas with rural industries and a higher tax base got financial support from both the government and rural industries. Why some poorest villages continued with CMS remains a puzzle. Despite the government edict in the mid-1980s to abolish the Cooperative Medical System, close to 10 percent of the rural villages continued to maintain their systems. This empirical evidence suggests that there is a significant amount of public support in many villages for establishing community-financing schemes. However, voluntary development of CMS is very limited even in affluent areas. For example, only about 6 percent of the villages have established CMS in Fujian, a high-income province in China. In our 30-county poverty study survey, 70 percent of villages that reinstated CMS did so at the request of the government. Experience from China and other countries demonstrated that government could play a significant role as initiator and enabler of community financing.

Why Do People Prefer to Have CMS?

Several large household surveys have found that a majority of Chinese peasants want cooperative financing established in their communities. The study of 30 poor counties involving 11,044 randomly selected households found strong support for reestablishing community-financed health care. Of the households not covered by community financing or maternal and child immunization prepayment schemes, 70 percent responded that they would like to see an improved scheme established, similar to the Cooperative Medical System. Of those covered by community-financing schemes, 88 percent stated that they would like those schemes to continue.

Several possible reasons could explain why people wish to maintain the CF schemes. We briefly enumerate the major ones.

Financial barriers reduce access to primary health care for rural populations. Another reason is physical supply especially since 80 percent of the rural poor live in mountainous areas. The number of medical personnel, including barefoot doctors and township and village health workers, have been reduced significantly. The 30-county study also showed that the number of villages with functioning health stations dropped from 71 percent in 1979 to 55 percent in 1993. Between 1983 and 1993, the costs of health care also rose at an average of 10 to 15 yuan per year, twice the average growth rate of farmers' disposable income in China.

The change to a fee-for-service system brought several changes, which factored heavily into increased costs, limiting access in the process. Under the current fee-for-service system, the income of village doctors and health facilities depends on the profits they can earn on drugs. The government sets very low prices for services; in compensation, practitioners are allowed to mark-up the wholesale price of drugs by 15 to 20 percent, which provides an incentive to overprescribe drugs. Moreover, user fees charged for previously free preventive services have had detrimental effects on public health through reduced demand for, and supply of, preventive services. The Epidemic Prevention Service workers shifted their attention to services for which high fees could easily be charged—such as cosmetic product inspection and food safety—which were not necessarily the highest priority or the most cost-effective activities.

The average charge per outpatient visit for uninsured patients is almost three times that of the patients under CMS. Community-financing schemes can exercise their bargaining power in demanding discounted prices or providers can be paid on a partial capitation basis. The increase in cost from the new fee-for-service system created a financial access barrier for people. In the 30-county study, 28 percent of seriously ill farmers did not seek health care, and 51 percent of rural patients refused hospitalization, mainly for financial reasons. The financial burden can be illustrated by one fact. A poor farmer would have to spend 1.2 years of his disposable income to pay for one episode of hospitalization at a county hospital.

The higher cost of health services and drugs impoverished many families. Eighteen percent of the households using health services incurred health expenditures that exceeded their total household income in 1993. Of the households interviewed, 24.5 percent borrowed or became indebted to pay for health expenses. Another 5.5 percent sold or mortgaged properties to pay for health care. High health expenses are a major cause of poverty in rural areas. In our 30-county survey, 47 percent of the medically indebted households reported having suffered from hunger. This interaction between health and income could start a vicious cycle of illness, poverty, and more illness.

Quality of care also suffered. The interconnection and cooperation among different rural health facilities weakened or disappeared after reforms. Under CMS, county hospitals and township health centers provided regular technical assistance and supervision to the lower level organizations, with a referral system that managed patients at a lower level when possible. After the collapse of CMS, however, these health care organizations became independent institutions, often competing for patients to increase revenue. This disintegration of the three-tier system may also have implications for the quality of services provided by uncoordinated rural health workers. In addition, the collapse of CMS led to the overprescribing of drugs and the overuse of injections and profitable tests.

Who Should Control and Manage CMS?

There was a clear preference for community control in the management of CMS. Of the households without coverage that favored reestablishing community-financing schemes, about 62 percent of the peasants wanted the village residents to have a strong voice. Only 17 percent trusted the government to manage it independently. About one-fourth preferred that the scheme be managed by the village, one-fourth preferred township management, and the rest preferred joint management by the township or village and the health facility.

How Much Are People Willing to Pay and for What?

Responses to the household surveys indicated a wide range of preferences for services, from drugs and village doctors to township health centers. There was also a preference for coverage of hospital inpatient services (catastrophic expenses), with a willingness to accept coinsurance.

World Health Organization study. To learn how to improve organization, financing, and service delivery, the World Health Organization studied community-financing schemes in 14 counties in Beijing, Henan, Hubei, Jiangsu, Jiangxi, Ningxia, and Zhejiang. In each county, a research team interviewed 540 households and surveyed health services.

The study found that a typical community fund might collect 5 yuan (US$0.63) per person from families, 1 yuan per person from the village's social welfare fund, and 1 yuan per person from the township. Patients typically must pay a deductible (for example, 100 yuan) and make a copayment on expenditures above the deductible. The schemes limit drug coverage to 120 kinds of medicines, including traditional Chinese medicines, and set a limit on reimbursement for diagnostic tests.

Rand experiment. In the Rand experiment, premiums were set at 1.5 percent of average income. Insured individuals could freely visit village and township facilities but could visit county hospitals only in an emergency or with the approval of the township health center. More than 90 percent of households in the test areas voluntarily joined the program, and 95 percent reenrolled after the first year. Administrative costs were kept low (8 percent of total reimbursements). The study also found that

- Coinsurance (or copayment) exerted a significant negative effect on demand for care across different population groups. There were no interactions between the effect of coinsurance and age, income, or health status.

- Users in all but one village reported high satisfaction with the insurance arrangement (Mao 1995, p. 16).

- Services were used less when there was no functioning village health station, underlining the importance of an adequate supply of basic services (Mao 1995).

As in other countries, a small share of the population (about 11.5 percent) accounted for a large share of total health expenditures (70 percent), underscoring the need for catastrophic insurance.

In most rural areas, particularly poor areas, adequate revenues for any organized financing scheme cannot be derived solely from households. Funding must come from multiple sources. According to the *Study of Thirty Poor Counties,* about half the financing for existing community-financed health plans came from household contributions, about 20 percent from village social welfare funds, and about 16 percent from the government (see table 3.8).

Affordability of Hypothetic Basic Benefit Packages

Whether community financing is feasible for rural China will depend first of all on its benefit structure: a low benefit package (for example, covering only cost-effective preventive services) is affordable but may not meet the rural population's

---

TABLE 3.8   Community Health Financing by Source in Selected Counties and Provinces, 1991 and 1993 (percent)

	Government	Village social welfare fund	Households	Other
Funds surveyed in Study of Thirty Poor Counties *(1993)*	16.1	20.3	48.1	15.5
Funds surveyed in Five Province Survey *(1991)*	8.0	30.3	58.7	3.0

Source: China Network and Harvard School of Public Health (1996); World Bank (1993).

need for protection from catastrophic medical expenses. Yet a high benefit package, though desirable, may not be feasible because people's willingness and ability to pay is limited. Illnesses are uncertain, and thus the payoff from participating in community-financing schemes is also uncertain for the households. We found that about 11 percent of the rural population consumed 70 percent of the total medical expenditure. This finding illustrates the need for catastrophic insurance and the potential problems of adverse selection and risk selection under a voluntary insurance program. The core issue in designing an appropriate and feasible basic benefit package is the balance among three considerations: the cost-effectiveness of the services covered, people's desired coverage, and the financial constraints on those paying for the coverage.

For illustrative purposes, we developed several basic benefit packages for the low-income rural population, based on data from the 30-county poverty survey. We used the following principles and assumptions in designing the benefit packages: (a) first cover the most cost-effective services, but take into account the fact that health care delivery is not organized by disease; (b) coinsurance should vary for different services depending on demand elasticity; and (c) people are risk-averse and demand coverage for catastrophic expenses. From a societal perspective, the coverage of catastrophic medical expenses also reduces the poverty rate.

The simulation results are shown in table 3.9. Depending on the coinsurance level, the estimated per capita cost is between 28 yuan and 31 yuan (about US$4 to US$5) to provide a basic benefit package that includes specified maternal and child health care services and a stop-loss provision of about 500 yuan to 600 yuan for patients in 1993.

TABLE 3.9   Two Prototype Benefit Packages for China's Rural Poor (benefit structure and costs)

Type of expenses covered	Level of coinsurance	
	High	Low
Village post—		
service fees	20%	10%
drug expenses	50%	40%
Township health center—		
outpatient service fees	30%	30%
outpatient drug expenses	50%	40%
inpatient	35%	30%
County hospital—		
outpatient service fees	40%	35%
outpatient drug expenses	50%	40%
inpatient	45%	35%
Catastrophic protection—		
cap patient's payment at	600 yuan	500 yuan
Estimated per capita costs	31 yuan	28 yuan

TABLE 3.10   Current Financing of Health Spending by Source in China's Poverty Regions

Source of payment	Expenditure per capita in 1993 (yuan)	Percent
Household	23.41	59.32
Government for public employees	13.18	33.40
Community financing	2.31	5.85
Welfare fund	0.31	0.80
Other	0.25	0.63
Total	39.46	100.00

Can the low-income population afford these basic benefit packages? In poverty areas, households already spend a significant amount of their income on health care. According to our survey, annual medical expenditures by such households were 23 yuan per capita in 1993 (see table 3.10). However, it would be unrealistic to expect that people are willing to prepay this amount to support an organized financing scheme. Although the majority of individuals surveyed expressed their support for CMS, their willingness to prepay into the system was only about 5 yuan per capita. Per capita contributions to existing community-financing schemes range from 1.05 yuan to 6.14 yuan. With effective social marketing, it might be expected that 10 yuan per capita could be obtained from households.

Therefore potentially 12 yuan could be collected from individuals and local communities, covering less than half the expected costs of a comprehensive package. The rest of the resource gap would have to be filled by public assistance. Without government support, community-financing schemes in the poverty regions can finance only a limited package for low-income households.

Why Did Most Communities Not Have a CMS?

When asked about the major reasons for the lack of community-financing initiatives, 53 percent of the community leaders cited financial difficulties. However, about two-fifths of the interviewed leaders listed nonfinancial reasons, such as lack of organizational capacity and lack of policy support from higher level government (see table 3.11).

TABLE 3.11   Percentage of 2,236 Surveyed Community Leaders Citing Major Reasons for Lack of Rural Community Financing

Inadequate organizational capacity	22 percent
Inadequate policy support	12 percent
No mass support	8 percent
Inadequate financial resources	53 percent

Indonesia's Dana Sehat and Health Card Schemes

Indonesia has the world's fourth largest population, around 210 million people, living on 5 major islands and 30 groups of small islands. In 1990, the urban-to-rural ratio was 30:70, placing the number of people living in the rural areas of Indonesia close to 145 million. In 1996, GDP per capita reached US$1,155; however, after the economic crisis of 1997, income per capita fell to US$380, impairing the people's ability to pay basic needs, including health services, family planning services, and food.

Since the early 1970s, the Ministry of Public Health (MPH) has encouraged the Dana Sehat (the Village Health Fund) program. The objective of this program has been to improve the coverage of health services in Indonesia by accelerating community participation in financing and maintaining its own health. In 2000, the total membership of Dana Sehat was 23 million people, about 11 percent of the total population. The Dana Sehat, a voluntary community-based, prepaid health care program is most common in the rural areas of Indonesia. The prime movers are health centers, local government, and NGOs such as cooperatives and pesantrens (Muslim teaching units). The people covered are primarily farmers, fishermen, and students.

Contributions come from local economic activities; some schemes generate funds through co-ops of crops or handicrafts, while others are paid in cash. Every household is obliged to pay the premium either in-kind or in cash to the bank or the committee of the Dana Sehat. Open management, trust, and community leadership form the basic culture of the Dana Sehat. Vision, mission, objectives, and program identification are based on deliberation and agreement among community members. Community control comes primarily from its members through periodic meetings to discuss the program, for which the government provides tools and guidance such as Dana Sehat operation, monitoring, and supervisory procedures.

There are many levels of Dana Sehat. On the smallest scale, the Dana Sehat operates with simple management organized by the village and often run by various local institutions. Membership is between 50 and 499 households, the premium is relatively low, and the highest contribution is Rp 100 per household per month. The health benefits are limited to Health Center Services because of the low contribution of the community. On a larger scale, Dana Sehat has a larger membership and is run by a consolidated organization, organized by several villages (that is, a township). It has an organizational structure and job description for the providers. The premium is about Rp 500 per household per month. At this level, Dana Sehat can provide more health benefits, including primary care as well as inpatient services. Payments to the providers are based on the number of consultations (Rp 700 per consultation).

Government officials usually initiate the process by organizing meetings between health providers, local authorities, religious organizations, and key persons in the community and also community-wide meetings. For community surveys, government officials help to train surveyors and assist with analysis and presentation of the results to the community. At a second round of community meetings facilitated by government authorities, community members choose the services to be covered by the fund, balancing their needs against their ability and willingness to finance the package. Poor rural communities often choose a package of basic outpatient and curative care, combined with free preventive services. Continued government supervision and monitoring, combined with monthly or bimonthly community meetings, guide fund management.

Indonesia Health Card

The Health Card program, begun in 1996, is a national commitment to assure health care access for the indigent. The target population is eligible people in villages. In 1999, the estimated number of participants was 11,096. The Health Card program is administered by the Municipality Health Office (MHO). The premium is fully subsidized; the beneficiaries do not have to pay any premiums or fees. Services at the health center and certain services in public hospitals are covered. Payment to the providers is Rp 10,000 per year by capitation of the designated poor. The basic funding comes from the Social Protection Sector Development Program (SPSDP) and MHO: 580,000,000 per year and public hospitals 600,000,000 per year. The government seems to be in charge of this program.

Several factors explain Dana Sehat's success. The community is heavily involved in the supervision and monitoring of health care activities of the Dana Sehat. However, at the village level, there are insufficient management capabilities, risk-pooling capacity, and ability to monitor the technical quality of services. As a result, many village-managed Dana Sehat rely more on fee-for-service than on prepayment.

Dana Sehat performs better at the township level. At this level, the managerial capacity improves and the larger population base allows greater risk-pooling. Centralized management has more resources and can offer more benefits and more providers.

One major barrier to establishing Dana Sehat is the absence of government subsidy. The poor community simply cannot afford the scheme. Only communities with rural enterprises or producer cooperatives have the potential to obtain funds to subsidize the very poor and perhaps the poor and near-poor as well to induce them to join.

Thailand's Health Card

The population of Thailand is estimated at 59 million, of whom 31.5 percent are urban, hence the ratio of urban to rural population is about 1:2. Income distribution has worsened; in 1992, the highest income quintile held 59.5 percent of the national income while the lowest income quintile held merely 3.8 percent. The 1994 per capita income was US$2,410.

The Health Card program was implemented in 1983 as a voluntary scheme, primarily to promote maternal and child health. Purchase of the card meant prepayment of a certain fixed premium, capitation to the provider, in return for free services for one year. Proceeds from the card sale went into the health card fund and was managed by a village committee. The program's primary objective at inception was to improve health among rural populations, with an emphasis on primary health care, including health education, environmental health, maternal and child health, and provision of essential drugs. The system incorporated a referral system from primary care to tertiary care. The program was also intended to involve local villagers in self-help as well as in managing the health card fund.

As time went by, various cards were introduced for different purposes, but by 1991 they had been discontinued, and only family cards priced at 500 Baht were offered. A major change in the program since 1994 is the explicit contribution of the MPH: an equal contribution of 500 Baht. In addition, no limits were imposed on the number of episodes or the cost of coverage per visit. Flexibility was built into the referral system, and each province could impose any conditions deemed appropriate for particular situations. Health care funds also became managed by a committee at the district level in coordination with village-level bodies, a move that was aimed at expanding the enrollment base to the district level. As for the share of funds, 80 percent of the card price was earmarked for providers for medical care, and the remaining 20 percent was to be retained for marketing and sales incentives. The health card project has evolved over the years and can now be considered a kind of social welfare program, since it now receives an explicit contribution from the government equal to the contribution of the cardholder.

In 1994, free health cards were given to community leaders and village health volunteers to provide free health care for their families. The voluntary cardholders consumed more health care than other types of cardholders. The compulsory community leader cards and health volunteer cards provided better risk pooling and compensated for the deficit on operating the voluntary health cards. Considering costs per card in relation to population coverage, provinces with low coverage of health cards were more likely to face higher utilization rates and health expenditure per card than provinces with high population coverage. Therefore, the health card fund provided on average only a 50 percent subsidy to the regional and general hospitals while providing 80 percent subsidy to the community hospitals and the full cost to health centers.

Initially, individuals with a monthly income below 1,000 Baht were eligible. Now, health card eligibility extends to families with monthly incomes lower than 2,800 Baht per month and individuals with monthly incomes below 2,000 Baht, primarily farmers and informal sector workers at the community level. The cards entitle holders to free medical care at all government health facilities operated by the Ministry of Public Health, the Bangkok Metropolitan Administration, the Red Cross Society, Pattaya City, and the municipalities. Each card is valid for three years. The government provides block grants to health facilities based on the expected distribution of the eligible population and past records.

Health centers are the cheapest source of health care, but inpatient care is available at community, general, and regional hospitals. Specifically, the budget allocation is based on the number of low-income people living in the designated less-developed villages. However, the budgetary allocation is invariably insufficient to cover the cost of providing services.

The health card fund has been changed so it can be managed like a revolving fund. In 1995, the Ministry of Finance set up an accounting system for the central and provincial health card funds that complies with the regulations of the government's revolving fund. Risk pooling at the central level facilitates portability of benefits and risk sharing among provincial funds, allowing for cross-boundary services used in different provinces and high-cost services within the same or different provinces. Now there are no benefit limits, and the program is targeted to the subgroup of the population with no health benefit coverage.

Those factors explain the success of the Thai Health Card: The health card is able to cover a large part of its target population, the near poor, because the government's subsidy is given directly to the eligible household. The subsidy is relatively large—100 percent matching for what the household pays. Currently, it covers about 3 million people.

The enrollees have unlimited access to free services at the public facilities. Thus it also offers a high degree of risk pooling.

Local or Target Population Schemes

Bangladesh Community-Financing Schemes

In Bangladesh, community participation in health care is increasing.[15] NGOs and the private sector actively organize and finance health care delivery. Community health insurance schemes have emerged as a mechanism for paying providers and mobilizing resources. Examples in Bangladesh include the Grameen Health Program (GHP), the Gonoshasthaya Kendra (GK) Health Care System, and the Dhaka Community Hospital Insurance Program. This section briefly describes the three schemes.

The Grameen Health Program

The Grameen Bank, internationally known as a successful group-based credit program, provides credit to the rural poor, particularly women, who own less than a half acre of land or whose assets do not exceed the value of one acre of land. At present, Grameen has 2.3 million members and covers almost half the villages in the country through 1,167 branches. The GB is an institution for financial intermediation, and it also supports social development programs for poverty alleviation. The Grameen has more than 20 years of operational experience as a financial intermediary. It started a health program only in 1993.

GB became involved in health care mainly because illness was identified as the single largest cause of loan default. A study found that 44 percent of the loan defaults were due to illness. Poor health prevented borrowers from carrying out their economic activities and therefore from repaying their loans because of limited access to health care and limited capability to pay for health services when health needs occur. Thus illness and its financial consequences are serious threats to the Grameen borrowers and the long-term viability of the GB itself. The Grameen Health Program (GHP) was established to provide basic health care services to its members as well as nonmembers living in the same operational area and to provide insurance to cover the cost of basic care. The GHP thus functions as an insurer as well as a health care provider.

The GHP started with five Grameen Health Centers in 1993. Each center is staffed with a doctor, who also acts as the center director, and with a paramedic, a lab technician, and an office manager. Each center is attached to a Grameen Bank branch and covers the branch's operational area, which normally has 2,500 GB families and 3,500 non-GB families. Some centers have subcenters, usually staffed with one paramedic and two health workers (Grameen Bank 1995).

A health center provides outpatient services, routine pathology, and basic drugs. A television is provided in the waiting room and shows various health education programs. Health workers provide door-to-door services on health education and health promotion.

The GHP's prepaid health insurance program is open to everyone covered by a GB branch, regardless of whether they are GB members. The insurance scheme utilizes the organizational structure of the GB credit program. The subscription of the insurance scheme for GB members is based on groups of a minimum of five families, the same requirement as for borrowing. In general, GB members participate in the health insurance program in the same groups as their loan groups. The GHP charges an annual premium of 120 taka (about US$2.60) per family for GB members and 150 taka (US$3.30) for non-GB members. However, if non-GB members can organize into a group of five, they pay the same rate as members. The benefit package covers unlimited outpatient visits with a copayment of 2 taka (about US$0.05) per episode; 50 percent of the cost of basic pathology tests and 15 essential drugs; 15 percent of other drugs sold at the health center; 50 percent of the cost of a specialist consultation and more sophisticated tests in referral hospitals; and reimbursement of up to 500 to 1,000 taka per year for hospitalization.

The number of Grameen health centers grew from 5 in 1993 to 10 in 1997. The number of insured families increased from 13,000 in 1994 to 25,935 in 1996. About 85 percent of the subscribers are GB members. This ratio has changed little over the years.

The Gonoshasthaya Kendra Health Care System

The Gonoshasthaya Kendra (GK) Health Care System is an NGO-run local health care system. It operates in Savar, a rapidly industrializing area with a population of 271,448, 40 kilometers from Dhaka, the capital city of Bangladesh. GK started as a health project in 1971 with donor support and gradually expanded into a two-tier health care system with a 70-bed hospital and 4 subcenters. Each sub-center covers 25,000 to 30,000 inhabitants with a team of 8 to 10 paramedics. A paramedic usually provides door-to-door services, including preventive and simple curative care and health education, to inhabitants under his or her coverage, usually 600 to 700 families. A doctor from the GK hospital visits a subcenter twice a week to see patients referred by the paramedics, and the severely ill are referred to the hospital. The GK system also runs other programs: a pharmaceutical factory, a workshop producing furniture, and a small credit program.

The GK initiated the first community insurance scheme in 1975 to increase the poor's access to health care. GK subscribers pay a premium for a package of benefits, including primary health care and some portion of hospital care.

The GK scheme classifies the population into four socioeconomic groups, and the premium and copayment schedules are set based on these groups. The criteria for determining households' socioeconomic status are not accurate measurements of income, but communities' perceptions of poverty. The communities in the catchment areas participated in the exercises for defining socioeconomic groups, and the final classifications were generally accepted by the population in the communities. The sliding fee structure was designed to reflect ability to pay. A household subscribing to the insurance scheme receives a registration card that indicates the household's socioeconomic group. The premium and copayment are charged according to the fee structure for that group. People who are not insured would pay fees based on market prices.

The sliding premium rates are differentiated according to the four socioeconomic status groups in the area. Group 1 encompasses destitute single-headed households (most of them widowed or divorced women) and the disabled. Group 2 consists of households that cannot afford two meals a day for all household members, landless farmers (less than an acre of land), and daily wage earners. Group 3 includes households that can afford minimum needs but have no savings, such as farmers with small landholdings (two to three acres), small shop owners, and industry labor workers. Group 4 covers households with savings, farmers with more than three acres of land, owners of big shops or businesses, middle- and upper-class civil servants, and professionals (Desmet and Chowdhury 1996).

The GK insurance scheme covers 12,393 member families, about 33 percent of the target population.

Dhaka Community Hospital Health Insurance Program

Dhaka Community Hospital (DCH) offers an innovative approach in health service provision. The DCH differs from other private hospitals in its mission and setup. A group of devoted senior medical practitioners organized a nonprofit trust in 1989, which later developed into a system with a 24-bed referral hospital, 19 rural health clinics, 12 school health clinics, and 24 industrial health clinics. Their mission is to provide quality health care services at low cost, so most of the poor people can afford them. In its system, DCH attempts to integrate the provision of primary, secondary, and tertiary care.

The DCH itself operates on a fee-for-service basis and provides walk-in services at fixed rates lower than those of equivalent private, for-profit hospitals. The DCH offers a special program called After Payment, which allows patients who cannot pay at the time of treatment to pay the medical bill in installments after treatment. The patient's community guarantees payment. The After Payment Program is very small, only two to three cases per clinic per year. Since communities take the responsibility for making sure the fees are paid, no default has thus far occurred. The DCH is self-reliant and receives no funds from the government or donors.

At its clinics, the DCH system operates as a health insurance scheme, known as a health card program. There are five types of health cards. The Family Health Card, intended for rural households, costs 40 taka per month (about US$1) for an initial enrollment and 20 taka for renewal, and covers up to 12 members per household, including servants living there. This plan entitles the whole household to consult the clinic doctor at any time and to receive monthly home visits by health workers who are trained by the DCH. Patients with the health card do not pay additional fees for consulting a doctor but have to buy medicines outside of the clinic. The School Children Card, free to schoolchildren living near the health clinics, offers children free physical examinations and health education. The Worker Health Card, for workers at enterprises near the clinics, costs 2 taka per month per worker. Premiums are paid by the companies or the owners' associations. The benefit package includes free consultation but no monthly home visits by health workers. The Sports Card, for professional sports players, is intended mainly as a means of publicizing the clinics. No premium is charged for enrollment, and medical consultations are free. Poor families in the communities receive a special Destitute Card at no cost, which allows household members to visit the clinic at 5 taka per visit. The community committees decide which families in the village are considered poor and should receive Destitute Cards.

Some services are provided by field health workers: preventive care, health education, and simple checkups such as measuring blood pressure and urine sugar levels. Specialists from the DCH visit clinics periodically to treat villagers. The rural health card scheme does not cover inpatient care or the costs of drugs or medical tests. Doctors in the clinics refer patients to the DCH, and patients pay for hospital care at DCH rates. The DCH has begun to provide health cards covering inpatient care at the DCH to some companies in urban areas.

As presented above, many communities in Asia have long-established community-based financing schemes for health care. Their sponsors vary, ranging from the government to the community itself, when it perceived the need for an organized way to finance and provide basic health care. These varied schemes offer different benefits and cover different populations; some are more affordable than others. After first classifying the different types of community-financing schemes, then evaluating them, we can discover the major factors that determine the success or failure of each type.

Acknowledgments: The authors are grateful to the World Health Organization (WHO) for having provided an opportunity to contribute to the work of the Commission on Macroeconomics and Health and to the World Bank for publishing the material in this chapter as an HNP Discussion Paper.

NOTES

1. This chapter was prepared as a part of the Commission on Macroeconomics and Health's Working Group 3 studies on mobilizing resources for households not employed in the formal sector (hereafter referred to as the "informal sector"). To state the obvious, they are not a homogenous group. Their occupations range from peasant, peddler, day laborer, taxi driver, and informal sector employee to shop owner and self-employed professional, such as a physician or a lawyer. Some of them are rich, but most are poor. Some live in the city, but most live in rural communities. This chapter focuses on mobilizing resources for the residents of rural communities, who make up more than 70 percent and 50 percent, respectively, of the population in low- and middle-income nations. The chapter also gives some attention to mobilizing resources for the urban poor.

2. Close to 50 percent of the total national health expenditure for most low-income nations comes from direct out-of-pocket payment by patients (WHO 2000).

3. The industrial nations (except the United States) use general revenue or compulsory social insurance to pay for health care for citizens working in the informal sector.

4. Funding maybe inadequate, but public funds usually go first to pay health workers, regardless of whether they deliver satisfactory services and whether drugs and other supplies are adequate. This practice has created a public employment program, not a health delivery program to meet patients' needs and demands.

5. There are exceptions, situations in which private nonprofit providers charge reasonable prices and deliver quality primary health care, such as the PROSALUD does in Boliva.

6. This confusion is exacerbated by studies that examine the community-financing schemes from a particular point of interest and then label them by that single unitary factor. Several widely circulated documents have used new terms such as *rural health insurance* (U.S. Agency for International Development and the World Health Organization) and *microinsurance* (International Labour Organization) for community-financing schemes.

7. *Community* is defined as a group of households living in close proximity to each other, such as a village or a neighborhood. Often for risk pooling and managerial purposes, the villages might be grouped. In addition to geographic proximity, a community must include organizations in which people who share common interests come together, as in producer and consumer cooperatives or women's banks.

8. Prepayment can be for two types of health expenses: high cost and low frequency; and low cost and high frequency. The former involves much greater risk pooling (insurance) than the latter. Insurance literature has long documented that most people lack the appreciation for the benefit of insurance, a fact that led to a common saying: "Insurance is sold not bought." In advanced economies, voluntary private health insurance is being sold to the affluent risk-averse households, but this is not the case in low-income countries.

9. *Affordable* is defined as reasonably priced as judged by historical precedents or by common sense.

10. The currently favored policy of separating financing from provision can work only when there are several competing providers. This condition seldom exists in villages and towns. In the United States, the major industry in many isolated towns organized the staff-model health maintenance organization (HMO) in which financing and provision are integrated. They have proven that this organizational form, controlled privately, can produce high quality health services at lower cost. Low-income countries have had similar experiences. More important, low-income countries have few qualified practitioners working in villages and towns. Where public health services are absent or operate inefficiently, peasants rely on indigenous doctors, drug peddlers, or private practitioners whose competence varies widely but who charge high prices. The local community can improve the efficiency and quality of basic health care by organizing health posts and clinics and by recruiting qualified health workers and practitioners and assuring them that they will have a steady, reasonable income. This requires, however, a prepayment financing arrangement.

11. Even in advanced economies in which people are better educated and buy other types of insurance, insurance companies initially found little willingness to buy health insurance. From the 1930s to the 1960s, it was often said that health insurance has to be sold, not bought.

12. In several countries, particularly in Africa, church-sponsored and -managed hospitals have enjoyed the people's confidence and have been successful in starting hospital-based prepayment plans.

13. *Community* is defined as a group of households living in close proximity to each other, such as a village or a neighborhood. Often for risk pooling and managerial purposes, the villages might be grouped. A community can also be a group of people formally organized to advance some common interest (for example, agricultural and consumer cooperatives).

14. Prepayment can be for two types of health expenses: high cost and low frequency; and low cost and high frequency. The former involves much greater risk pooling (insurance) than the latter. In advanced economies, voluntary private health insurance is being sold to affluent risk-averse households, but this is not the case in low-income countries.

15. This section is taken largely from the paper by Shiyan Chao (1998), *Community Health Insurance in Bangladesh: A Viable Option?*

REFERENCES

Atim, C. 1998. *Contribution of Mutual Health to Financing, Delivery, and Access to Health Care: Synthesis of Research in Nine West and Central African Countries.* Technical Report 18. Partnerships for Health Reform Project; Abt Associates Inc., Bethesda, Md.

Bennett S., A. Creese, and R. Monasch. 1998. *Health Insurance Schemes for People Outside Formal Sector Employment.* ARA Paper 16. WHO, Geneva.

Bitran, R. 1995. "Efficiency and Quality in the Public and Private Sectors in Senegal." *Health Policy and Planning* 10 (3): 271–83.

Carrin, G., and M. Vereecke. 1992. *Strategies for Health Care Finance in Developing Countries with a Focus on Community Financing in Sub-Saharan Africa.* New York: St. Martin's Press.

Chao, Shiyan. 1998. *Community Health Insurance in Bangladesh: A Viable Option?* Unpublished report. World Bank.

China Network and Harvard School of Public Health. 1996. *Study of 30 Poor Counties.*

Gilson, L. 1995. "Management and Health Care Reform in Sub-Saharan Africa." *Social Science and Medicine* 40(5): 695–710.

Gilson, L., P. D. Sen, S. Mohammed, and P. Mujinja. 1994. "The Potential of Health Sector Non-Governmental Organizations: Policy Options." *Health Policy and Planning* 9(1): 14–24.

Grameen Bank. 1995. *Preparatory Report on the Establishment of the Grameen Health Program.* Dhaka.

Hsiao, W. C. 1995. "The Chinese Health Care System: Lessons for Other Nations." *Social Science and Medicine* 41(8): 1047–55.

Liu, Y. 2001. *Demand for Community Pre-Payment Schemes in Health Care.* Unpublished.

Mao, Z. 1995. "Findings from the Rand Experiment in China. *Chinese Health Economics Journal* 11(3): 16.

McPake, B., K. Hanson, and A. Mills. 1992. *Experience to Date of Implementing the Bamako Initiative: A Review and Five Country Case Studies.* London: London School of Hygiene and Tropical Medicine.

Narayan, D., and L. Pritchett. 1997. *Cents and Sociability: Household Income and Social Capital in Rural Tanzania.* Washington, D.C.: World Bank.

Putnam, R. 1993. *Making Democracy Work: Civic Traditions in Modern Italy.* Princeton, N.J.: Princeton University Press.

Saurborne, R., A. Nougtara, and E. Latimer. 1994. "The Elasticity of Demand for Health Care in Burkina Faso: Differences across Age and Income." *Health Policy and Planning* 9: 186–92.

Stinson, W. 1982. *Community Financing of Primary Health Care.* Washington, D.C.: American Public Health Association.

World Bank. 1993. *World Development Report 1993: Investing in Health.* Washington, D.C.

———. 2001. *World Development Report 2000–2001: Attacking Poverty.* Washington, D.C.

WHO (World Health Organization). 2000. *The World Health Report 2000: Health Systems—Measuring Performance.* Geneva.

Zere, E., D. McIntyre, and T. Addison. 2001. "Technical Efficiency and Productivity of Public Sector Hospitals in Three South African Provinces." *South African Journal of Economics* 69(2): 336–58.

CHAPTER 4

Experience of Community Health Financing in the African Region

Dyna Arhin-Tenkorang

Abstract: Studies and literature reviews of health insurance schemes targeting rural or informal sector populations in developing countries (often called community insurance schemes) frequently conclude that schemes have design weaknesses, yet do not explore in detail the effect of design features on performance. This chapter presents a conceptualization of how performance in the areas of risk protection and resource mobilization is determined by the interaction of design features with institutional and technical factors. Design features refer to scheme specifications (for example, required contribution) and to operating modalities (for example, procedures for enrollment or obtaining benefits). Performance, with respect to risk protection and resource mobilization, of several potential high-population schemes for the informal sector in Africa, is assessed. The outcome suggests that the design of community health insurance schemes may be improved by (a) design specifications that utilize data on willingness to pay (WTP) of the target population and projected health care costs; and (b) incorporating modalities of operations that facilitate cost-effective exchange between a formal organization and individuals acting in an informal environment.

Increasing the access of African populations to health care is one of the formidable challenges facing the global community. During the 1980s and 1990s, African governments, with the endorsement of their international and bilateral donor partners, implemented health sector reforms intended to improve the efficiency of health systems and the quality of care. In many countries, these reforms included the introduction or consolidation of cost-recovery mechanisms, in particular out-of-pocket fees, paid at the time of illness *(user fees),* which had the unintended effect of decreasing the poor's access to health care (Bethune, Alfani, and Lahaye 1989; Booth and others 1995; Nyonator and Kutzin 1999). Since the mid-1990s, the increasing incidence and prevalence in low-income countries of HIV/AIDS, tuberculosis (TB), and other communicable diseases have contributed to the widening of the gap between the need for, and the utilization of, health services among poor individuals.

At the time of ill health, households in Africa do not have recourse to mechanisms that will protect the financial resources required for basic consumption needs, such as transportation, education, and food not produced by the household. As most functional health insurance schemes in Africa are associated with formal sector employment—requiring regular contributions compatible with formal sector earnings—the majority of individuals are not insured. Vogel (1990) and Abel-Smith and Rawal (1994) conclude that the formal sector schemes effectively cover only members of the relatively small upper and middle classes.

Uncertainty about the timing of illness, the unpredictability of health care costs during illness, and the low and irregular income of individuals mean that it is virtually impossible for households to make financial provision for illness-related expenditures. User fees constitute a major part of such expenditures. As a consequence, user fees have been, and still are, a major contributing factor to the high incidence of out-of-pocket payment by individuals and households at the time of illness. Furthermore, most households cannot obtain credit from the formal banking system. Thus user fees, in addition to having been largely unsuccessful in raising significant resources, have contributed significantly to increasing the exposure of poor households to financial risks associated with illness.

Individuals are subject to illness-related financial risks correlated with health care prices and their disposable incomes. As ratios of health care prices to incomes rise, households' probabilities of illness-related loss of wealth and assets increase. Health care must often be consumed in complete packages and is therefore a discrete, rather than a continuous, variable in the health production function. Furthermore, components of packages (for example, consultations, laboratory tests, prescribed drugs) will vary in quantity and type, giving rise to complex relationships between the quantities consumed, the costs, and the health outcomes.

As a result of the complexity of these relationships and the variations in the type and course of illnesses, identical household budget constraints often have disparate impacts on the consumption of effective health care. In poor communities, this complex relationship also leads to identical health status outcomes for households, irrespective of the income groups to which they belong. Although people in the high-income groups, obtained by ranking, have the economic means to purchase a greater proportion of health care packages, providers are often unwilling to offer an incomplete package—as in the example of "half a surgical procedure." If an incomplete package is offered, it is usually ineffective in improving health, as in the case of a partial course of antibiotics. Consequently, in many situations of low per capita incomes, ranking households into income groups is of little use for policy formulation aimed at providing universal access to effective health care. Rather, public provision of financial protection becomes a crucial element of strategies to reduce poverty for all households in poor communities such as those in rural areas and slums, irrespective of their incomes relative to others in those areas.

Over the long term, health investments that make *preventive* health care available will lead to improved health and productivity of the people, hence to higher incomes. In the short term, provision of access to *curative* health care is needed to limit income shocks from illness that might otherwise push people into poverty. Households can frequently prevent illnesses, but they are unequipped to treat many illnesses effectively. To prevent malaria, for example, a farming mother in a village in Ghana can build up her immunity system and her child's by eating high-protein, homegrown foods and by breastfeeding. She can also take actions to repel mosquitoes. These measures enable her to dramatically influence the frequency and prognosis of malaria episodes suffered by her child. In contrast, because households cannot treat severe malaria, society considers accessible treatment of this disease a high priority among the functions expected of its health system.

A premise of this chapter is that in poor African countries, individuals in the informal sector—regardless of their income rank—cannot access appropriate health care, particularly curative care, at the time of need. In one study, expenditure for 70 percent of inpatient episodes exceeded 6 percent (in the fourth income quintile) and 4 percent (in the highest quintile) of the average annual income for individuals (Arhin 1995b). In this environment, insurance schemes that provide financial protection to households in the informal sector would constitute an important poverty-reduction measure. Another premise is that attempts to stratify informal populations by income, so as to target financial protection just to those in the lower ranks, will be only partially effective in achieving access to health care for the very poor.

Establishing subnational health insurance schemes, each targeting households in defined poor communities such as villages or districts, is an option for providing immediate financial risk protection (FRP) to a significant number of households. It also offers the potential of eventually achieving universal coverage and high cross-subsidization between high- and low-income households through the future linking of schemes for the informal sector to each other and to schemes for the formal sector. The alternative strategy of attempting to provide universal coverage on a national scale by implementing a single national scheme at the outset would be problematic because of the diversity in African populations and the absence of appropriate administrative infrastructures.

Studies and literature reviews of subnational health insurance schemes (often referred to as *community-financing schemes* or *microfinancing schemes*) targeting rural or informal sector populations in developing countries frequently conclude that such schemes have design flaws that impair their performances (Bennett, Creese, and Monasch 1998). As the reviews do not explore in detail the relationships between design features and specific dimensions of performance, this chapter focuses on the design-related issues of subnational health insurance schemes for the informal sector in sub-Saharan Africa. It examines, in particular, the functions of risk protection against the financial consequences of ill health and the mobilization of significant resources for the health sector. Resource mobilization is examined with reference to the fiscal impact of the insurance on health care provision rather than from an accounting perspective focusing on meeting the financial obligations of a given scheme. Therefore cost recovery is considered a variable related to resource mobilization rather than a prime indicator of performance.

The first part of the chapter presents a conceptual framework intended to inform readers about the design of a health insurance scheme that focuses on the characteristics of schemes and factors influencing their performance. It presents key technical and institutional factors that, together with the design features, determine scheme performance in resource mobilization and financial protection. Emphasis is placed on dimensions of these factors that are particularly relevant to schemes targeting individuals and households in the informal sector in low-income countries. The technical factors relate to the data (its nature and quality) and the methodology used to specify the contribution levels, the benefit package, and the level of external financial subsidy. The institutional factors include the congruence between principles underlying the scheme's operations and norms of the participating population. Other institutional factors include experiences of health providers with third-party contractual arrangements and payments. These institutional factors have a crucial influence on the nature and extent of community participation in the scheme, and on the quality of scheme management and monitoring. Although regulatory factors—such as the guidelines produced by responsible government agencies and laws governing insurance and health care provision—also determine the insurance and health care quality, they are not considered here.

In the second part of the chapter, evidence is reviewed about the effectiveness and efficiency with which selected health insurance schemes for the informal sector population have achieved resource mobilization and risk protection. The evidence is presented mainly from schemes judged to have the necessary—though often insufficient—design and implementation features that would permit expansion to achieve high primary or secondary participation rates.[1] Logically these features exist because, at the minimum, the calculation of contribution levels reflects the ability and willingness to pay (economic demand) of the target population. The proposed scheme is described to potential buyers in terms of benefit package and management structure, and the demand is the ability and willingness to pay (WTP) the annual contribution in the required installments.

Although relatively few schemes for Africa's informal sector populations have based their contribution calculations on WTP data, some, through a variety of approaches, have arrived at affordable or near-affordable premiums for their target populations. Some schemes have also obtained sufficient external resources to potentially fund the type and quality of health care benefits their enrolled members expect. Such potentially large population schemes include the Carte d'Assurance Maladie (CAM) program (Burundi), Community Health Fund (CHF, Tanzania), Abota Village Insurance Scheme (Guinea-Bissau), Nkoranza Community Financing Health Insurance Scheme (Ghana), Bwamanda Hospital Insurance Scheme (Democratic Republic of Congo), and Dangme West Health Insurance Scheme (Ghana).

Of the examples of potentially large population schemes studied in this chapter, two of them, CAM in Burundi and the Health Card Fund in Tanzania, are in some respect national schemes. These two schemes have significant central government involvement. Other schemes may be considered district-based schemes from the outset, while the Abota Scheme, for example, evolved into a form of a district scheme and is still expanding, through an institutionalization process, toward national dimensions and characteristics. Criel (1998) uses two main features to characterize three schemes in Africa as district-based health insurance schemes (DBHIS): first, a prominent role of the local health service administrators in its operations, and second, an expectation that the scheme will eventually cover the entire population residing in the health administrative area or district. Evidence is presented from several schemes (including the Nkoranza Scheme in Ghana and the Bwamanda Scheme in Democratic Republic of Congo), which under Criel's framework are examples of DBHIS. These are effectively single-facility provider schemes (in both cases the facility being a hospital) and are susceptible to the problems of low participation because benefits are accessible at only one location, discouraging enrollment by people who live far from the provider.

When the inclusion of all levels of facilities (health post, health center, and district hospital) as providers is used in addition to Criel's two characteristics to categorize DBHIS, the only true example in the chapter is the Dangme West Health Insurance Scheme (Dangme Hewami Nami Kpee) in Ghana (Arhin and Adjai 1997). The outpatient (OPD) benefit package provided by lower level providers (health centers) in the Dangme Scheme encourages insured patients to present illnesses early, when treatment resource requirements are minimal. In addition, the absence of financial incentives for insured patients to obtain inappropriate admissions has the potential to foster proper functioning of the referral system. Finally, the availability of OPD and emergency care as part of the benefit package has proven a critical factor in decisions to participate in a scheme. Although the schemes studied have large target populations, provide a comprehensive package in some cases, and are geographically readily accessible to enrolled members, the evidence shows that enrollment is often relatively low. Many institutional factors interact with design features either to enhance or to limit the performance of all schemes.

Based on the evidence from the selected schemes, the third part of the chapter discusses those institutional and technical factors that appear to influence performance. In the absence of established best practices in the scheme design, an argument is made for experimentation, guided by lessons from these schemes. Suggestions are also made of broad national and international policy measures to support the implementation of risk-protection schemes for populations in the informal sectors.

CONCEPTUAL FRAMEWORK

Health Insurance, Risk, and Willingness to Pay

Health insurance is a mechanism for spreading the risks of incurring health care costs over a group of individuals or households. This definition is not dependent on the nature of the administrative arrangements employed, but on the outcome of risk sharing and subsequent cross-subsidization of health care expenditures among the participants. An arrangement designed to provide risk sharing for illness-related events, and which is accessible to households in the informal sectors in low-income countries, is a health insurance scheme regardless of the orthodoxy of its operational modalities. In such an arrangement, an insured individual acquires "a state-contingent income claim" before the state of the world is known and is entitled to resources, income, or both to address the event for which he or she is insured if the event occurs.

Some studies have reported that low-income households are initially reluctant to join insurance schemes because they do not readily accept the idea of "paying" for services they might not use (Brown and Churchill 2000). Interpreting such findings as evidence that these households have risk attitudes nonsupportive of insurance (risk neutral or risk-loving attitudes) would predict limited potential for insurance schemes targeting these households. In contrast, three studies in Ghana, Burundi, and Guinea-Bissau suggest that households in rural areas are risk-averse with regard to health care (Arhin 1996a, p. 629). Such differences in population attitude and WTP for health insurance would theoretically lead to predictable variation in insurance scheme enrollment. Therefore WTP information for a target population would facilitate scheme design and implementation.

Currently, limited theoretical constructs and empirical evidence are available to guide WTP studies undertaken in developing countries for the purpose of pricing goods and services, as in the case of providing pricing inputs for the design of goods supplied publicly rather than privately. Consequently, published data on the demand of population groups for health insurance, as indicated by their willingness and ability to pay premiums, pertain to a limited number of countries (Arhin 1996b; Mathiyazhagan 1998; Asenso-Okyere and others 1997).

In many developing countries, ensuring the reliability and validity of WTP studies of insurance goods presents many problems, partly because of the population's limited experience with insurance policies. For example, this limited experience increases the probability that inappropriate discourse may be used to ascertain perceptions and result in an erroneous conclusion of reluctance to pay for uncertain consumption. As a consequence, inept strategies of basic education may be adopted, instead of marketing approaches, to provide information on modalities and build trust. Exploratory discussions before introducing a scheme in a rural part of Ghana found that the term *health insurance* was not associated with risk sharing and instead referred to an unfamiliar product purchased mainly by the urban elite. Risk-sharing arrangements that were familiar to the rural communities were described as *solidarity groups,* associations of people who assist each other when events associated with specific needs occur (Arhin 1995c).

Relevant Scheme Models

Health insurance schemes are arrangements in which officials formally hold funds that consist of payments by insured participants and use the resultant resource pool to finance all or part of members' health care costs. In African countries that have schemes for the informal sector, most plans fall into the first three of the following four models. Where the officials are members of an identifiable group whose contributions make up the pools, and are responsible for management activities such as determining benefits and contributions, the model is a mutual benefit society model. Atim provides an example and defines a *mutual health organization* as "a voluntary, nonprofit insurance scheme, formed on the basis of an ethic of mutual aid, solidarity, and the collective pooling of health risks, in which the members participate effectively in its management and functioning" (Atim 1998). In *provider insurance models,* the officials originate from the health care provider institution (or from the ultimate provider organization such as the government or mission health administration) and manage both the insurance and the health care aspects of the scheme, similar to health maintenance organizations (HMOs). In a variant of these mutual and provider models, the officials are responsible for managing the insurance product and providing health care, and are drawn from members of a mutual society as well as a health care provider organization. Such a model may be termed a *mutual-provider partnership model* and correlates in general to the concept of community-based insurance put forward to test the hypothesis of feasibility of insurance for households in the informal sector (Arhin 1991). *Third-party insurance* has not been a feature of insurance schemes for the informal sector in Africa.[2]

Each of the four design models is associated with incentive structures that influence the behavior of the actors in the models. For example, mutual models encourage greater accountability to the individuals who make up the pool but also generate a significant requirement for committed time, skill, and knowledge from these individuals. Mutual-provider partnership models reduce the level of these requirements from the informal insured group. The integration of insurance management and health care provision in a scheme offers strong motivation for providing health promotion services and preventive care to limit benefit claims. Yet where health care is provided to members by a separate insurance entity, the threat of nonpayment or contract termination may result in a higher quality of service. The skills and management capacities of the different actors, resource availability, the nature of the existing power balance, and the prospects for positive change will influence the appropriateness of a model for a given setting.

In Africa, schemes intended for the informal sector are confronted with the target populations' low and irregular incomes and consequently negligible profit-making potential. Of necessity, therefore, schemes for the informal sector have social welfare dimensions rather than commercial characteristics. This is made more apparent in mutual models since they involve actions by social institutions, communities, and the state (the latter through regulation and legislation). The mutual schemes represent public action taken to reduce human deprivation and eliminate vulnerability (Burgess and Stern 1991). They facilitate explicit or implicit participation by communities in scheme design and implementation. Depending on the community's composition and cultural norms, emphasis will be placed either equally or preferentially on achieving the schemes' social and financial functions. Although they are intrinsically linked, the social and financial functions performed by a social welfare-oriented health insurance scheme may be considered separately. The social function affects risk protection for the individual, whereas the financial function leads to resource mobilization for the group.

Risk-Protection Function of Schemes

Risk protection, in the health context, is the shielding of an individual from critical income losses as a result of illness or injury. In sub-Saharan Africa, *critical income* is the resource required for needs such as food not grown on the household farm, housing construction material that cannot be produced by the household (for example, corrugated iron sheets for roofing), and basic formal education. Health-related financial risk protection is inversely related to the percentage of income required to meet expenditures related to treatment for an illness episode. To illustrate, a household survey finding that out-of-pocket expenditure for 20 percent of inpatient episodes exceeded half the mean annual household income for people in the lowest income quintile suggests that risk protection is nonexistent for a significant proportion of Africans (Arhin 1997). Insurance schemes that provide 100 percent coverage for illness episodes provide the highest levels of protection, and those involving copayment provide lower levels of protection.

Protection is a function of income, the price of health care and other goods, the illness incidence, and the completeness of an insurance benefit package. Therefore data on all these aspects of illness and economic activity are necessary to assess the financial protection afforded by a health system. Using the system's ability to safeguard individuals' critical income in the event of illness as a measure of risk protection allows cross-country comparisons of schemes' risk-protection performance under different economic circumstances. Other measures of risk protection such as differences in the out-of-pocket payment between scheme members and nonmembers permit comparisons only between schemes operating in similar economic situations. For example, two schemes whose benefit structures require members to pay the same flat fee per prescription will provide different risk protection if the incomes and living costs of members of the two schemes are dissimilar.

To provide FRP, a scheme must offer an insurance product that is accessible to the target population and either eliminates payments associated with receiving care, as in the case of a zero copayment rate, or reduces the payment to a level that has negligible impact on critical consumption. Accessibility in this context will be high when a scheme's premium does not exceed targeted individuals' noncritical income. The compatibility of the collection schedule with the target households' cash flow patterns, for example, taking into account the seasonality of agricultural workers' cash income, will also enhance accessibility.

Since the process of obtaining health care in most low-income settings is a "bad" rather than a "good" (often associated with long journeys on foot and relatively expensive and uncomfortable travel by road, long hours of queuing, and loss of production for most of the day), there is little justification for including measures such as copayments to reduce possible moral hazard. In addition, the completeness of the benefit package is a design feature that has a major influence on FRP. Schemes in which the benefit package excludes commoner expensive care or both will, as in the case of copayments, frequently entail significant payments for the care that is covered, and therefore limited financial risk protection.

In many instances, the data on illness incidence, incomes, and prices required for direct assessment of the protection offered by an insurance scheme will not be available, as scheme implementers rarely collect population-based data. As an alternative, from the information commonly collected about community health insurance schemes, a set of "second-best" markers may be combined and used to provide an approximate evaluation of a scheme's financial risk protection. These markers are composed of, first, process indicators of a scheme's accessibility and the likelihood of payment associated with receipt of care, and second, outcome indicators of increased accessibility to care. They include the following: affordability of premiums charged by a scheme; appropriateness of payment schedules to their target population, particularly rural dwellers and informal workers; absence of copayments or affordable copayments; completeness of the benefit package; and increases in the population's utilization of health care services as a result of a scheme.

In the absence of risk protection, the cost of care becomes a barrier to seeking and obtaining health care. Thus health insurance not only provides protection for the income consequences of ill-health, but also removes financial barriers to obtaining health care at the time of illness, enabling prompt access to treatment. Several African studies have demonstrated that many typical households cannot utilize formal health services effectively for lack of cash to make the immediate cash payments involved (Arhin-Tenkorang 2000). Sick individuals have to postpone visits to the health facilities until their conditions become critical. Yet delayed emergency treatments can lead to serious health and financial consequences resulting in further impoverishment of the household. The financial barriers to care from the formal health system often lead would-be patients to resort to self-medication and other practices that sometimes injure their health.

The risk protection provided by insurance also improves health equity in a community. Equity is enhanced as the healthy, at lower risk of illness, subsidize the health care costs of less healthy, higher risk individuals. Although this may be regarded as income redistribution, the more critical interpretation is that health insurance promotes equity because, irrespective of economic status, individuals who have equal *health care needs* (that is, capacity to benefit from care) are assisted in obtaining comparable care. All participating members of an insurance scheme benefit from the removal of uncertainty about their claims to health at the time of ill health. In addition to the private benefits, health insurance, by promoting the optimal consumption of health care by individuals in society, maximizes the public benefit accruing from the positive externalities associated with healthier populations.

Resource Mobilization Function of Schemes

A health insurance scheme functions as a financial arrangement for mobilizing and pooling funds to cover all, or (in government-subsidized schemes) part, of the cost of health care for contributors to the pool. The existence of a pool facilitates the realization of economies of scale and reduces the tendency to *micropurchase* (spend for a few isolated cases as revenue becomes available from, for example, user fees). Thus the pool enables providers to increase efficiency and cost-effectiveness. A scheme's financial performance is a function of contributions, the cost of health care consumed by the insured, the level of external subsidy, the size of the pool, and the extent of economies of scale achieved.

For a scheme to produce net financial benefit to society in a given period, the pool of funds should represent resource mobilization in excess of that which would otherwise be achieved for health care expenditure by the population. This is true if, in the absence of insurance, some of the funds in the pool would not have been used for health activities (for example, the contributions of members who do not become sick during the period). From the perspective of the public sector, insurance-mediated resource mobilization can also be a consequence of shifts from private sector health expenditure of the participating population. Measuring the resource mobilization effect of a scheme necessitates an estimation of percentage increases in resources for health expenditure among the target group, and this will be heavily influenced by people's willingness and ability to pay or contribute.

In the absence of direct measures of resource mobilization, an approximation can be obtained by ascertaining if the ratio of health care expenditure to scheme revenue from contributions is positive and greater than unity in the presence of evidence of increased overall utilization rates (that is, for both insured and uninsured). Alternatively, positive and greater than unity ratios of "average expenditure on an individual" to "the average individual contribution" will also imply net positive resource mobilization. Where the average individual contribution approaches the average expenditure per individual member of the scheme, it suggests that the scheme is functioning as a medical savings scheme. A medical savings scheme enables its members to prepay for their health care and significantly limits the net resource mobilization benefit to the society. From the above conceptualization, net positive resource mobilization will be associated with the following outcome indicators of financial performance, which may be used as second-best markers: positive and greater than unity ratios of "health care expenditures" to "revenue from contributions," and significantly greater than unity ratio of "average expenditure on an individual" to "average individual contribution."

The financial performance of schemes can be considered adequate if they raise enough revenue from contributions to cover the target or stipulated percentage of the costs of delivering care, plus all administrative costs. Yet schemes may have poor financial performance because of an excess of high-risk members in the scheme *(adverse selection)* or as a consequence of targeting to fund from contributions a percentage of costs incompatible with the willingness and ability of members to pay. Although in theory, irrespective of a net benefit in resource mobilization terms, a scheme may be unable to fund the target percentage of the health care claimed by its insured because members make inappropriately high demands for care as a response to being insured *(moral hazard)*, as already argued, moral hazard is not a major problem among poor populations.

Design and Institutionalization

A consultative and inclusive process of scheme design will facilitate positive and optimal interactions between the scheme and entities that constitute its stakeholders. Effective consultation requires the specific identities of all the major stakeholders to be established at the outset of the design process. Because a statement of the scheme's mission defines its business in terms of client groups, client needs, and implied organizational competence, early adoption of a mission statement will assist early identification. As stakeholders, these entities have a claim, or interest, in the scheme, and in what it does and how well it performs. Among the local entities, some (health workers, health facility managers, and advisory committee members) will be internal stakeholders. Others will make up the external stakeholder group—insured members, suppliers, local supporting government and donor institutions, and the general public. As stakeholders are, or will be, the providers of present and future resources to the scheme as represented in figure 4.1, they form relationships with the scheme in which resources are exchanged in the expectation that interests will be satisfied by inducements (Hill and Jones 1998). Like any other organization, a health insurance scheme must therefore have as part of its objectives the provision of satisfactory returns on stakeholder investments and the satisfaction of their interests to maintain

FIGURE 4.1   Relationships between Stakeholders and the Scheme

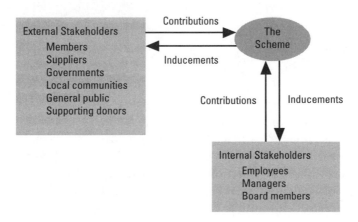

Source: Hill and Jones (1998).

TABLE 4.1   Scheme Design Options

Dimension	Choices	Strengths	Weaknesses
Utility functions	Access maximization Revenue maximization Cost recovery	Encourages affordable premiums and hence high participation Encourages community-rated premiums and enhances cross-subsidization between scheme members	Discourages affordable premiums (based on WTP)
Operation level	Single-facility based (a hospital scheme) Provider-network based (scheme consisting of participating clinics and referral hospitals)	Encourages wider geographic spread of participants and greater range of benefits, and permits effective referral system	Discourages participation by distant populations, and limits range of benefits
Range of providers	Restricted to public and not-for-profit private Includes or limited to for-profit private	Absence of profit motivation and use of existing structures may lower premiums	Profit margins may lead to high premiums
Range of benefits	Full basic package (outpatient plus inpatient care) Partial packages		Encourages high enrollment, prompt attendance to health problems Discourages early treatment until illness is severe or complications arise that are covered by scheme, leading to high costs

Note: WTP = willingness to pay

the exchange of resources. As a consequence, a critical component of a scheme's governance will be mechanisms to ensure that the actions of scheme officials are consistent with the interests of the different stakeholder groups.

By undertaking a situation analysis in which information is collected about proposed or existing target populations and about care providers, the potential contributions of stakeholders to the functions of a scheme can be factored appropriately into the design. Participation of stakeholders in the design will help ensure that the interpretation of the information obtained is based on an understanding of societal norms and expectations, as these will have a bearing on the skills and resources that stakeholders may wish to make available to the scheme. The approaches for collecting the relevant detailed information include focus group discussions, household surveys, and health facility costing studies. A situation analysis of a proposed or an existing scheme will reveal for consideration design options in several dimensions. Table 4.1 sets out the main options available

TABLE 4.2   An Example of Goals Matched to Design Options

Goal	Matching design option
Financial access—affordable contributions	Public and not-for-profit private
	No or partial cost recovery
Physical access to providers	Provider-network based
Efficiency	Full package benefits

when designing a health insurance scheme for the informal sector in Sub-Saharan Africa. Ultimately, a match between the selected goals and options is the intent.

For most schemes in Sub-Saharan Africa, an analysis of the situation reveals, in addition to information about stakeholders and design options, the following contextual factors: inadequate budget allocation to the health sector coupled with financial barriers to use resulting from out-of-pocket fees; and inadequacies of physical input and human resources resulting in poor quality of health care. An additional feature of this context is a crisis of management and administrative skills within the health sector. This is manifested by micropurchasing and an inadequate referral system, which in turn lead to internal inefficiencies. These contextual factors are the main determinants of the goals that have been selected for schemes. These and other situational findings relating to the target population's economic profiles and their health-related needs have, in most cases, led scheme designers and operators to adapt implicitly or explicitly one or more of the following goals: (a) provision or improvement of financial access with high participation and risk protection, (b) provision or improvement of physical access to health care providers, (c) improvement of supply of services, and (d) improvement of quality of care.

Scheme designers' challenge is, in consultation with stakeholders, to identify the design options that will achieve the group's goals. Table 4.2 gives an example of a set of design options that could be used to meet goals in physical and financial access and efficiency.

Tasks to be Accomplished by Designs

As stated above, in pursuit of its goals, a health insurance scheme for the informal sector—like other organizations—must accomplish the primary task (sometimes referred to as "buffering" by Hatch) of resource (material, services, and money) transfer between it and the entities that make up its stakeholders (Hatch 1997). In particular, a scheme relevant to this discussion must first effect the efficient transfer of contribution funds from its members in the informal sector to an organization that operates largely in the formal sector. The majority of members will be limited to transactions in cash, and therefore potentially efficient payment mechanisms are not options (for example, checks, installments by standing bank orders, payments in response to regular bills, and credit card payments). The scheme must then realize transfer of health care resources, in some cases cash from or via the scheme, to health care providers or members of the scheme who have limited mobility or transportation possibilities.

Another major task of all organizations is the transfer of information across the boundaries that separate it from its environment *(boundary spanning)*. In a health insurance scheme, information transfer is required between scheme officials and elements in the environment such as insured members, health care providers, and the government. This activity is crucial in establishing an understanding of the obligations and benefits between members and the scheme. Additionally, by capturing shifts in the scheme members' demand preferences and willingness to pay, transfer of information helps to minimize differences in perceptions of these obligations and benefits over time.

A set of economic and financial specifications will be required to facilitate the primary task, and specific administrative and management structures—including business and legal processes—will be the basis for realizing the information-related task. For a given benefit structure, the following economic variables must be specified: amount of contribution (may be cash or in-kind), unit of contribution (may be per individual, household, or village), and schedule of contribution (may be per month, half-year, or year).

For financial viability and the meeting of financial obligations, expenditures must be less than the revenue from contributions. These factors have a bearing on resource mobilization, as explained above, while financial protection of the target population will be increased by a unit contribution that does not exceed the target group's WTP.

A trade-off is required in setting these specifications when the contribution that leads to desired financial viability is greater than the contribution that optimizes risk protection. Alternatively, both financial performance and high-risk protection can be maintained by lowering financial obligations through subsidies to the scheme.

Administrative and management structures to realize the task of information transfer provide the data to monitor financial performance and risk protection. Their monitoring depends on continuous predictions of expenditure, based on detailed data on the target population and provider activities. With regard to the target population, the specific data include the level of utilization, pattern of illness, and care-seeking behavior. Data required about the care provider include cost per unit of care for different services and the financing or income source. Similarly, monitoring will rely on continuous assessment, prediction of revenue, or both, as determined and influenced by WTP, health insurance perceptions and preferences, quality-of-care perceptions and preferences, and the target population's socioeconomic characteristics. Hence this secondary function translates into consumer-oriented research and marketing and also leads to internal analysis of the scheme by its officials. The goal of an internal analysis is to understand the scheme in depth: its strengths, weaknesses, resources, and constraints. Information from such an analysis can be used to develop responsive strategies that either exploit strengths or compensate for weaknesses. This process must be ongoing to facilitate the institutionalization process.

Institutionalization of the scheme's operational modalities involves a lengthy process of innovation, political lobbying, and geographic expansion. The process permits civil societies to gradually tailor the modalities of operation to local socioeconomic conditions and align their operations with prevailing cultural norms relating to collectivism. This is less likely to happen if a scheme starts as a detailed project proposal, created by a development professional. Development initiatives that have detailed plans at the outset often have limited opportunities for communities to participate fully. *Participation,* as used here, refers to a "process of empowerment of the deprived and the isolated" (Ghai 1988). It implies an increase in the ability of social groups to exercise economic and political power and to make decisions, both private and public. Community involvement in the scheme for the informal sector should therefore extend beyond the mobilization of local material and labor resources. The willingness of the formal health sector to engage in dialogue and collaborate with potential patients as a collective, rather than as individuals, is a crucial determinant of the success of the institutionalization process. The organizational culture of the health providers in the scheme will determine the ease with which effective dialogue and collaboration evolves between scheme members (through their official representatives), health managers, and health care workers. In addition, functional collective solidarity schemes in most African societies usually involve the provision of benefits produced in the informal sector and in the control of ordinary people rather than professional groups. Examples of this are associations that provide member households with funeral assistance or periodic payments from member contributions.

EVIDENCE

This section presents information from the literature and personal experience about the performance of schemes, particularly the provision of financial protection to their target populations and mobilization of resources for health care. Because data on this topic are limited, the focus is on indirect measures of performance with reference to specific schemes. The literature about existing "potentially large population" schemes illustrates a diversity of benefits, organizational structures, administrative arrangements, and paths of evolution (see table 4.3).

Carte d'Assurance Maladie, Burundi

This is a national health card insurance scheme introduced by the government of Burundi in 1984. The scheme has the characteristics of the provider insurance model in which the government is the organization responsible for both managing

TABLE 4.3   Features of "Potentially Large Population" Schemes for Informal Sector Households

	Policy and legal context	Organizational structure	Contributions estimation: method and data
Carte d'Assurance Maladie (CAM) program, Burundi (provider insurance model, by government)	❑ Part of national strategy ❑ Revenue collected and controlled by local government	❑ Financial control by local government (communes) ❑ Care provided by public health facilities	❑ Fixed nationally by central government ❑ No information on method or data
Community Health Fund (CHF), Tanzania (mutual-provider partnership model)	❑ Governed by district council bylaws ❑ Political support from central government	❑ Management and decisions by district CHF board and CHF ward committees	❑ Inconclusive information on method ❑ No evidence of use of data
Abota Village Insurance Scheme, Guinea-Bissau (mutual benefit society model)	❑ Village committees control with oversight by donors, government, or both	❑ Village management ❑ Suppliers from central MOH	❑ Trial and error by community to limit periods of drug stock-outs
Nkoranza Community Financing Health Insurance Scheme, Ghana (provider insurance model, by hospital)	❑ Religious health sector rules by hospital staff and external donor oversight and regulations	❑ 3-tier: Advisory board Management team Voluntary registrars	❑ Subjective judgment of affordability by hospital staff
Bwamanda Hospital Insurance Scheme, Dem. Republic of Congo (provider insurance model, by hospital)		❑ Enrollment and accounting by health staff ❑ Scheme assisted by NGO	❑ Selection of premium and copayment options by community
Dangme West Health Insurance Scheme (Dangme Hewami Nami Kpee), Ghana (mutual-provider partnership model)	❑ Government by decentralized district and regional MOH ❑ Planned registration of association as an NGO	❑ Community association and the District Insurance Management Team	❑ Based on simulation applying data on WTP and costs and illness rates from survey

the insurance scheme and providing health care. Purchase of a Carte d'Assurance Maladie (CAM) card by a household entitles its members (restricted to two adults and all children under 18 years of age) to free health care at all public health facilities. The card is sold at a fixed price, irrespective of household size (in June 1992, the price of the card was 500 FBu [Burundi franc] [US$1.85]). Persons without cards must pay user charges for government health care. The user charge per episode of illness treated is determined by the health worker at his or her discretion and generally varies with the age of the patient and the quantity and type of treatment received. All health services provided by the government are covered by the CAM scheme, and therefore, in theory, CAM cardholders who seek health care at government facilities should not incur out-of-pocket

Premium level and membership unit	Payment schedule	Benefits package
❏ Purchase of CAM card, 500FB (US$1.85) per household in 1992 ❏ Household defined as 2 adults and all dependent children	❏ Annually	❏ All care at government clinic and hospitals
❏ Flat rate per household irrespective of size ❏ Rate carries by ward	❏ Annually	❏ All care provided by facility where registered ❏ No upper limits on value
❏ Cash or in-kind per household or individual	❏ Determined by village, usually annually or biannually	❏ Outpatient care by village health worker ❏ Free referral care
❏ c450 (US$1) in 1991 per individual enrolled by family	❏ Annual registration October–December	❏ Inpatient care ❏ Refund of referral expenses
❏ Cash = price of 2 kg soy beans + copayment per individual	❏ Annually (normally in March)	❏ All hospitalization and chronic care in health centers
❏ Membership by households ❏ Contribution per individual	❏ Planned to be annually	❏ Outpatient care at any district facility ❏ Inpatient care when referred to regional hospitals

expenses. However, due to the shortage of drugs and other inputs, CAM holders, like fee-paying patients, are sometimes given prescriptions to purchase drugs on the open market.

The names of household members entitled to use a card are written on the card at the time of purchase, making it difficult for individuals from other households to use it. The card is valid for one year and may be purchased from a community representative at any time of year. This makes it possible for a non-CAM patient to pay a user charge at a health center and, on referral to a hospital, to purchase a CAM card to obtain free hospital care. The cards are not accepted by nongovernmental health facilities, such as mission and for-profit clinics and hospitals.

The revenues from CAM card sales and user charges are retained by commune committees.[3] These committees have some financial responsibilities for the health centers in their localities and are expected to fund recurrent expenditures such as stationery, fuel for refrigerators, linen, and in some cases, capital projects such as construction of new health centers. However, revenues from CAM and user charges are not designated to be used in the provision of health care, and therefore, in practice, only a small fraction is allocated by communes to health. In 1990, 8 percent of the revenues of communes in Muyinga Province came from the sale of CAM cards, whereas an average of only 1 percent of commune revenues were used to finance health care (McPake and others 1992). The government, through the Ministry of Health budget, funds the salaries of health workers and drug costs.

CAM: Risk Protection

Affordability of premiums and copayments. A study in Muyinga Province, undertaken in 1993, reported that women had limited access to cash, and therefore, by eliminating cash payment at the point of care, CAM empowered them to decide the need for—and timing of—health care consumption by household members. (Women in CAM households do not require money, and hence permission, from male household heads to seek health care [Arhin 1994].) Cash had become less of a barrier to obtaining curative treatment for cardholders, and it appeared that women, being the main carriers, derived additional utility from the knowledge that, if a child were to fall ill, treatment would be available even in the absence of cash in the household. Large households were more likely to purchase a CAM card than small households, and therefore illness episodes per household were significantly greater for CAM households than for non-CAM households. This situation may be described as "adverse household selection," and possible results would be lowered risk sharing among households.

The same study also found that approximately 27 percent of households gave "financial inability" to purchase a CAM card as one of the main reasons for nonmembership. However, in practice, non-CAM patients referred from health centers to higher level facilities often purchased cards prior to, or on arrival at, the referral center, thus manipulating the scheme to reduce their financial barrier to expensive curative care without prior participation as members. The conclusion of the study was that a CAM card provided significant financial protection to the communities studied.

CAM: Resource Mobilization

Relationships between premiums and benefits. A public treatment rate of 0.91 per household per month and a mean value of drugs of 134.1 FBu per formal treatment at the time of evaluation by the author implied that an average household consumed 1,464.4 FBu of outpatient drugs annually. The price of the CAM card could therefore cover 34.1 percent of the drug costs, suggesting that the ratio of "average expenditure on an individual" to "average individual contribution" may have been less than unity. (In practice, revenue from CAM did not appear to be used to purchase drugs or medical supplies required for patient care at the health center.) In general, the target population for the scheme assessed the quality of care provided to members to be inadequate. As a consequence, women who participated in the focus groups were willing to pay a higher CAM contribution to improve the benefits provided. In particular, they were willing to pay a higher price for the CAM card on the condition that more drugs would become available at government facilities.

Adverse selection and moral hazard are major causes of inefficiencies in the functioning of health insurance schemes and therefore have consequences for financial viability (Arrow 1963; Pauly 1963; Lohr and others 1986; Manning 1987). The rate of illness per person was found to be almost identical for members of CAM as for non-CAM households, and therefore adverse selection of individuals did not seem to be a problem. In the absence of adverse selection, it can be inferred that capitalizing on WTP for improved benefits would result in a significant increase in resource mobilization. Even so, this chapter omits an evaluation of the level of resource mobilization actually achieved because other indicators of financial performance could not be obtained.

Community Health Fund, Tanzania

In Tanzania, the Community Health Fund (CHF) strategy for financing rural health services was piloted in Igunga District in 1996, and by 1999 it had been initiated in nine other districts. Currently, schemes comprising the CHF are governed by district council bylaws and are also guided by a coordinator located in the headquarters of the Ministry of Health. Partly as a consequence of receiving funding and external technical assistance through a government–World Bank funded project, the CHF represents a national initiative and thus has the central government's political support.

Three financing mechanisms are employed in the CHF: national user fees (introduced by the central government in 1993), insurance contributions, and matching subsidies from the government (funded by a World Bank project). A team of expert consultants designed the CHF and its schemes in 1995. Subsequently, some aspects of the design were modified following consultations with communities in the first pilot district. In particular, the level of pooling was changed from districts to subdistricts (wards), although a central management role was retained at the district level by the district CHF board. Decisions about the use of funds are made at ward level and are reflected in ward health plans and budgets for their public health facilities and outreach services. Employees of government health facilities have management roles in the CHF. They may be members of the ward health committee, may be selected by the community to collect contributions, or may be part of a consultative group representing community groups and health facility management that meet to review progress. The model of the CHF is therefore a mutual-provider partnership model.

All households in a participating district are eligible to enroll in the scheme and are required to pay a flat rate contribution per household irrespective of household size. The level of contribution is determined by the community (at the ward level), and the decisionmaking process is in the hands of the CHF ward committee. Contributing households are registered with a public health facility in the ward where the household resides, and household members are entitled to all the health services provided by the facility.

CHF: Risk Protection

Affordability of premiums and copayments. One study found that "over 50 percent of members were considered to be poor," suggesting high affordability (World Bank 1999). In addition, the CHF schemes include exemption mechanisms for households that are determined by the ward committee, and certified by the district board, as too poor to pay a flat insurance contribution or the user fees. In contrast, some health workers in Igunga District reported that the majority of participants of the insurance component of the CHF are salaried workers, and the procedure for obtaining exemption status is sometimes inaccessible by those whose incomes and socioeconomic status are very low. The care provided as a benefit is not subject to an upper ceiling of value and copayments are not required.

Resulting level of access to health care among the population. About 5 percent of the target population is enrolled, and insured individuals constitute 75 percent of patients who receive care in the provider facilities (Musau 1999). By inference, the increased funding of government health facilities provided by the scheme's revenue (contributions and matching funds) will increase the supply of, and hence the access to, care for the target population.

CHF: Resource Mobilization

By 1999, the total funds of the scheme for the participating district were US$371,000, consisting of 95 million shillings (35 percent) insurance contributions, 81 million shillings (30 percent) user fees, and 95 million shillings (35 percent) matching government funds. The existence of matching funds makes it almost certain that the scheme resulted in increased resources for health care for the target population and hence a high level of resource mobilization.

Abota Village Insurance Scheme, Guinea-Bissau

The Abota system entails prepayment for essential drugs and the provision of primary health care at the village level by trained villagers. The system comprises many hundreds of autonomous Abota schemes at the village level. Health care is provided voluntarily by members of the village, village health workers known as *Agentes de Saude de Base*, and by birth attendants at the village health post (*Unidad de Saude de Base* [USB]). The USBs were constructed from local building materials by the villagers and furnished with basic equipment (such as a metal storage cupboard, an obstetric stethoscope, a lantern, and a kit of teaching aids) by the Ministry of Health. Administration of the Abota system in each village is the responsibility of the village committee, the lowest level of the country's decentralized political system. This is an example of a mutual benefit society model, in which the officials are community members participating in the scheme.

The earliest Abota schemes began in 1980 in a few villages as part of a general village health care program (Chabot and Savage 1984). Villages in the program adopted and modified an indigenous payment mechanism, originally used to collectively finance ceremonies to fund inputs for primary health care. Chabot and others describe the process of trial and error used by these villages over a three- to four-year period, to determine the frequency and level of prepayments that would ensure the availability of drugs throughout the year.

Since 1983, patients referred by village health workers to the public health facilities have been exempt from payment of consultation fees upon showing evidence, usually a receipt, of having contributed to Abota. Growth of the scheme was continuous (in 1991, 462 villages participated). By the time of the author's study, the Abota system was widespread, forming an integral part of the country's health system. Furthermore, the Guinea-Bissau government's 10-year health plan (1984–93) emphasized the role of village-based primary health care, thus making the efficient functioning of the Abota system critical to the country's health strategy (World Bank 1987). The Abota revenue is used to purchase essential drugs and bandages from nearby government health centers or sectoral hospitals. The ultimate supplier is the central medical store in the capital. In each village, the village committee decides the procedures for collecting contributions, purchasing drugs, and monitoring the system overall. As a consequence of this autonomy, prepayment terms vary substantially from one village to another. In 1988, the annual contributions per adult male varied from PG 20 to PG 500 (at 1988 exchange rates, US$1 = 1,129 Guinea-Bissau pesos). In 2 of 18 villages surveyed by Eklund and Stavem (1990), only men paid; and in another 2 villages contributions were by household. Other villages accepted in-kind contributions of agricultural produce.

Since the mid-1990s, the country's economic difficulties have threatened the survival of the Abota. Problems such as inadequate recurrent budget allocations, drug shortages, and low health worker salaries plague the public health system (Tanner 1990). Ramifications include a decreasing capacity of government health workers to train and supervise village health workers and difficulties in resupplying village health posts, even when their Abota revenues are sufficient to fund their requisitions. In a few cases, Abota funds have been misappropriated (Knippeneberg and others 1991) either by village health workers or Ministry of Health staff.

The published and unpublished literature drawn upon to provide the description of the Abota also permits a limited evaluation of the scheme. Again, the criteria of affordability, payment schedules, revenue and expenditure, and associated access to health care were used. The results are described below.

Abota: Risk Protection

Affordability of premiums. Studies of the Abota do not provide direct information on affordability, but since the contribution was set by the members of the village, it is likely that the majority could afford the amount set. The fact that many individuals were willing to increase their contribution also supports this general conclusion.

Appropriateness of payment schedules. The number of times prepayment contributions were collected in a year varied: some villages collected twice yearly, others once. Because the villages themselves determined the frequency of payments, it is reasonable to assume the schedule was the most appropriate for the community.

Resulting level of access to health care among the population. The fact that participating villages had basic health care made available within the village implies significant increases in access. Near-universal membership in participating villages excluded adverse selection, and the watchfulness of health workers and local communities appeared to prevent moral hazard (Eklund and Stavem 1990).

Abota: Resource Mobilization

Relationship between premiums and benefits. In the first year of operation, the villages' drug supply was depleted within three months because the revenue from contributions was exhausted. The scheme appears not to have held reserve capital to ensure the quality of the insurance policy.

Nkoranza Community Financing Health Insurance Scheme, Ghana

Started in 1992, the scheme, an example of a provider insurance model in which management and health care are provided by hospital personnel, is administrated by a three-tier structure:

- Insurance management team (IMT) in the hospital, consisting of the medical officer in charge of public health and the hospital management team. This is the scheme's decisionmaking body.

- Insurance advisory board made up of traditional, political, religious, and administrative leaders in the community and district health leaders (Ministry of Health and nongovernmental organizations).

- Zonal coordinators and field workers—each of the 11 health zones is managed by a team of three zonal coordinators. They supervise voluntary fieldworkers who register families into the scheme.

The premiums are calculated per person and thus vary with the size of the family. The scheme ensures access to care at St. Theresa's Hospital in Nkoranza District (Ghana) by providing free admission in the medical, surgical, and maternity wards. However, admissions for normal deliveries are excluded. In addition, insured persons who are referred to other health institutions may claim refunds

FIGURE 4.2   Percentage of Community Enrolled, by Distance

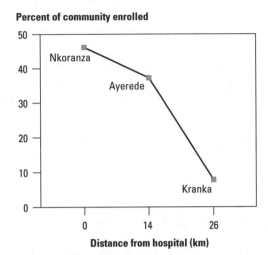

Percent of community enrolled

Distance from hospital (km)

equal to the cost of an average admission at St. Theresa's. The scheme is available only to families living in the Nkoranza District, and every family member must register. Members have to travel various distances to the hospital, and a relationship has been observed between the distance of a community from the hospital and the enrollment of members in that community (see figure 4.2). Registration is renewable annually, during the last two months of the year only.

Nkoranza: Risk Protection

Appropriateness of payment schedules. In the first year of operation, 72 percent of fieldworkers and 65 percent of household heads stated that "people find it difficult to register because they are short of money between October and December" (Dept. of Insurance 1993). Sixty-five percent of fieldworkers and 75 percent of household heads were of the opinion that "more people will register if registration is between January and March." Later evaluations of the scheme, including one undertaken in mid-1999, have continued to report a mismatch between the registration period and the time of highest cash availability among district households (Atim and Sock 2000).

Resulting level of access to health care among the population. The findings suggested that the scheme had removed a barrier to admission for people in the district. Utilization, in terms of admissions per 100 person-years, was greater than the uninsured by a factor of 2.4. Among the insured population, an estimated 9 percent of admissions was due to factors such as earlier reporting of patients and more liberal admission policy of staff; without the insurance policy this would not have occurred.

Nkoranza: Resource Mobilization

Revenue from premiums and expenditure for benefits. During the first year of operation, admission cost data for the insured population indicated that income obtained from premiums was 55 percent of the expenditure for insured inpatients. At that time, the premium was set at c450 per person (approximately US$1 at 1992 exchange rates). Premium increases of between 40 percent and 70 percent relative to the preceding year occurred annually. In 1998, the premium had risen to c5,000 per person (approximately US$1.90 at 1998 exchange rates). Since the mid-1990s, the ratio of revenue to expenditure has been approximately one, implying significant resource mobilization. In addition, the ratio of the average cost per benefit (inpatient costs) to premium was 17.5 in 1998, also suggesting that resource mobilization among those enrolled was substantial.

Bwamanda Insurance Scheme, Democratic Republic of Congo

Bwamanda Health Zone is linked to a development project, Center for Integrated Development (CDI), started in 1969 and supported by Belgian volunteer workers. Impetus for the insurance scheme came from the zone's medical staff, concerned about the barrier to access caused by user fees and the low recovery of hospital costs from fees. Although the zonal hospital (a 156-bed reference hospital) had recovered 48 percent of its operating costs in 1985, this was a lower rate than that of eight comparable hospitals in the country (Bitrab and others 1987). The parameters of the insurance plan, set by hospital staff, were explained to the community, and preferences between two options of premium and copayment levels were obtained. Enrollment of members was carried out by health center staff, mainly nurses, who received 3 percent of the premiums they collected as commission. Zone administrative staff made frequent supervisory visits to health centers during the enrollment period to monitor payment records, distribute membership stamps, and transfer premiums to the hospital. They also managed the plan at the hospital by verifying the membership status of admitted patients and keeping administrative and accounting records. Members of the Bwamanda insurance plan are covered for hospitalizations, including deliveries, dental extractions, and outpatient surgery. The cost of illness treatment at health centers is also covered. A 20 percent copayment is charged, but some groups are exempt.

Information in a World Bank report was used to assess the social and financial functioning of the Bwamanda health insurance plan in Democratic Republic of Congo (Shaw and Ainsworth 1995). The assessment results pertaining to the affordability criteria, payment schedules, revenue and expenditure, and associated access to health care are presented below.

Bwamanda: Risk Protection

Affordability of premiums and copayments. Absolute unaffordability did not appear to be a problem. It was reported that, in setting the premiums, the health staff used the price of two kilograms of soybeans as a measure of affordability. In addition, only 16 percent of 21 nonmembers stated that they had not joined the plan because of inadequate cash. However, the combined costs of the travel and premium may have been unaffordable for some households: when in 1988 the copayment rate was lowered for those living more than 25 kilometers from the hospital, the enrollment declined less with distance than in other years. In 1987–95, the percentage of the target population enrolled ranged from 41 percent to 66 percent (Criel and Kegels 1997).

Appropriateness of payment schedules. Communities elected to pay premiums during the months that followed the second harvest period (March to April). The explanation provided by the authors was that after the first harvest, cash was needed for school expenses and therefore appropriateness of time of collecting was ensured by consulting the community.

Bwamanda: Resource Mobilization

Revenue from premiums and expenditure for benefits. The financial data for the insurance plan showed that in 1987 and 1988, premiums and interest were equivalent to 145 percent of the expenditure on care for beneficiaries. As a consequence, the share of the hospital's operating costs recovered rose from 48 percent in 1985 to 79 percent in 1988.

Resulting level of access to health care among the population. It was reported in the World Bank study that insured persons were 6.7 times more likely than the uninsured to be hospitalized, implying that access to care was greater for the former group. The fact that more than 60 percent of the zone's population was insured implies a significant increase in access to care as a result of the insurance plan. Even so, households living close to the hospital were also more likely to be insured, and therefore their high access and utilization may have been due to good physical access rather than the insurance plan. The combined effects of adverse selection and moral hazard were also felt to account for the high utilization. Even so, the prevalence of adverse selection and moral hazard was likely reduced by the inclusion of copayments and the requirement that all household members join the plan. However, other researchers working in Democratic Republic of Congo reported the rate of hospitalization among the insured to be only slightly higher than that of the uninsured (Moens 1990).

Dangme West Health Insurance Scheme (Dangme Hewami Nami Kpee), Ghana

Empirical research initiated by the Ministry of Health[4] and undertaken from 1993 to 1995 in a rural district in southern Ghana concluded that household preferences and WTP were compatible with high membership in, and satisfactory performance of, a proposed health insurance scheme. The research findings led a health ministry team to work with households in Dangme West District to design and implement the Dangme West Health Insurance Scheme (Dangme

Hewami Nami Kpee). The scheme is a collaboration between a mutual society and government health providers at the district level, and therefore it is a mutual-provider partnership model. The scheme was part of research carried out to improve the quality of health care provided by Ministry of Health facilities and increase access of households, and to evaluate the outcome of the intervention and draw policy-relevant lessons. Quality-related objectives were to be addressed in three ways. The first was by providing in-service training of health workers to improve technical competence in patient diagnosis and treatment, drug supply and management procedures, and interpersonal skills. The second was supportive supervision to ensure the use of skills acquired during training. The third was the refurbishment of health ministry facilities to ensure that basic physical and laboratory investigations could be carried out. The health insurance scheme was the main strategy to increase access by eliminating user fees for participating households.

As a result of consultations with the district assembly (the local government for the district) and a series of durburs (community meetings) attended by approximately 4,250 adults (7 percent of the district's adult population), a mutual-provider partnership model for the scheme emerged. The model consists of: (a) a solidarity association named Dangme West Hewami Nami Kpee (literally translated, "a good health group"; registered members of the scheme become association members); (b) the Dangme West District Ministry of Health responsible for providing health care in the district through the public health facilities; and (c) the district insurance management teams (DIMTs), ultimately consisting of staff of the district health ministry and elected members of the association. The DIMT is responsible for financial and administrative matters, including allocating insurance funds to health centers and hospitals using an approved formula and monitoring performance to ensure that paid-up members of the association have access to good quality health care at hospitals and clinics without paying fees. Prior to the election of members of the association to the DIMT, implementation and management is the responsibility of an interim team consisting of the district assembly members and the district health administration members.

The first registration period for the scheme was October 2000 to January 2001. Enrollment was by household and the contribution for a household was calculated using a flat rate per adult (12,000 cedis [approximately US$1.80]) and per child (6,000 cedis). As adjustments were not made for increased earnings and cost of living, in real terms the contribution rate was lower than households' WTP in 1998. Members are entitled to outpatient care at any of the district health centers and clinics and to inpatient care at secondary hospitals in the regions and nearby hospitals. Although the implementation team (with the assistance of a local information technology [IT] group) developed software to integrate registration and identification of members with an information management system, plans to install appropriate inputs were abandoned due to resource constraints. Two local donors declined to support a proposal endorsed by Ministry of Health headquarters for US$28,560 to fund the required physical inputs and training for four years of operations (Arhin-Tenkorang 1999). The goal of the proposal was to provide effective management and IT solutions with respect to compatibility with existing processes, hardware affordability, and technical skill requirements. The inputs included hardware and specialized ID software. Consequently, registration with manual production of registration booklets was carried out using a Polaroid camera. Immediately following the first registration period, it became evident that a manual system of registration, identification of members at health facility centers, and collection of claim information would be inefficient and not cost-effective.

Dangme West: Risk Protection

Affordability of premiums. The data obtained from the target population in 1998, 18 months before the first premium collection, indicated that 35 percent of households would be willing and able to pay the contribution rate. The first collection of premiums was undertaken between October and January—a time when cash is tight in farming households. The resulting enrollment rate of 5 percent of the target population is evidence that financial protection was subnormal, due in part to the low affordability of premiums.

Appropriateness of payment schedules. The period for collecting the first premiums, determined by scheme officials, appeared to be incompatible with cash availability at that time. However, the officials' decision to have contributions paid annually was in line with the preferences found in a household survey conducted prior to implementing the scheme.

Dangme West: Resource Mobilization

Revenue from premiums and expenditure for benefits. As of July 2001, six months after the first premium payments by enrolled households, officials of the scheme had yet to compile and analyze the financial data. However, in view of the modest enrollment rate, it is reasonable to assume that resource mobilization will be appreciable but suboptimal.

Performance Overview of Selected "Potentially Large Population" Schemes

Table 4.4 provides information relating to the second-best indicators of financial risk protection (as proposed in the conceptual section) for the selected schemes. The final column contains the author's assessment of financial risk protection (FRP) provided by the scheme, as inferred from the information. The assessments are based on these indicators because data were unavailable on illness incidences, incomes, and the prices of health care and other goods faced by targeted populations conceptualized as necessary for direct assessment of FRP. One scheme (the Community Health Fund) was assessed as providing modest financial risk protection. The risk-protection performance of two schemes (the Abota Village Insurance Scheme and

TABLE 4.4 "Potentially Large Population" Schemes' Financial Risk-Protection Performance

	Indicators of Financial Risk Protection (FRP)				Assessment of Financial Risk Protection (FRP)
	Affordability and % of target population enrolled	Appropriateness of payment schedules	Completeness of package	Level of access	
Carte d'Assurance Maladie (CAM) program, Burundi (provider insurance model, by government)	• Affordable to about 77% • 54% ever enrolled (in 1 province studied in 1992)	Generally appropriate	Full clinic and inpatient care when referred	Increased—insured/uninsured illness episodes	Significant FRP provided
Community Health Fund (CHF), Tanzania (mutual-provider partnership model)	• Affordable to majority—includes exemption mechanism • 5.3% (in 2 districts studied in 1999)		Variable—dependent on the services at facility	Increased—75% of patients receiving care are uninsured	Modest FRP provided
Abota Village Insurance Scheme, Guinea-Bissau (mutual benefit society model)	• Affordable to majority—level determined by villagers	Appropriate—determined by villagers	Full clinic and inpatient care when referred	Increased—primary health care available in villages	Significant FRP provided
Nkoranza Community Financing Health Insurance Scheme, Ghana (provider insurance model, by hospital)	• Premiums assessed as unaffordable by two-thirds of households and health workers • approx. 27%	Inappropriate—low cash availability between November and December	Inpatient care	Increased—insured/uninsured admissions = 2.4 responsible for 9% increase in admissions	Suboptimal FRP provided
Bwamanda Hospital Insurance Scheme, Dem. Republic of Congo (provider insurance model, by hospital)	• Affordable premiums but copayment unaffordable to households living far from hospital • 41%–66% (1987–1995)	Appropriate—time chosen by community	Inpatient care	Increased—insured/uninsured admissions = 6.7	Suboptimal FRP provided
Dangme West Health Insurance Scheme (Dangme Hewami Nami Kpee), Ghana (mutual-provider partnership model)	• WTP data (in 1998) implies affordable to approximately 35% of households enrolled • Approx. 5% of households (first enrollment period 2000)	Inappropriate—low cash availability at time of first enrollment	Full clinic and inpatient care when referred		Suboptimal FRP provided

the Carte d'Assurance Maladie) was assessed as being superior to that of the CHF as they provided significant protection. Common to these three schemes are benefit packages that include outpatient and inpatient care, although the range of inpatient provision in the CHF depended on the facility with which an insured member was registered. These schemes also set premium or contribution levels that appeared to be affordable to a high percentage of their target populations and can be interpreted as being compatible with the populations' WTP. Two of the three schemes also involved significant decisionmaking by the target population.

In the literature on the selected schemes, increases in the resources for health care that resulted from the insurance schemes (postulated to be the appropriate direct measure of resource mobilization in the framework presented earlier) were unavailable for the selected schemes. With the exception of information permitting estimation of the ratio of expenditure to revenue, information about the second-best indicators of resource mobilization (notably, combined changes in utilization rates of insured and uninsured and the ratio of "average expenditure on an individual" to "average individual contribution") was incomplete or absent. Therefore, assessments of resource mobilization of these schemes were not attempted.

DISCUSSION

Institutional and Technical Influences on Scheme Design

The schemes selected for review in this chapter increased the consumption of health care by insured persons relative to the uninsured. The levels of increased consumption, when combined with affordable premiums, suggest that for three of the schemes, the financial risk protection provided is modest to significant. The low participation rate of the target populations in all the schemes strongly suggests that the level of resource mobilization achieved is below the potentially attainable. Some of the evidence supports the conclusion that the low performance in resource mobilization may be traced to institutional factors that influenced the design of these schemes and their modalities of operation. Secondary data on household preference and WTP were not available, and with the exception of the Dangme Scheme, primary collection of such data was not undertaken. Contribution calculations were based largely on assumptions, and consequently, in almost all the schemes, low affordability among the target population was a major hindrance to participation.

In general, WTP data are rarely collected or used as part of the process of designing health insurance schemes in developing countries. Yet contingent valuation theory and empirical evidence suggest studies could be undertaken in developing countries to obtain valid and reliable health-related WTP data (Russell, Fox-Rushby, and Arhin 1995). Measures that may be important in increasing the validity and reliability of WTP studies of the demand for health insurance in developing countries include the following items (Arhin 1999).

First, a careful questionnaire design to limit the problems of hypothetical and strategic bias. In addition to the respondents' contingent demands, two other areas of inquiry must be included in a WTP questionnaire. These are past practices and expenditure for similar and substitute goods and respondent socioeconomic characteristics. A plausible description of the hypothetical market must precede contingent demand questions. In this regard, guidelines emerge on the appropriate structure and content of open-ended and closed questions that would create realistic scenarios.

Second, the undertaking of an initial qualitative study to ensure that the WTP questions use words and phrases that are consistent with the discourse on health, health care spending, and financial transactions used by the study subjects.

Third, the careful training of interviewers to administer the questionnaire accurately. Differences between the interviewers and the respondents in their level of exposure to, and the discourse about, insurance may compromise validity and reliability. The problem is most acute if the interviewer must translate questions from an official language in which the questionnaire is written into a local dialect.

Respondents should be given adequate time to consider the hypothetical good. Where possible, questions should be asked and repeated in an interview subsequent to that in which the hypothetical good was first described to the respondent.

Whereas the concept of achieving compatibility between WTP and contribution levels has not been a driving force in scheme design, achieving financial sustainability through cost-recovery goals appears to have been a major influence among designers and implementers when estimating contributions and designing benefits. Greater emphasis on the social functions of risk protection provided by the insurance would have dictated lower contribution rates, more comprehensive benefit packages, and measures to increase physical access to benefits. Low participation among the target population of the Nkoranza hospital scheme in Ghana suggests that hospital-based schemes may have the problem of being attractive mainly to people living close to the hospital and, as a result, achieve low enrollment. The subscription to the scheme appears not to depend on income disparity but on the differences in the direct and indirect costs of traveling to the one district hospital operating the scheme (Noterman and others 1993). As predicted by theory, achievement of financial and social goals in these reported schemes appears to mirror enrollment rates. Enrollment rates, in turn, reflect the target population's WTP for insurance plans offered by the schemes.

Setting priorities for risk-protection objectives is not incompatible with goals that relate to increased resources for the supply of services. Detailed costing of health care provided by government and not-for-profit private facilities, and subsequent comparison of costs with government funding and user fee revenue, may be undertaken to provide information on the resource gap to be filled by contributions. In planning the Dangme Scheme and in evaluating the CAM scheme, analyses of this type were undertaken. The findings suggested that mobilization of resources through contributions would exceed, or exceeded

FIGURE 4.3   Premiums, Participation, and Revenues: Predictions for Option C

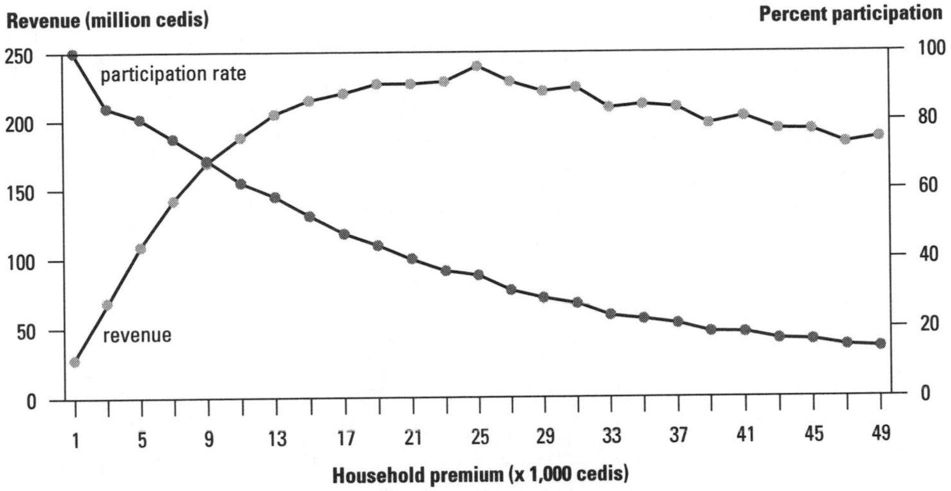

respectively, that realized by user fees, even when the majority could afford the premiums. Given recent accelerated rises in health care costs as a result of the HIV/AIDS crisis and the sharp decline in real earnings of households in low-income countries, such predictions of revenues and costs will become critical in the design of schemes.

The demand curve and revenue curve estimated by initial research that guided the Dangme Scheme illustrate the relationship between affordability of premium enrollment rates and revenues. Figure 4.3 shows the expected participation rates for a benefit package that combines inpatient and outpatient coverage (referred to as option C; options A and B are, respectively, inpatient and outpatient packages). The figure provides the predicted revenues (assuming a district population of 150,000) at different levels of household contributions based on the demand curve from WTP data. The highest revenue is predicted at a premium level of approximately c25,000 and corresponds to a low participation rate of 35 percent of the population. Above this premium level, both total revenue and the participation rate start to decline. If both revenue from the scheme and utilization of health care by individuals (hence participation) enter into the utility function of decisionmakers, setting the household contribution level above c11,000 would not be rational. The fall in participation would not be compensated by the rise in revenue, and total utility would start to fall. However, below this level, a particular utility may be obtained with different premiums and therefore different participation rates. The optimum premium will then depend on the relative values of revenue and utilization and hence the relative revenue and participation. Introducing a concern for consumers' utility and taking into account their income constraints will further lower premiums.

FIGURE 4.4   Willingness to Pay for Adult Insurance

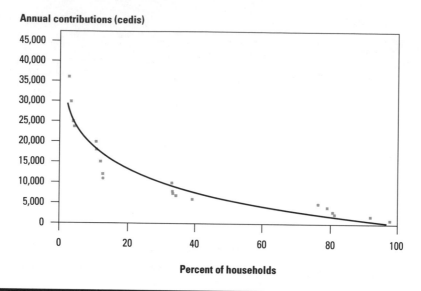

Institutional factors also have a bearing on the technical methods used to design and simulate the scheme performance. The access to, and the tradition of consulting, reports, and documents on technical issues relating to insurance are examples of factors. The disciplines from which the implementers originate will also influence the rigor with which health, epidemiological, social, and economic data will be sought and analyzed to influence design and management of the scheme. Simulation of revenue outcomes of a proposed scheme is an example of an activity that will be more readily undertaken if appropriate disciplines are used in the design and management process. Figure 4.4 illustrates an example of simulation activity that relies on planner and economic disciplines. For a proposed scheme in a district in Ghana, contingent evaluation techniques provided estimates of the maximum amounts that household heads would be willing to pay as an annual health insurance premium per adult and per child.

Taking into account consumers' tendency to understate the maximum, in the hope that their contribution will be low, estimates were based on a contribution rate of c10,000 per adult per year. Deducting administration costs of c2,500 gave an estimated net annual scheme revenue of c250,200,000 (55.9 percent of 1998 district expenditure). In 1998, government health services in the study district were funded from two sources: the government of Ghana and user fees obtained from patients, known as internally generated funds (IGF). IGF accounted for 3.21 percent of total funds utilized. The net revenue estimate from the moderate contribution rate would be equivalent to the IGF that would be obtained from 64,584.41 episodes of outpatient care (in 1998 the actual number of outpatient episodes treated was only 11,124).

Institutional Factors and Policy Environment

Institutional factors influencing health care providers' behavior, national policy formulation, and donor reactions to local initiatives appear to be important determinants of scheme performance. In several schemes, the initiator was external to the community to which the target individuals or households belonged, leading often to increased external financial support but also to increased pressure to implement the scheme quickly to conform to the project time frame. In these circumstances, primary data collection about illness experience and health care costs required to simulate the operations of the scheme were not carried out. The Dangme Scheme, however, is an example of local initiation and conceptualization complemented by substantial primary data collection and analysis. Work was undertaken by the implementation team with the support of a full-time economist and health planner and illustrates the time-consuming nature of activities required to support innovative schemes.

The familiarity of donors with the subject of health insurance is decisive in determining the outcome of schemes. Unfamiliarity may lead a local donor to underestimate the complexity of inputs required to support an emerging scheme, particularly technical advice and data management systems, as in the case of the Dangme Scheme.

As available evidence for best practice is scarce, donor funding procedures and regulation need to be flexible to support experimentation by communities, local governments, and local NGOs. These actors will require support to implement, monitor, and evaluate schemes. An external agency's inability to support both intervention (implementation) and research (monitoring and evaluation) of schemes adds significant transaction costs, as local actors must secure additional support from another donor.

Although the existence of user fees gives people a strong incentive to enroll in insurance schemes, the institutionalization of user fees within health care providers' practices presents an obstacle to the effective implementation of insurance schemes. Introduction of a scheme is likely to alter the power relationship between the provider and the individual consumer and requires changes in organizational culture and behavior. The provider may have to negotiate and contract with patients who interact with health care institutions as a collective group and as direct sponsors. How an implementing team manages such changes will determine the level of trust between actors in the scheme. Orientation periods will be required to introduce health workers to their new or additional roles arising from an insurance scheme.

Institutional factors in the policy formulation arena may hamper systematic progress in obtaining consensus about national or local priorities and objectives for health insurance. In particular, the absence of a culture of consumer dialogue and marketing is a major disadvantage for policy formulation in this area, as consumer reactions govern the success or failure of a policy. A mismatch between the expectations of policymakers and of the general public will result from institutional emphasis on resource mobilization at the expense of financial protection.

Organizations and institutions formed to provide health insurance to households in the informal sector ideally should be accountable not only to scheme members, through officials of relevant mutual groups, but also to civil society in general. Civil society in this case refers to groups that already provide social services, including health care, internationally or nationally—for example, church-related health providers. In many African countries, mission health facilities are major health care providers, especially to low-income households and rural areas. As a result of their devotion and convictions, these faith-based health providers have proven to be accountable to the people, and their reputations are untarnished by corruption.

Policy Implications

By the early 1990s, despite considerable involvement in health-financing policy formulation in Africa, many of the international agencies had failed to encourage appropriate insurance-based alternatives to fee payment at the point of use. In particular, the 1993 *World Development Report* did not make recommendations for low-income countries that would change the situation in the short to medium term. By the end of the decade, the situation had changed significantly, leading to several international meetings focusing on health insurance for low- and middle-income countries. Following published data in the late 1990s, there is now increasing recognition of the vital role of insurance mechanisms in health systems (WHO 2000). Many national and international departments and agencies now accept that the principles of health insurance are applicable to low-income populations and are willing to study examples of insurance initiatives for poor and informal households.

The priority placed on health insurance within national health policy will partly determine the stage of financial protection attained, as illustrated in figure 4.5. In the figure, the triangular area represents "total population" health-related financial protection. The area below each of the levels approximates the magnitude of the population effectively protected from the financial risks of ill health as a consequence of the level. For example, at the level of "predominance of out-of-pocket payments" for personal health services, common in low-income Sub-Saharan countries, a very small percentage of the population has protection. Conversely, true universal insurance coverage, as in Scandinavian countries, corresponds to virtually "total population" protection. Policy thrusts placed below the level are those that will facilitate attainment of the level and those placed above will support efficiency and equity within the level.

The appropriateness of launching a given policy thrust to establish health insurance schemes will be determined by the socioeconomic context. The role of national policymakers and donor agencies includes establishing the principle of disassociation between utilization or access and financial contributions. This will pave the way for strategic policies aimed at providing financial protection through insurance schemes. Policies supporting the substitution of health insur-

FIGURE 4.5   Stages of Financial Protection and Supporting Policies

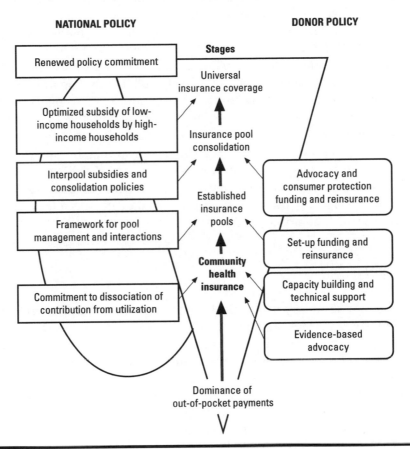

ance for out-of-pocket fees are therefore an initial requirement. Given the socio-economic diversity among low-income populations, in the short term, contributions into subnational insurance pools offer the greatest possibility of financial and administrative feasibility (Arhin 1995a).

HMO-type arrangements should be the goal, rather than third-party schemes, since the former has the potential to stabilize health care costs and thus maintain low premiums. Nevertheless, in many low-income countries, voluntary contributory schemes will not have the revenue potential to fund all the health service costs for their members. Significant central government funding (fiscal transfers and budget allocations) must therefore be reinstituted in some cases, for example in China, or maintained in others, as in Ghana. Being key stakeholders in many schemes, donors can be instrumental in establishing subnational schemes by providing start-up funding and reinsurance guarantees, where appropriate.

Subnational insurance schemes, in which solidarity organizations form partnerships with providers, and that meet cost containment and quality requirements, will represent important collaboration with civil society. Policy to support such collaboration must provide the regulatory framework (legal, financial, and informational) for scheme management and interactions with other parts of the health system. This includes enabling acquisition of appropriate human resources to counteract "capture" tendencies by health workers and profit-driven private investors and to monitor financial and social outcomes of the individual schemes. Donors have significant roles to play in capacity building to support these goals.

Where logistical inadequacies hinder active promotion of progressive contributions, as in informal sector schemes, the overriding objective should be maximization of enrollment rather than revenue, and sanctioning community-rated premiums that most of the targeted households can afford. These considerations and the inability to consolidate pools into a few large pools will necessitate reinsurance for some subnational schemes. Donors as external stakeholders have crucial roles in assisting low-income countries to meet the need for reinsurance through sectorwide approaches.

CONCLUSION

In the foreseeable future, it is unlikely that either centralized government or large commercial schemes, as found in rich countries, can provide near-universal health insurance cover for people in Africa, most of whom live in rural areas. Yet despite the endorsement of community health financing by many African countries with the support of international agencies, few large-scale community-based health insurance schemes have been attempted. Therefore there are only a small number of experiences of "potentially large population" health insurance schemes in Africa upon which to base conclusions about their performance. Nevertheless, the performance of the schemes studied suggests that insurance mechanisms in some situations, have, or may eventually have, a significant membership rate among the population and therefore are capable of increasing access to health care and, to a limited extent, mobilizing resources.

Constraints that have hindered attempts to design appropriate community insurance schemes include the policy environment, inadequate administrative infrastructures, and a shortage of trained staff to manage schemes. This underscores the need for information on the feasibility of schemes designed for rural populations. Data on WTP will be a critical part of such information since WTP will determine demand and the relationship between revenue and expenditure, hence social and financial performance. Affordability of premiums and appropriateness of payment schedules of existing rural health schemes suggest that WTP is substantial for such schemes.

Prospects for achieving resource mobilization effects that are significant relative to total health care costs are declining because of decreasing purchasing power in developing countries and the rising incidence of HIV/AIDS, TB, and other infectious diseases. Recognizing that the low income of households in the informal sector will

---

BOX 4.1   GHANA'S POLICY THRUSTS TO ENABLE EVOLUTION OF COMMUNITY HEALTH INSURANCE

". . . expediting the establishment of health insurance or prepayment mechanisms will be critical to providing financial access."

". . . the health policy goals are best served by a multischeme health insurance system."

Ghana's Programme of Work 2000–02
Ministry of Health, 1999

After two decades of intent to include insurance in its health financing strategy, during which several policy-oriented research projects and feasibility studies were commissioned, a Ministry of Health policy framework has emerged promoting a "multischeme health insurance system." The goal is a system that embraces both the formal and informal sectors, providing affordable health insurance to the majority of Ghanaians and exemptions for indigents. Insurance schemes for the rural population present the greatest challenge. The framework envisages that "community-based health insurance schemes and mutual health organizations for the informal rural sector" will be a component of the multischeme health insurance system that will meet this challenge.

The Planning, Monitoring, and Evaluation Department of the MOH is charged with facilitating and supporting districts and regions that wish to establish insurance and prepayment schemes for the populations they serve. In this new policy framework, prospects have magnified for a district initiative in Dangme West, for example, to provide policy lessons that will inform the process of developing and implementing health insurance in Ghana. In addition, the availability of technical expertise to achieve this aim has permitted the initiative to undertake baseline studies that will be used to evaluate the scheme. These include household surveys of willingness to pay (WTP) for health insurance, studies of district health accounts, and studies of drug prescribing and stock levels of district health insurance. Future health policy on insurance will have the benefit of evidence from this and other subnational schemes.

---

result in WTP insufficient to fund all the health care costs for scheme members, central government support of these schemes in the form of fiscal transfers and budget allocations will be required. Furthermore, schemes in which solidarity organizations form partnerships with providers create incentives for increased efficiency and accountability and should be supported by national government policies through appropriate legal, financial, and informational mechanisms. In the absence of established best practices in the design of schemes, donor-funding procedures and regulations need to be flexible to assist experimentation by communities, local governments, and local nongovernmental organizations. Schemes operated by NGOs (especially church-related providers or civil society in partnership with local authorities, such as district health authorities) may be effective and efficient recipients of donor funds (for example, matching funds) in the short term and may provide the basic structure for future national insurance schemes in the medium term.

Acknowledgments: The author is grateful to the World Health Organization for having provided an opportunity to contribute to the work of the Commission on Macroeconomics and Health and to the World Bank for publishing the material in this chapter as an HNP Discussion Paper.

NOTES

1. The *primary participation rate* is that of the individual reference scheme; the *secondary participation rate* refers to the total membership of a reference group of linked schemes as in the case of insurance funds of several small schemes.

2. In third-party insurance, scheme officials are neither pool members nor providers of health care benefits, as in the case of a company whose sole function is to collect contributions and pay claims to patients or directly to hospitals and clinics.

3. The commune is the country's lowest unit of local administration.

4. The principal investigator was a health economist from the Ministry of Health, seconded to an academic health economics group in the United Kingdom. The head of the ministry was one of the research advisers.

REFERENCES

Abel-Smith, B., and P. Rawal. 1994. "Employer's Willingness to Pay: The Case for Compulsory Health Insurance in Tanzania." *Health Policy and Planning* 9(4): 409–18.

Arhin, D. C. 1991. "Community Health Insurance in Developing Countries and Its Feasibility in Ghana." Research proposal submitted to UNICEF and the International Development Research Centre (IDRC).

———. 1994. "The Health Card Insurance Scheme in Burundi: A Social Asset or a Non-Viable Venture?" *Social Science and Medicine* 39(6): 861–70.

———. 1995a. "Health Insurance in Rural Africa." *The Lancet* 345: 44–45.

———. 1995b. "Health Insurance in Sub-Saharan Africa: What Are the Options?" Paper presented at the Symposium on Health Care Financing at the European Conference on Tropical Medicine, October 22–26. Hamburg, Germany.

———. 1995c. *Rural Health Insurance: A Viable Alternative to User Fees?* Public Health and Policy (PHP) Departmental Publication 19. London School of Hygiene and Tropical Medicine (LSHTM).

———. 1996a. Book review of "Community Participation in Primary Health Care," by E. Alihonou, S. Inoussa, L. Res, M. Sagbohan, and C. M. Varkevisser. *Social Science and Medicine* 42(4): 629.

———. 1996b. "Health Insurance Demand in Ghana: A Contingent Valuation." Paper presented at the International Health Economics Association (IHEA) Conference, May 19–23. Vancouver, Canada.

———. 1997. "Are People in Ghana Willing to Pay for Health Care?" Paper presented at the Fifteenth Annual Conference of the German Association of Tropical Paediatricians, January 23–25. Kiel, Germany.

———. 1999. "Using WTP Instruments for Health Insurance in Low Income Countries." Unpublished paper. Health Economics and Financing Programme at LSHTM.

Arhin, D. C., and S. Adjai. 1997. *A National Health Insurance System for Ghana: A Concept Paper and Proposal.* Health Research Unit, Ministry of Health, Accra, Ghana, and LSHTM, London.

Arhin-Tenkorang, D.C. 1999. "A Proposal to Set Up an Integrated Registration and Information Management System and Train Health Facility Staff and MOH District Administration Staff in Its Application." Submitted to the Ministry of Health (MOH), Ghana.

———. 2000. "Mobilizing Resources for Health: The Case for User Fees Re-Visited." Paper prepared for the Third Meeting of the Commission on Macroeconomics and Health (CMH), November 8–10. Paris.

Arrow, K. J. 1963. "Uncertainty and the Welfare Economics of Medical Care." *American Economic Review* 53(5): 941–73.

Asenso-Okyere, W., I. Osei-Akoto, A. Amun, and E. N. Appiah. 1997. "Willingness to Pay for Health Insurance in a Developing Economy: A Pilot Study of the Informal Sector of Ghana Using Contingent Valuation." *Health Policy* 42(3): 223–37.

Atim, C. 1998. *Contribution of Mutual Health Organizations to Financing, Delivery, and Access to Health Care: Synthesis of Research in Nine West and Central African Countries.* Technical Report 18. Partnerships for Health Reform Project, Abt Associates Inc., Bethesda, Md.

Atim, C., and M. Sock. 2000. *An External Evaluation of the Nkoranza Community Financing Health Insurance Scheme, Ghana.* Technical Report 50. Partnerships for Health Reform Project, Abt Associates Inc., Bethesda, Md.

Bennett S., A. Creese, and R. Monasch. 1998. *Health Insurance Schemes for People Outside Formal Sector Employment.* ARA Paper 16. WHO, Geneva.

Bethune, X. de, S. Alfani, and J. P. Lahaye. 1989. "The Influence of an Abrupt Price Increase on Health Services Utilization: Evidence from Zaire." *Health Policy and Planning* 4(1): 76–81.

Bitrab, R., and others. 1987. "Health Zones Financing Study Zaïre." Report prepared for the Resources for Child Health Project, USAID, Arlington, Va.

Booth, D., J. Milimo, G. Bond, and others. 1995. *Coping with Cost Recovery.* Report to the Swedish International Development Authority, Development Studies Unit, Dept. of Anthropology, Stockholm University, Stockholm.

Brown, W., and C. Churchill. 2000. *Insurance Provision in Low-Income Communities: Part II—Initial Lessons from Micro-Insurance Experiments for the Poor.* Calmeadow, Microenterprise Best Practices (MBP) Project, Development Alternatives Inc.

Burgess, R., and N. Stern. 1991. "Social Security in Developing Countries: What, Why, Who, and How?" In E. Ahmad, J. Drèze, J. Hills, and A. Sen, eds., *Social Security in Developing Countries.* Oxford: Clarendon Press.

Chabot, J., and F. Savage. 1984. *A Community Health Project in Africa.* St. Albans, U.K.: Teaching Aids at Low Cost (TALC).

Criel, B. 1998. *District-Based Health Insurance in Sub-Saharan Africa.* Antwerp: IGT Press.

Criel, B., and G. Kegels. 1997. "A Health Insurance Scheme for Hospital Care in Bwamanda District, Zaire: Lessons and Questions after 10 Years of Functioning." *Tropical Medicine and International Health* 2(7): 654–72.

Department of Insurance at St. Theresa's Hospital. 1993. "Evaluation of First Year of Health Insurance for Nkoranza District." Unpublished report. Ghana.

Eklund, P., and K. Stavem. 1990. "Prepaid Financing of Primary Health Care in Guinea-Bissau: An Assessment of 18 Village Health Posts." Working Paper Series 488. World Bank, Africa Technical Department, Washington, D.C.

Ghai, D. 1988. "Participatory Development: Some Perspectives from Grass-Root Experiences." Discussion Paper 5. United Nations Research Institute for Social Development (UNRISD), Geneva.

Hatch, M. J. 1997. *Organizational Theory: Modern Symbolic and Postmodern Perspective.* New York: Oxford University Press.

Hill, C. W. L., and G. R. Jones. 1998. *Strategic Management: An Integrated Approach.* Boston: Houghton Mifflin.

Knippeneberg, R., and others. 1991. "Joint Report on Progress Assessment of BI in Guinea Bissau." Unpublished draft. UNICEF and WHO.

Lohr, K. N., R. H. Brook, C. J. Kamberg, G. A. Goldberg, A. Leibowitz, J. W. Keesey, D. M. Reboussin, and J. P. Newhouse. 1986. "Use of Medical Care in the Rand Health Insurance Experiment: Diagnosis and Service-Specific Analysis of Randomized Controlled Trial." *Medical Care* 24 (supplement): S1-87.

Manning, W. G. 1987. "Health Insurance and the Demand for Medical Care: Evidence from a Randomized Experiment." *American Economic Review* 77: 251–77.

Mathiyazhagan, K. 1998. "Willingness to Pay for Rural Health Insurance through Community Participation in India." *International Journal of Health Planning and Management* 13(1): 47–67.

McPake, B., and others. 1992. *Experiences to Date of Implementing the Bamako Initiative in Africa.* London: Health Policy Unit of the LSHTM.

Moens, F. 1990. "Design, Implementation, and Evaluation of a Community Financing Scheme for Hospital Care in Developing Countries: A Pre-Paid Health Plan in Bwamanda Health Zone, Zaïre." *Social Science and Medicine* 130(12): 1319–27.

Musau, S. N. 1999. *Community-Based Health Insurance: Experiences and Lessons Learned from East and Southern Africa.* Technical Report 34. Partnerships for Health Reform, Abt Associates Inc., Bethesda, Md.

Noterman, J., B. Criel, G. Kegels, and K. Isu. 1993. "A Prepayment Scheme for Hospital Care in the Masisi District in Zaïre: A Critical Evaluation." *Social Science and Medicine* 40(7): 919–30.

Nyonator, F., and J. Kutzin. 1999. "Health for Some? The Effects of User Fees in the Volta Region of Ghana." *Health Policy and Planning* 14(4): 329–41.

Pauly, M. V. 1963. "Taxation, Health Insurance, and the Market Failure in the Medical Economy." *Journal of Economic Literature* 24: 629–75.

Russell, S., J. Fox-Rushby, and D. C. Arhin. 1995. "Willingness and Ability to Pay for Health Care: A Selection of Methods and Issues." *Health Policy and Planning* 10(1): 94–101.

Shaw, R. P., and M. Ainsworth, eds. 1995. *Financing Health Services through User Fees and Insurance: Lessons from Sub-Saharan Africa*. World Bank Discussion Paper 294. Washington, D.C.

Tanner, K. 1990. *Impact of Structural Adjustment and Policy Choices for Promoting the Welfare of Children and Women in Guinea*. Bissau: UNICEF.

Vogel, R. J. "Health Insurance in Sub-Saharan Africa: A Survey and Analysis." 1990. Africa Technical Department of the World Bank (Working Paper Series 476), Washington, D.C.

World Bank. 1987. *Health Sector Memorandum*. May 21.

———. 1999. *Community Health Fund in Tanzania*. Washington D.C. Video.

World Health Organization. 2000. *World Health Report 2000: Health Systems—Improving Performance*. Geneva.

PART 2

Country Case Studies Using Household Survey Analysis

CHAPTER 5

Analysis of Community Financing Using Household Surveys

Melitta Jakab, Alexander S. Preker, Chitra Krishnan, Pia Schneider, François Diop, Johannes Paul Jütting, Anil Gumber, M. Kent Ranson, and Siripen Supakankunti

Abstract: *Objective:* to provide empirical evidence regarding the performance of community-based health care financing in terms of social inclusion and financial protection. *Methods:* five nonstandardized household surveys were analyzed from India (two samples), Rwanda, Senegal, and Thailand. Common methodology was applied to the five data sets. Logistic regression was used to estimate the determinants of enrolling in a community-financing scheme. A two-part model was used to assess the determinants of financial protection: part one used logistic regression to estimate the determinants of the likelihood of visiting a health care provider; part two used ordinary least-squares regression to estimate the determinants of out-of-pocket payments. *Findings:* Social inclusion— our findings suggest that community financing can be inclusive of the poorest even in the most economically deprived context. Nevertheless, this targeting outcome is not automatically attributable to the involvement of the community; rather it depends on key design and implementation characteristics of the schemes. Financial protection— community financing reduces financial barriers to health care as demonstrated by higher utilization and simultaneously lower out-of-pocket expenditure of scheme members controlling for a range of socioeconomic variables. *Conclusions:* Social inclusion—design and implementation characteristics of community-financing schemes matter in achieving good targeting outcome; community involvement alone does not guarantee social inclusion. Further research is needed to delineate which design and implementation characteristics allow better inclusion of the poor. Financial protection—prepayment and risk sharing, even on a small scale, reduce financial access barriers.

Community-based health financing (CF) has been attracting increasing attention as a potential instrument for protecting low-income populations from the impoverishing effects of health care expenditures. Proponents argue that communities have incentives as well as instruments to reach the poor and the socially excluded. In contrast, general tax- and social insurance-funded health care structures often lack instruments to achieve close targeting of the poor and ensure their financial protection at the time of illness. Market-based organizations, however, lack incentives to promote their insurance products to rural populations as high transaction costs would translate into high and unaffordable premiums for the poor (Preker and Jakab 2001; Wiesmann and Jütting 2001; Dror and Jacquier 1999; Jütting 2002).

However, many observers point out that community structures are not inherently inclusive of the poor either. Community structures may not necessarily reflect the views of the wider population, critical decisions may not take into account the interests of the poorest, and the poorest may not be involved in the decisionmaking (Gilson and others 2000). As recent thinking related to social capital suggests, communities can be as exclusive creating a gap between the "in-community" and "out-community" groups as they can be inclusive and provide a bridge for the disadvantaged (Narayan1999).

The literature on community financing provides some insights into this debate, although the evidence is far from conclusive. A recent review of 45 articles on community financing found that fewer than a dozen provided some indication of whether the reviewed schemes were inclusive of the poor and whether they were effective in protecting them from the impoverishing effects of illness (Jakab and Krishnan 2001).

These studies suggest that CF is effective in reaching a large number of low-income populations who would otherwise have no financial protection against the cost of illness (Desmet, Chowdhury, and Islam 1999; Diop, Yazbeck, and Bitran 1995; Arhin 1994; Liu and others 1996; DeRoeck and others 1996; CLAISS 1999; Hsiao 2001). At the same time, several studies demonstrate that the very poorest are excluded from the financial protection benefits of CF schemes. The main reason appears to be that the schemes are not able to reduce the financial access barrier for the lowest income groups (McPake, Hanson, and Mills 1993; Criel, van der Stuyft, and van Lerberghe 1999; Atim and Sock 2000; Arhin 1994; Supakankunti 1998).

Nonetheless, it is difficult to make far-reaching systematic conclusions about the impact of CF on preventing impoverishment based on these studies. Most of the reviewed studies did not have access to household data to assess the impact of scheme membership on beneficiaries. In the few cases in which household data were used, the studies faced methodological difficulties. The most important difficulty in a cross-sectional setting is that the variation in membership status is endogenous. This is due to the fact that enrollment in voluntary health insurance is driven by both observable and unobservable characteristics, and the latter are likely to be correlated with the observable explanatory variables. In most of the available studies, these issues are not properly addressed. In addition, the large variety of indicators reported prevents comparability. Furthermore, many studies report indirect measures of social inclusion and impoverishment due to health expenditures. Because of these limitations, there continues to be a need to provide empirical evidence explaining who is covered by CF schemes, why those are covered and not other groups, how effective CF is in terms of financial protection, and what structural characteristics make certain schemes more inclusive and more effective than others.

This study is an attempt to address some of these shortcomings. The study analyzes household data from four countries (India, Rwanda, Senegal, and Thailand) with a common methodology. The study addresses two principal questions: Are the surveyed CF schemes in these four countries inclusive of the poor? Are the surveyed CF schemes in the four countries effective in providing financial protection from the impoverishing effects of illness?

This opening section of the chapter summarizes the methodology, synthesizes the results, and discusses the reasons behind commonalities and differences in findings. It is followed by sections presenting the country reports. The second section provides background about the four countries, their health systems, and the surveyed CF schemes. The third section describes the methodology used in the analysis. The fourth section presents the results. The fifth section discusses the findings.

BACKGROUND

The chapter synthesizes findings from five household surveys conducted in four countries: India, Rwanda, Senegal, and Thailand. Despite their varied socioeconomic and cultural contexts, all four countries have sizeable poor populations—many in the informal sector—who lack access to government and social insurance-funded health care services. Community-financing schemes are present in the four countries and aim to fill the gap in financial protection for the poor against the impoverishing effects of illness. This section reviews the socioeconomic background of the four countries, their health systems, and characteristics of the community-financing schemes surveyed.

Socioeconomic Background

Three of the four countries surveyed are classified as low-income countries with a per capita gross national product (GNP) ranging from US$250 in Rwanda to US$510 in Senegal. Thailand is a lower middle-income country, with a per capita GNP of US$1,960. The four countries have varied sociodemographic characteristics (see table 5.1).

All four countries are characterized by sizeable poor populations. Rwanda, one of the world's poorest countries, counts 70 percent of its population as falling below the national poverty line. In Senegal, 26 percent of the population (2.4 million people) lives in absolute poverty on less than a dollar a day. In India, 44 percent of the population (439 million people) lives in absolute poverty. Even in Thailand, the only middle-income country in the sample, 13 percent of the population lives below the national poverty line, and about 1 million people still live in absolute poverty

Health System

There are similarities in the health system of the four countries: a large proportion of the population is not covered by prepayment schemes, and access problems are

TABLE 5.1   Socioeconomic Characteristics of Rwanda, Senegal, India, and Thailand, 1999

	Rwanda	Senegal	India	Thailand
Population (millions)	8.3	9.3	997.5	61.7
Urban population (percent of total)	6	47	28	21
Labor force (percent of total population)	48	43	44	60
Adult illiteracy rate	29 (m)	55 (m)	33 (m)	3 (m)
(percent of people 15+)	43 (f)	74 (f)	57 (f)	7 (f)
GNP per capita (US$)	250	510	450	1,960
Population living below US$1 per day (percent)	—	26.3	44.2 (1997)	< 2 (1998)
Population below national poverty line (percent)	70 (1997)	— (1995)	35 (1994)	13.1 (1992)

Source: World Bank (2000).

reported. With the exception of Thailand, the countries are classified as high child and high adult mortality rate stratum by the World Health Organization (WHO). Health spending in the three low-income countries is US$13 to US$23 per capita. Despite the much higher level of per capita spending, Thailand channels comparable amounts of resources through out-of-pocket payments (see table 5.2).

Rwanda

The Rwandan health sector has a three-tier structure, consisting of the Ministry of Health (MOH) at the central level, 11 health regions, and 38 health districts. Medical care is provided in two public referral hospitals and one private hospital, 28 district hospitals, and 283 health centers. On average district hospitals cover an area of 217,428 inhabitants, and health centers serve a population of 23,030 individuals. The Rwandan government remains the major provider of health services, with religious organizations as partners, especially in rural areas. The role of private providers is limited. There are only two health insurance companies. They insure about 1 percent of the Rwandan population, including 6 percent of the formal sector employees. Most employers contract with providers directly to ensure care for their employees. Financial barriers restrict access to medical care for the poor, who are excluded from formal sector employment. The Rwandan health sector is financed by foreign assistance (50 percent) and by private out-of-pocket spending (40 percent); the government contributes only 10 percent of total funds.

The genocide in 1994 was followed by a period of humanitarian assistance. During this time, public health care services were provided free to patients, financed by donors and the government. In 1996, the Ministry of Health reintroduced prewar-level user fees in health facilities. By 1999, utilization of primary health care services had dropped from 0.3 in 1997 to a national average of

0.25 annual consultations per capita. This sharp drop in demand for health services combined with growing concerns about rising poverty, poor health outcome indicators, and a worrisome HIV prevalence among all population groups motivated the Rwandan government to develop community-based health insurance to assure access for the poor to the modern health system.

Senegal

In Senegal, as in most other African countries, large proportions of people are not covered by formal health insurance, and access problems are reported in terms of financing and geographic outreach. Social health insurance, introduced in 1975, extended coverage to private sector employees and their families. The added coverage of social insurance and the partial coverage of civil servants and their dependants, however, still leave most of the population in the urban informal sector and rural sector underprotected against the financial risks associated with illness.

The Senegalese health care system has three different levels: health district, regional, and central level. The health district has a health care center as well as health posts. Senegal has 50 health districts run by a chief health doctor (1998). The regional level is attached to the administrative division of a region, and the central level is attached directly to the Ministry of Health. The Senegalese health sector is financed by the central government (about 50 percent), user fees (about 10 percent), local government (about 6 percent), and donors (about 30 percent).

In Senegal, the private sector plays an important part in the health care system due to both its size and its geographic distribution. Private providers are a mix of for-profits, serving urban high- and middle-income groups and charging relatively high fees, and nonprofits, mostly church-run facilities, serving rural and poor populations and charging only modest fees. Company clinics are also important. In Senegal there are about 40 private clinics (1994), about three-quarters of them located in Dakar; half of these private facilities are mainly maternity clinics. There are also about 14 diagnostic labs, 11 of them in Dakar.

In the nonprofit sector, the Catholic Church health posts (about 70, mainly in rural areas) and the Catholic hospital (St. Jean de Dieu in Thiès) play an important role. The church deliberately put most of its nonprofit services in the rural areas to reach the otherwise excluded populations and the poor. The church network developed mostly in the 1950s and 1970s. Church-based providers are especially important in reaching rural areas with preventive services.

India

Health care in India is provided through general tax-funded public providers and insurance for the formally employed, and increasingly through nongovernmental organizations (NGOs) and charitable institutions.

Public system. There are concerns about access and use of subsidized public health facilities. Most of the poor households, especially rural, reside in remote regions where neither government facilities nor private medical practitioners are available. These people must depend heavily on services provided by local, often unqualified, practitioners and faith healers. In addition, wherever accessibility is not a constraint, the primary health centers are generally either dysfunctional or provide low-quality services. The government's claim to provide free secondary and tertiary care does not stand; in reality there are charges for various services (Gumber and Kulkarni 2000).

Voluntary insurance. Only 9 percent of the Indian workforce is covered by some form of health insurance—the majority of those covered belong to the formally employed sector. Public insurance companies so far have paid very little attention to voluntary medical insurance because of low profitability and high risk as well as lack of demand. From the consumer point of view, the insurance coverage is low because information about the private health insurance plans is lacking, and the mechanisms used by the health insurance providers are not suitable to consumers.

Nongovernmental organizations. NGOs and charitable institutions (not-for-profit) have played an important role in delivering affordable health services to the poor, but their coverage has remained small. The issue is how to reach the socially excluded and, more recently, how to ensure that the uninsured get minimum affordable quality services.

Thailand

Health insurance schemes in Thailand can be classified into three types: welfare and fringe benefit, compulsory, and voluntary health insurance.

Surveyed Community-Financing Schemes

In all four countries, community financing plays a role in raising resources for health care and providing financial protection. In India, Senegal, and Thailand, community financing has had a relatively long tradition, while in Rwanda, it is a new phenomenon. The community-financing arrangements surveyed in the four countries are similar in that they are based on prepayment and risk sharing. Using the categorization developed by Jakab and Krishnan (2001), India, Rwanda, and Senegal fall under modality 2—community health funds and mutual health organizations—while Thailand belongs to modality 4—community financing with substantial government or social insurance involvement.

Rwanda

In early 1999, the Rwandan MOH in collaboration with local communities, and the technical and financial support of Partnerships for Health Reform (PHR), started the process to pilot test prepayment schemes in three health districts. At the end of the first operational year, the 54 schemes had enrolled more than 88,000 members.

Under Rwandan law, the schemes are deemed mutual health associations, headed by an executive bureau with four volunteers, elected by, and among, the scheme members during a community-based health insurance (CBHI) general assembly. On a district level, the schemes have formed a federation. Six members have been elected by, and among all, prepayment schemes' (PPS) executive bureau representatives in their general assembly to constitute the bureau of the district federation of prepayment schemes. The federation is the partner to the district hospital as well as to the health district and other authorities. Each prepayment bureau has signed a contract with the affiliated health center, and each federation with the district hospital, defining in 17 articles the rules of collaboration between the insurer and provider. According to the schemes' bylaws, members are invited, at least once a year, to attend the prepayment scheme's general assembly.

The CBHI schemes promote group membership. Households that would like to be insured pay, at the time of enrollment, an annual premium of 2,500 francs[1] per family of up to seven persons to the CBHI affiliated with their "preferred" health center.[2] An individual pays 2,000 francs upon enrollment. PPS membership entitles members—after a one-month waiting period—to a basic health care package covering all services and drugs provided in their preferred health center, including ambulance transfer to the district public or church-owned hospital, where a limited package is covered.[3] Group enrollment and the one-month waiting period are designed in the voluntary CBHI schemes of Rwanda to minimize adverse selection. In case of sickness, members contact first their preferred health center, which is usually the nearest public or church-owned facility. Members pay a 100 francs[4] copayment for each health center visit. Health centers play a gatekeeper function, and hospital services are covered for members only if they are referred by their preferred health centers. This is done to discourage members and providers from frivolous use of more expensive hospital services.

Senegal

Senegal has had a long tradition of mutual health insurance schemes. The first experience began in the village of Fandène in the Thiès region in 1990. From the beginning, the movement in Senegal has been supported by a local health care provider, the nonprofit St. Jean de Dieu Hospital. Sixteen mutual health insurance schemes operate in the area of Thiès. The schemes' main features are:

- They are community based.

- Ninety percent of the schemes operate in rural areas.

- With the exception of one mutual—Ngaye Ngaye—the schemes cover only hospitalization.

- The mutuals have a contract with St. Jean de Dieu Hospital, where they get a reduction of up to 50 percent for treatment.

- In general, the household is a member of a mutual and participates in the decisions. The insured has a membership card on which he or she can list all or selected family members (beneficiaries). The membership fee is per person insured.

India

The Self-Employed Women's Association's (SEWA's) Integrated Social Security Scheme was initiated in 1992. SEWA is a trade union of more than 2 million women, all workers in the informal sector. This integrated income-protection scheme provides life insurance, medical insurance, and asset insurance. Women who pay the annual Social Security Scheme premium of 72.5 rupees—30 rupees of which is earmarked for the Medical Insurance Fund (herein referred to as the Fund)—are covered to a maximum of 1,200 rupees yearly in case of hospitalization in any registered (private or public) facility.

Women between the ages of 18 and 58 are eligible for membership in the Fund. Women also have the option of becoming lifetime members of the Social Security Scheme by making a fixed deposit of 700 rupees. Interest on the deposit is used to pay the annual premium, and the deposit is refunded when the woman reaches 58 years of age. Upon discharge from the hospital, members must first pay for the hospitalization out-of-pocket. They submit receipts and doctors' certificates to SEWA, and if the insurance claim is approved, they are reimbursed by check. Excluded from Fund coverage are certain chronic diseases (for example, chronic tuberculosis, certain cancers, diabetes, hypertension, piles) and "disease caused by addiction" (SEWA brochures, 2000).

Throughout the 10 districts of Gujarat where it operates, the Fund had 23,000 members in 1999–2000 (this compares with coverage of roughly 150,000 women under the broader SEWA trade union, statewide).

Thailand

The Health Insurance Card Scheme was introduced in 1983. Its three main objectives are to promote community development under the primary health care program, foster the rational use of health services via a referral system, and increase health resources based on a community-financing concept.

The target population is the near-poor and middle-income classes in rural areas or people who can afford the premium. The health insurance card costs bath 1,000 (US$40) per year per household of up to five members. A household contributes half of the price, and the other half is subsidized by general tax revenue through the Ministry of Public Health. The benefits include outpatient care for illness and injuries, inpatient care, and mother and child health services. There is no limit on utilization of the services. However, the beneficiaries can go only to health care provider units under the Ministry of Public Health. The first

TABLE 5.2   Health Outcomes and Expenditures in Rwanda, Senegal, India, and Thailand, 1999

	Rwanda	Senegal	India	Thailand
Health outcomes				
U5MR	189 (m)	134 (m)	97 (m)	40 (m)
	163 (f)	126 (f)	104 (f)	27 (f)
Life expectancy	41.2 (m)	53.5 (m)	59.6 (m)	66 (m)
	42.3 (f)	56.2 (f)	61.2 (f)	70.4 (f)
Health expenditures				
Total (percent of GDP)	5	4.5	5.2	5.7
Total per capita (US$)	13	23	23	133
Out-of-pocket (as percent of total)	49.9	44.3	84.6	65.4

Note: U5MR means under-five mortality rate.

Source: WHO (2000). Health expenditure figures for Rwanda: Schneider and others (2000).

contact is at either the health center or the community hospital; patients must then follow a referral line for higher levels of care.

There is a specific time for card selling at each health card cycle. At present the cycle is one year, and the specific time for card selling depends on the seasonal fluctuations in income. The premium is collected when cash incomes are highest (for example, when crops are harvested). In 1992, the population coverage by the health card program was 3.6 million, about 5 percent of the total population.

METHODS

Data Sources

The use of standardized and nationally representative surveys (Living Standard Measurement Surveys [LSMS], Demographic and Health Surveys [DHS]) was explored, but they did not prove to be useful for the purpose of this study. Though preferred for their representative sampling and standardized measures of socioeconomic status, these large-scale surveys did not allow us to identify households with access to community-based health financing. Even where the survey included health-financing questions, coverage through community financing could not be separated from other health-financing instruments such as private insurance or social insurance. The appendix provides the complete list of survey instruments reviewed in 21 countries as well as the variables predefined as selection criteria.

Eleven smaller scale nonstandardized surveys matched the requirements for the core list of variables. The five available for further analysis were included in this report. The other six were either impossible to access for further analysis (four), data collection was incomplete (one), or authors were not available to collaborate within the short time frame of the project (one).

TABLE 5.3   Characteristics of 5 Survey Instruments

	Name of scheme	Year of data collection	Sample size # of observations (households)	Organization associated with the survey
Rwanda	54 prepayment schemes in 3 districts of Kabutare, Byumba, and Kabgayi	2000	11,583 individuals 2,518 HH	Partnerships for Health Reform (PHR) in collaboration with National Population Office
Senegal	4 Mutual Health Insurance Schemes (Thiés Region)	2000	2,987 individuals 346 HH	Center for Development Research (ZEF Bonn) in cooperation with the Institute for Health and Development
India (1)	Self-Employed Women's Association (SEWA)	1998–99	1,200 HH	National Council of Applied Economic Research (NCAER)
India (2)	Self-Employed Women's Association (SEWA)	1998–99	1,200 HH	London School of Hygiene and Tropical Medicine
Thailand	Voluntary Health Card Scheme (HCP)	1994–95	1,005 HH	National Statistics Office

The five household surveys identified and accessible for analysis for the purposes of this report represent nonstandardized, relatively small scale data collection efforts with a sample size of 346 to 1,200 households. The surveys were not nationally representative but were rather random samples of the local population. With the exception of Thailand's, the surveys are very recent. Table 5.3 summarizes the key characteristics of these surveys. The individual country sections provide more detailed information about the survey instruments.

Rwanda

The Rwanda household survey was carried out by PHR in collaboration with the Rwandan National Population Office (ONAPO). Data collection took place during 40 days in October–November 2000 in three pilot districts. The household survey includes 2,518 households (11,583 individuals) successfully interviewed in the three pilot districts. The sample was based on the same sampling frame as the Rwandan Demographic and Health Survey (DHS) 2000, covering 11 health regions in Rwanda.[5] Households for the prepayment household survey in the three districts were sampled at random from a list of primary sample households from sample cells identified in the national DHS sample, rendering the household survey sample representative to the district level.

The prepayment household survey used three structured questionnaires for data collection: a socioeconomic household questionnaire, a curative care questionnaire, and a preventive care questionnaire. The household questionnaire collected information on households' and individuals' sociodemographic and economic characteristics, including household expenditures for consumption goods, health and education, and participation in CBHI. The curative care questionnaire was addressed to household members who were sick two weeks prior to the interview, and the preventive care questionnaire was used to interview women of childbearing age who had delivered a child in the past five years or who were pregnant during the year preceding the interview (Diop and Schneider 2001).

Senegal

The Senegal household survey was carried out by the Institute for Health and Development (ISED) in Dakar in cooperation with the Center for Development Research in Bonn between March 2000 (pretest) and May 2000 (final survey). Households were randomly selected in four villages of Fandène, Sanghé, Ngaye Ngaye, and Mont Rolland in the Thiès region of Senegal where mutual health organizations are in place. A total of 346 households were surveyed, 70 percent of which are members of the mutual health organizations (MHOs). The data set consists of 2,987 persons, 60 percent of them members (some households did not insure their whole families). The participation rate in the interviews was very high, more than 95 percent.

India (1)

The first household survey for India was carried out by the National Council of Applied Economic Research (NCAER). A primary survey of 1,200 households was conducted in the Ahmedabad District of Gujarat, India, between December 1998 and December 1999. The survey included households from four types of health insurance enrollment status in rural and urban areas:

- 360 households belonging to a contributory plan known as Employees' State Insurance Scheme (ESIS)

- 120 households subscribing to a voluntary plan (Mediclaim)

- 360 households belonging to a community- and self-financing scheme run by an NGO called Self-Employed Women's Association (SEWA)

- 360 uninsured households purchasing health care services directly from the market (control group).

The survey sample came from eight localities (about 90 households each) dominated by slum populations in the city of Ahmedabad and six villages (about 60 households each) in the neighborhood.

India (2)

The second survey of India also surveyed the SEWA population. This was a cross-sectional cohort study; respondents were interviewed at only one point in time, and we fixed in advance the number of SEWA and uninsured households (the two "cohorts"). Two-stage, random cluster sampling was used. The primary sampling units (PSUs) were villages. Twenty villages were selected randomly (using random-number tables); the probability of selection was equal for all villages regardless of size. The secondary sampling units were households. Within each village, insured were randomly selected from lists compiled by SEWA and uninsured were randomly selected from census or voting lists. In 10 villages, 14 SEWA households and 14 uninsured households were sampled, and in 10 villages, 14 SEWA households and 28 uninsured households were sampled (20 villages × 14 SEWA households = 280 SEWA households; 10 villages × 14 controls + 10 villages × 28 controls = 420 controls; therefore 700 households are included in this analysis).[6]

Thailand

The Thailand survey was conducted in 1994–95 in the Khon Kaen Province of Thailand, which had experience with the voluntary health insurance scheme or the Health Card Program dating to 1983. The pilot study was implemented in six districts, where a sample of 1,005 households was selected and categorized into four groups:

- Those who did not have a health card between 1993 and 1995 (495 households)
- New health cardholders in 1995 (297 households)
- Continued card purchasers (132 households)
- Health card dropouts (81 households).

Secondary data (National Statistics Office) statistics of card usage rates and utilization rates, reimbursement from providers, and the number of insured and uninsured in the province before and after the implementation of the program by the type of insurance scheme was also used in the study.

Empirical Methods

This section describes the general methods applied to the data sets. Since each of the five data sets is different, some variations in methodology exists and are reported in the individual reports.

Determinants of Inclusion in Community Financing

To assess the determinants of social inclusion in community-financing schemes, we assume that the choice of whether to enroll is influenced by two main determinants: individual and household characteristics, and community characteristics.

Individual and household characteristics such as age, gender, income, and health status shape individuals' preferences toward health risks as well as their ability to pay membership fees and thus influence their demand for insurance.

We hypothesize that individual choice about whether to enroll in a prepayment scheme is moderated through certain social characteristics of the community. Social, ethnic, and religious values may shape peoples' preferences and attitudes toward health, risk, and solidarity. This may alter the outcome of the rational choice process for two individuals with similar individual and household characteristics. They may decide differently about joining depending on encouragement from community leaders, availability of information, ease of maneuvering unknown processes, and the like.

To estimate the weight of these determinants, a binary logit model was applied to four of the data sets, and a binary probit was applied to the Senegal data set. The model can be formally written as follows.

(5.1) $\text{Prob (membership} > 0) = X_1\beta_1 + X_2\beta_2 + \epsilon$

The independent variable takes on a value of 1 if the individual is a member of a community-financing scheme and 0 if he or she is not. X_1 represents a set of independent variables that are characteristics of the individual and the household, such as income, gender, age, marker on chronic illness, or disability. X_2 represents a set of independent variables that approximate the social values in the communities: religion, marker on various communities where appropriate. Other variables specific to the surveys as well as interaction terms were included where appropriate. β_1 and β_2 are vectors of coefficient estimates, and ϵ is the error term.

The two variables of primary interest are income and marker on different communities.

Income. Income is the key variable in measuring the extent of social inclusion achieved by community-financing schemes. This assumes that income is a good approximation of social inclusion. Admittedly, this assumption ignores the fact that poverty and social exclusion have many dimensions and causes other than income such as ethnicity, religion, and mental and physical disabilities, to mention only a few. However, we hypothesize that effective demand for insurance is strongly determined by ability to pay. This hypothesis is supported by some of the literature on community financing, which suggests that the poorest and higher income groups are not included in pooling arrangements.

Community characteristics. Community-specific dummy variables are our key variables in picking up unobservable characteristics of communities, such as social values and solidarity, to see if those variables influence individual choice to enroll in a community-financing scheme. Our hypothesis is that the impact of the communities is a significant determinant of the probability of enrolling in a scheme.

Ideally, one would control for social values, social capital, and collective attitudes toward solidarity, risk, and health with more sensitive and direct variables. However, only the Senegal data set included a variable that directly measured the perceived level of solidarity among survey respondents. For the other surveys, community and district specific dummy variables were included. Admittedly, this is a crude measure to assess variation in social values, collective attitudes toward risk, health, and solidarity. Therefore a statistically significant finding regarding the community and district dummy variables will call for further examination of which community characteristics are really measured and picked up by these variables.

In addition to income and community-specific dummies, other control variables are also included: gender, age, disability or chronic illness, religion, and distance to the health center under the scheme. Some of these variables are important to control for the different probability of health care use (for example, age, health status, distance from provider). These variables also allow us to test the presence and importance of adverse selection to which all voluntary prepayment schemes are subject.

Other variables are included to control for the different individual and household attitudes toward investment in health at a time when illness is not necessarily present (for example, gender, religion). The literature has shown that distance gradient to the hospitals and local health centers and existence of outreach programs influence the decision to purchase membership in the scheme.

Determinants of Financial Protection Provided by Community Financing

To empirically assess the impact of scheme membership on financial protection, a two-part model was used.[7] The first part of the model analyzes the determinants of using health care services. The second part of the model analyzes the determinants of health care expenditures for those who reported any health care use.

There are several reasons for taking this approach. First, using health expenditure alone as a predictor of financial protection does not allow us to capture the lack of financial protection for those who choose not to seek health care because they cannot afford it. As the first part of the model assesses the determinants of utilization, this approach allows us to see whether membership in community financing reduces barriers to accessing health care services.

Second, the distribution of health expenditures is typically not a normal distribution. There are a large number of nonspenders who do not use health care in the recall period. The distribution also has a long tail due to the small number of very high spenders. To address the first cause of non-normality, we restrict the analysis of health expenditures to those who report any health care use. As the first part of the model assesses determinants of use, we will still be able to look into whether scheme membership removes barriers to care. To address the second part of non-normality, a log-linear model specification is used.

Part one of the model is a binary logit model for the India, Rwanda, and Thailand data sets and a probit model in the Senegal model. The model estimates the probability of an individual's visiting a health care provider. Formally, part one of the model can be written as follows:

(5.2)   Prob (visit > 0) = $X\beta + \varepsilon$

Part two is a log-linear model that estimates the incurred level of out-of-pocket expenditures, conditioned on positive use of health care services. Formally, part two of the model can be written as follows:

Log (out-of-pocket expenditure $\mid$ visit > 0) $= X\gamma + \mu$

where X represents a set of individual and household characteristics that are hypothesized to affect individual patterns of utilization and expenditures.

β and γ are vectors of coefficient estimates of the respective models; ε and μ are error terms.

The two variables of primary interest are scheme membership status and income.

Scheme membership status. The key independent variable of interest is membership status in community-financing schemes. The key question is that, controlling for a number of individual and household characteristics, do members of community-financing schemes have better access and a lower financial burden of seeking health care? Our hypothesis is that well-functioning prepayment and pooling schemes remove financial barriers to health care access demonstrated by increased utilization and reduced out-of-pocket spending of scheme members relative to nonmembers. Interaction terms between insurance membership status and income are also explored.

Income. Without the financial protection afforded by insurance, demand for health care is heavily determined by ability to pay, and for those who use health care, out-of-pocket expenditures are likely to mean a heavy financial burden. Through prepayment and pooling, we expect that financial barriers to care are reduced and income becomes a less significant predictor of health care utilization and out-of-pocket expenditures.

Other control variables were also included in the estimation model to control for the differences in need for health care (for example, age, gender), differences in preferences toward seeking health care (for example, gender, religion), and differences in the cost (direct and indirect) of seeking health care (for example, distance).

Limitations of the Methodology

The applied methodology has several limitations. First, the estimated coefficients might reflect bias due to adverse selection in the model trying to assess the inclusiveness of community-financing schemes. Adverse selection occurs because participation in the schemes is voluntary, and therefore those with greater than average health risk are more likely to enroll than those with lower than average risk. While multiple regression techniques can adjust for the observable characteristics that affect adverse selection, they cannot adjust for unobservable characteristics. This leads to biased coefficient estimates and thus undermines the internal validity of the results. We try to control for the adverse selection by including variables associated with health risk such as age, gender, and perceived health status.

Second, bias may also be present in part two of the model because of potential endogenity between the choice of whether to enroll in health insurance and health care use. Individuals who self-select into the insurance program have unobservable characteristics—related to preference or health status (adverse selection)—that make them more likely than others to join the program and which also influence their decision to use health care services. An observed association between health insurance affiliation and health care use and expenditure may therefore be due not to insurance but to the underlying unobservable characteristics. In the Senegal study, the Hausman test has been performed to control for the effects of the unobservable characteristics.

Third, the variables we use to approximate social inclusion and community characteristics are indirect. Social inclusion-exclusion is measured here only in terms of income, and other determinants, such as ethnicity or religion, are not taken into account. Social values, social capital, collective attitudes toward risk, health, and solidarity are not measured through direct variables—only through indirect community or district–specific dummy variables that measure all unobserved characteristics that vary across the surveyed communities. Both of these weaknesses can be addressed in the future by finding more appropriate and more sociology-driven measures for social exclusion.

Fourth, we do not have a direct measure of financial protection. Ideally, we would like to measure the impact of community financing on impoverishment directly. Such data were not, however, available within the time frame of this study. Our measures, utilization plus out-of-pocket spending, are indirect approximations of financial protection.

RESULTS

This section presents the key findings from the individual country analyses. Not all variables and findings that are important for the specific countries are included here. This section aims to present the findings with regard to the key variables of interest described under the methods section. The individual country chapters provide more comprehensive descriptions of regression results as well as discussion of those findings.

Determinants of Social Inclusion in Community Financing

The results in terms of the determinants of social inclusion through community financing are varied. Table 5.4 presents the determinants that were found statistically significant in the five household surveys.

Income and Other Socioeconomic Determinants

We had hypothesized that household income is a significant determinant of membership in a prepayment scheme as ability to pay influences demand for prepayment. The results of the five studies neither confirmed nor disproved this hypothesis. Household income was a significant determinant of membership in a prepayment scheme in Senegal and Thailand but not significant in India and Rwanda.

TABLE 5.4   Statistically Significant Determinants of Inclusion in Community Financing

	Rwanda	Senegal	India (1)	India (2)	Thailand
Model					
	Logit	Probit	Logit	Logit	Logit
Dependent variable					
Dependent variable	Proportion of population enrolled in 54 schemes in 3 districts	Proportion of population enrolled in 1 of 4 schemes	Proportion of population enrolled in SEWA insurance	Proportion of population enrolled in SEWA insurance	Proportion of population that purchased new health card, continued, dropped out, never purchased
Independent variables: individual and household characteristics					
Income/assets	No	**Yes**	No	**For the poorest fifth**	No
Age	No	No	**Yes**	**Yes**	No
Education	**Yes**	No	No	No	**Yes**
Gender	No	No	—	—	No
Health status	No	No	**Yes**	**Yes**	**Yes**
Household size	**Yes**	—	**Yes**	No	—
Marital status	—	—	**Yes**	No	No
Religion	—	**Yes**	—	No	—
Ethnic group	—	**Yes**	—	—	—
Membership in other organization	—	**Yes**	—	—	—
Distance of household from scheme provider	**Yes**	—	—	—	—
Independent variables: community characteristics					
Community marker for unobservable characteristics	**Yes**	**Yes**	—	—	—
Solidarity	N/A	No	N/A	N/A	N/A

Note: Yes: variable is significant at least at the 10 percent level. No: variable is not significant. (—) : not included in the particular model.

In the Senegal data set, the income variable was significant. Income was included in the model in three forms: as a continuous variable (significant at the 1 percent level) divided into terziles (significant at the 10 percent level for the lower terzile and at the 5 percent level for the upper terzile), and as a self-reported measure of being poor or nonpoor (poor significant at 1 percent). In all cases, income had a positive impact on the probability of being a scheme member. This indicates that ability to pay does make a difference in the decision to join: lower income households and the self-reported poor were less likely to join a scheme than higher income households.

In Rwanda, the income variable, divided into quartiles, was not a significant determinant of scheme membership. Of the two included asset variables, cattle and radio ownership, only radio ownership was significant and had a positive impact on the probability of membership. As further explored in the discussion section, the strong impact of radio ownership is more likely to measure the success of the information campaign than the impact of assets on the decision. These results are robust in alternative models: in particular, the results do not change as variables colinear with income were excluded.

Both household surveys in India had similar findings. SEWA membership was not strongly influenced by income or by household assets. In the first survey, household income was included as quintiles. Only being in the highest income quintile had any impact on membership status. Being in the top quintile increased the probability of membership in SEWA by 1.87 percentage points as compared with the lowest quintile. There is some indication, however, that the income variable is measured with error, and thus it does not pick up the true welfare characteristics of households. For example, large household size (six or more members) is a significant predictor of the probability of being a member. Households with more than six members are 2 to 7 percentage points less likely to join than households with fewer than four members. Similarly, activity status is also a significant predictor of the probability of membership. Members of any trade are 2 to 4 percentage points more likely to be members of SEWA than non-workers. The insignificance of the income variable remains when activity status is excluded from the model for colinearity reasons. To the extent that household size and employment status is a proxy for income and welfare, there is reasonable doubt as to whether the income variable is measured with error.

In the second survey, an asset index was developed to measure household wealth. The asset index was not found to significantly influence the probability of being a SEWA member.

Other Individual and Household Characteristics

Health status was included in the analysis of all five surveys. The hypothesis explored was that adverse selection was present: people with worse health status are more likely to join the prepayment scheme as their expected value from insurance is higher than those with better health status. The hypothesis was disproved in Senegal and Rwanda. In the other three studies, the hypothesis was confirmed.

In the Rwanda survey, households with a pregnancy over the past year were marked as well as households with children below the age of 5. Neither variable was significant.

In Senegal, two variables were introduced to capture health status: illness ratio, measuring reported illness in the previous six months, and hospitalization ratio, measuring the frequency of hospitalization in the previous two years. Both variables were found to have no influence on participation in a mutual scheme.

In the India (1) survey, three variables aimed to control for health status: whether the respondent had a chronic ailment, whether the respondent had been hospitalized over the recall period, and whether the respondent had given birth during the previous two years. The significance of the variables varied in the alternative three models. Childbirth was significant in two of the models, and reported hospitalization was significant in one. When significant, both childbirth and reported hospitalization increased the likelihood of SEWA membership threefold.

In the India (2) survey, the number of acute illness episodes reported over the previous 30 days was included to control for general level of health. The variable was significant at the 5 percent level. Those who reported illness over the previous 30 days were 68 percent more likely to be part of SEWA than those who did not.

In Thailand, there were several control variables for health status: presence of illness in the household in the previous three months, the number of sick members with chronic illness in the family, and economic problems during sickness of family members. The presence of illness was a significant determinant of purchasing a health card while the other two health status variables were not (co-linearity). Those reporting illness in the previous three months are 57 percentage points more likely to have ever purchased a health card compared with those who reported no illness over the previous three months.

Community Characteristics

To control for community characteristics and test the hypothesis of whether community characteristics modified individual decisionmaking, two models included a dummy variable to control for all the unobservable differences at the community level that may influence individual decisionmaking. In both cases, the dummy variables were significant predictors of the probability of enrolling in the prepayment scheme.

In Rwanda, three communities were surveyed, and the community dummies were found to be highly significant at the 1 percent level. Households from Kabgayi were 3.5 times as likely to purchase a prepayment plan and households from Byumba were 15.8 times as likely to purchase a prepayment plan as households from Kabutare.

In Senegal, different model variations show that the inhabitants of the villages of Sanghé and Mont Rolland have significantly lower probability of membership than people from Ngaye Ngaye and Fandène. These results indicate that the different types of health insurance provided—primary health care in Ngaye Ngaye and inpatient care in the other three mutuals—had no significant influence on the decision to participate. Instead, specific village factors such as the management of the mutual seem to play a role. The mutual of Sanghé has faced several financing and managerial difficulties that have led to a suspension of operations for some time. As a consequence, several people left the mutual. Efforts to reestablish the mutual have been successful; the mutual is functioning again today, but with a lower participation rate.

Determinants of Financial Protection in Community Financing

The results in terms of the determinants of financial protection through community financing are varied. Table 5.5 presents the determinants that were found statistically significant in four of the household surveys. The household survey conducted in Thailand does not permit analysis of the determinants of out-of-pocket payments and was therefore excluded from the analysis.

Insurance Effect

In three of the four household surveys, scheme membership was a significant determinant of the probability of using health care and the level of out-of-pocket payments. This confirms our original hypothesis that even small-scale prepayment and risk pooling reduce financial barriers to health care.

In Rwanda, scheme members are six times more likely to enter the modern health care system when sick than nonmembers. Scheme members who report any visit to a professional provider have lower out-of-pocket payments per illness episode than nonmembers.

In Senegal, scheme members are 2 percentage points more likely to use hospital care than nonmembers (marginal effect). Their out-of-pocket payment for hospital care decreased by 50 percent in comparison with nonmembers, with all other factors constant.

In India, the picture is mixed. Model one reports significant impact of SEWA membership on the probability of using health care but finds no impact on the total annual cost of health care utilization. In contrast, model two finds that SEWA membership has no impact on the likelihood of being admitted for hospital care but finds that membership reduces the total annual out-of-pocket payments for hospitalization.

Socioeconomic Determinants

Our second key hypothesis was that insurance coverage makes income a less significant determinant of health care utilization and out-of-pocket payments. This hypothesis is neither confirmed nor disproved by our findings, which are quite varied.

In Rwanda, income continues to be a determinant of the likelihood of using health care as well of the average out-of-pocket payment for the poorest quintile, with all other variables constant.

In Senegal, income is a determinant of using hospital care only for the richest third of the sample. Income is a significant determinant of the level of out-of-pocket spending on hospital care.

In India, model 1 reports that income is not a significant determinant of use and is a significant determinant of out-of-pocket payments only for the richest quintile. Model 2 confirms the finding that income is not a significant determinant of use and thereby confirms our original hypothesis. It also finds that income is a significant determinant of out-of-pocket expenditures for the richest quintile.

TABLE 5.5 Summary Findings: Statistically Significant (at least at 10 percent) Determinants of Utilization and Out-of-Pocket Expenditure Patterns

	Rwanda		Senegal		India (1)		India (2)	
	Utilization	OOPs	Utilization	OOPs	Utilization	OOPs	Utilization	OOPs
Model	Logit	Log-linear conditional on (use > 0)	Logit	Log-linear conditional on (use > 0)	Logit	Log-linear conditional on (use > 0)	Logit	Log-linear conditional on (use > 0)
Dependent variable								
Dependent variable	Proportion of sample w/ at least one visit to professional health care provider	Total illness-related out-of-pocket payment per episode of illness for the full episode	Proportion of sample w/ at least one hospitalization	Out-of-pocket spending on hospitalization	Proportion of sample reporting any health care use	Total annual direct and indirect cost of health care use	Proportion of sample w/ at least one hospitalization	Total annual out-of-pocket payment for use of hospital care
Independent variable: insurance effect								
Scheme membership	**Yes**	**Yes**	**Yes**	**Yes**	**Yes**	No	No	**Yes**
Independent variables: individual and household characteristics								
Income/assets	**Yes**	**For poorest quartile**	**For richest terzile**	**Yes**	No	**Yes**	**For richest quintile**	**Yes**
Age	**Yes**	No	**Yes**	**For < 26 group**	No	—	**For oldest group**	No
Education	No	No	No	No	No	—	No	**Yes**
Gender	No	**Yes**	**Yes**	No	No	**Yes**	—	—
Health status/severity of illness	**Yes**	No	No	No	**For very severe**	**Yes**	—	—
Household size	No	No	—	—	No	**Small household size**	No	**Yes**
Marital status	—	—	—	—	No	—	No	No
Religion	—	—	No	No	—	—	No	**Yes**
Distance of household from scheme provider	**Yes**	No	—	—	—	—	—	—

Note: Other control variables were included in some of the studies but as they are not discussed in this chapter, we did not include them in this table. OOPs: out-of-pocket payments.

Other Determinants

Where included, distance from the scheme provider was a significant determinant of the likelihood of using health care.

In Rwanda, people who live close to the health facility are significantly more likely to seek care (61 percent) than those who live farther away. Patients in the lowest income quartile are far less likely to seek care than those in the highest income quartile. This means that while the prepayment scheme has significantly increased access to health care for members, including those who are poor, the impact at the district level in increased access to health care for the poor remains an issue. The solution is to find mechanisms to increase enrollment of poor households in the prepayment schemes.

DISCUSSION

Determinants of Social Inclusion in Community Financing

Socioeconomic Determinants

We had hypothesized that household income is a significant determinant of membership in a prepayment scheme. Ability to pay would influence the demand for prepayment. Review of the literature suggested that this was the case for many schemes and that, for the very poorest, financial barriers to care remained even with the introduction of community financing.

The findings of this research suggest that financial barriers can be overcome by community-financing schemes even in a very poor context (India, Rwanda). In the case of two schemes, income was found not to be a significant determinant of membership status, suggesting that the poor were just as likely to be included in the schemes as the better-off community members.

This finding is no doubt due to the fact that, because all clients of community-financing schemes are poor, there is no large variation in the income variable. But this is true in all four countries and does not explain why the schemes in India and Rwanda have achieved inclusion of the poor while those in Senegal and Thailand have not.

In our interpretation, assuming that this finding is not due to methodological error, it indicates that certain design and implementation features allow poor communities to overcome the inability of their poorest residents to pay. In other words, how schemes are designed and implemented makes a difference in terms of their success in targeting the very poor. Further analysis is required to compare the structural, managerial, organizational, and institutional characteristics of the surveyed schemes to determine precisely which features contribute to better targeting outcomes.

Three design and implementation features of the Rwanda scheme stand out as potential explanatory factors that have allowed for the inclusion of the poorest:

participatory process, subsidies and facilitation of contribution payments, and information campaigns.

First, participatory design and democratic management of the scheme led to a sense of ownership and trust toward the health scheme. This has shaped the preferences and attitudes of households toward investment in their health care. Participation was achieved through community-level meetings and allowing community members to vote. This finding is consistent with the social capital literature that suggests that voice leads to empowerment, which in turn contributes to better sustainability.

Second, the poorest's ability to pay was given special consideration. Those who could not afford to pay a one-time enrollment fee were allowed to pay in installments. Furthermore, the community and the churches collected money to contribute for the enrollment fee of the indigent, the disabled, orphans, and other disadvantaged people. This finding is consistent with the literature that suggests that poorly designed contribution schemes often stand in the way of expanding enrollment. Flexibility in scheme design makes a difference, for example, allowing cash contributions or timing collection time to coincide with cash-endowed periods.

Third, information campaigns were conducted through 30 workshops in the three pilot districts. The information campaign in the districts of Byumba and Kabgayi was more intensive than in the control region. This may explain why the coefficient of the two variables marking these districts was a strong determinant of the likelihood of participation. Households in these two regions were 3.5 and 15.8 percentage points more likely to be members of the prepayment scheme than the inhabitants of the control Kabutare region.

An interesting question is whether the Rwanda scheme can maintain this high level of inclusion as the scheme ages and matures. A significant difference between the Senegal and Rwanda schemes is that the surveyed schemes in Senegal have been in existence for 10 years. In contrast, the Rwanda scheme is recent. As the years go by, will the Rwanda scheme become subject to the often-reported issues of adverse selection?

In the case of SEWA in India, successful targeting of the poor can potentially be attributed to the linkages that the prepayment scheme has to other social protection mechanisms SEWA has in place. The fact that SEWA's Social Security Scheme is nested within a larger development organization has undoubtedly been an important factor in ensuring inclusion of the poor. Other factors that have facilitated inclusion of the poor include: affordable premiums, village-level representatives who are themselves poor, self-employed women, and efforts to serve geographically isolated villages.

An interesting question requiring further exploration is: To what extent is better social inclusion due to explicit subsidies for the poor (through churches, government, or donors) versus participatory social structures? In other words: To what extent can income deprivation be overcome through giving voice to the poor? Participatory structures have their weaknesses as well. Because the rich always have the financial incentive to opt out of income-pooling arrangements if they can, achieving a high level of participation may be costly, especially for the poor.

In sum, further assessment is required to identify the factors that contribute to better social inclusion and which of them can be influenced at the household, community, and government levels.

Community Determinants

We found significant results for community variables. Individuals living in different villages or districts have a different likelihood of joining a prepayment scheme, holding all other facts constant. Our original intention was to attribute some of the variation in of the community dummies to the variation in social values and collective attitudes toward risk, health, and solidarity. Upon further reflection, however, many other factors differ across these communities that other variables do not control for.

Thus the community variables may measure some other aspects of the design and implementation of community financing. For example, the strength of the advertising campaign as in the case of Rwanda. In the Rwanda case, there was a considerable difference in terms of the advertisement campaign and the involvement of the local leaders in the three districts. It is likely that this is what is picked up by the variables.

In the case of Senegal, people in Fandène and Ngaye-Ngaye tend to enroll proportionately more than people living in the villages of Mont Rolland and Sanghé. For Fandène this is not surprising: its mutual is the oldest, it functions quite well, and it is closest to the hospital. For Ngaye-Ngaye, the interpretation is more difficult, as people have stated that they were not satisfied with the mutual's functioning. The scheme in Ngaye-Ngaye covers primary care and not hospitalization. Hence this result could also be interpreted as showing that there is also a demand for ensuring high-frequency, low-cost risks.

This suggests that community variables as they are crudely constructed pick up variations in the design and implementation of community-financing schemes that directly influence the value people get from being enrolled. This suggests that while community appears to be a significant determinant of enrollment, better measures are needed to assess which community characteristics encourage social inclusion and which characteristics tend to be more exclusive. Variables that better capture values, attitudes toward health, social cohesion, and solidarity would enable delineation of the community characteristics that create a fostering environment for community financing and those that do not.

From a policy perspective, this would contribute to our understanding about which characteristics can be influenced and which ones cannot and therefore need to be taken into consideration as a constraint when designing community-financing schemes. For example, attitudes toward health can be shifted through health education campaigns and information while social cohesion, or the lack thereof, is hard to foster if it is not present at the onset.

Determinants of Financial Protection in Community Financing

The results confirm our initial hypothesis that community financing through prepayment and risk sharing reduces financial barriers to health care, as demonstrated by higher utilization but lower out-of-pocket expenditure of scheme members.

At the same time, income still influences use and expenditure, although its influence is more pronounced for higher income groups than for lower income groups. This suggests that community financing has been particularly successful in reducing the financial barrier to access for the lower income groups in the surveyed population.

These findings confirm that risk pooling and prepayment, no matter how small scale, improve financial protection for the populations they serve. The policy implication of this finding is that it is critical to move away from resource-mobilization instruments that are based on point-of-service payments. If prepayment and risk sharing can be encouraged, it is likely to have an immediate poverty impact—directly, by preventing impoverishment due to catastrophic health expenditures, or indirectly, by ensuring access to health care, thereby improving health and allowing the individual to take advantage of economic and social opportunities.

In this, the critical question becomes: What form of community financing is better able to provide financial protection for its members? Those that include hospital care? Those that include primary care? Those that are based on some common professional characteristics? Those that have strong government support? Provider-based ones? Assessing what scheme characteristics will encourage financial protection is the next important research step.

CONCLUDING REMARKS

This study aimed to present initial findings from five household surveys regarding the social inclusion and financial protection impact of community-financing schemes. While the findings are preliminary, a number of common performance patterns have emerged.

First, successful inclusion of the poorest is not an automatic outcome of community structures. Community involvement can be exclusionary as well as inclusionary. This suggests that certain community characteristics as well as scheme design and implementation features are important determinants to achieve pro-poor targeting outcomes. These determinants and the direct causality are not well explored with regard to health financing, and further investigation is warranted.

In particular, the role of external financial support (such as government subsidies, donor funding, reinsurance) in encouraging social inclusion needs further exploration. So, too, does the role of participation, by providing the poor with a voice.

Second, community financing reduces financial barriers to health care, as demonstrated by higher utilization but lower out-of-pocket expenditure of scheme members relative to nonmembers. This suggests that prepayment and risk sharing—even on a small scale—lower financial barriers to health care.

APPENDIX 5A. LIST OF REVIEWED SURVEY INSTRUMENTS

An extensive search of available research instruments was undertaken during January–March 2001. The objective of the search was to identify household surveys that would allow us to test the impact of community-based health financing on social inclusion and household level financial protection.

Twenty-one countries were identified as likely candidates (those where we had prior knowledge of some kind of community-financing initiatives). In these countries, four survey instruments were reviewed:

Living Standards Measurement Surveys (LSMS)

Demographic and Health Surveys (DHS)

Household budget surveys

Other nonstandard surveys

The following set of variables was defined as minimum criteria for the survey to be useful for our project.

Key independent variable. Identifier for the type of prepayment scheme that covers the household. Of these, we looked for those in which we could separate households covered by community-based health financing from those either not covered or covered by formal (general tax, social insurance) mechanisms.

Control (independent) variables. Socioeconomic status, religion, age, gender, income level, and chronic illness or disability.

Outcome (dependent) variables of interest. Health outcomes, financial protection (that is, some sense of out-of-pocket spending *and* household income level), and consumer satisfaction.

Having initially reviewed four LSMS, nine DHS surveys, and six household budget surveys, we concluded that they did not allow us to identify households with access to community-based health financing. Even when the survey included health-financing questions, coverage through community financing could not be separated from other health-financing instruments such as private insurance or social insurance. As a result, not all available LSMS and DHS survey questionnaires were reviewed for the selected countries, and instead we focused on identifying small-scale nonstandardized surveys.

TABLE 5.6 Reviewed Surveys for 21 Countries

Country	LSMS		DHS		HH Budget Survey		Other Surveys			Status of Data
	Search	Useful	Search	Useful	Search	Useful	Search	Useful	Holder of data	
Asia										
India							✔	Yes	NCAER, India / Anil Gumber	✔
Bangladesh							✔	Yes	M. Desmet, Belgian Administration for Development	Could not contact
Philippines							✔	No		
China							✔	Yes	Harvard HSPH	Data collection is still in progress
Cambodia							✔	No		
Thailand							✔	Yes	Center for Health Economics / Chulalonkron University, Thailand / S. Supakankunti	✔
Nepal	✔	No	✔	No						
Africa										
Senegal			✔	No	✔	No	✔	Yes	Center for Development Research, Bonn / Johannes Jütting	✔
Niger	✔	No	✔		✔	No	✔	Yes	PHR	Data set not accessible for further analysis
Rwanda							✔	Yes	PHR	✔
Ghana	✔	No	✔	No			✔	Yes	PHR	Data set not accessible for further analysis
Tanzania	✔	No	✔	No	✔	No				
Mali					✔	No	✔	No	PHR	
Uganda			✔				✔	No		
Zambia			✔	No	✔	No	✔			
Nigeria			✔	No	✔	No	✔			
Benin			✔	No	✔	No	✔	Yes	UNICEF CREDESA	Data set not accessible for further analysis
Guinea							✔	Yes	UNICEF CREDESA	Data set not accessible for further analysis
Latin America										
Bolivia	✔		✔	No						
Ecuador	✔	No					✔	Yes	PHR	Data set not accessible for further analysis
Guatemala			✔	No						

Note: UNICEF CREDESA = Regional Centre for Health and Development.

Acknowledgments: The authors are grateful to the World Health Organization (WHO) for having provided an opportunity to contribute to the work of the Commission on Macroeconomics and Health and to the World Bank for having published the material in this chapter as an HNP Discussion Paper. Valuable guidance on methodological issues was provided by Adam Wagstaff.

NOTES

1. July 1999: RWF 2,500 = US$7.50.

2. Premium rates were set by taking into account existing user fees and by assuming that utilization rates would increase by 25 percent over baseline levels. See TR 45: chapter 3.1.1.

3. The Kabgayi PPS covers full stays at the hospital for caesarian sections (C-sections), malaria, and nonsurgical pediatrics, whereas the Kabutare PPS and Byumba PPS cover C-sections, physician consultation, and an overnight stay at the district hospitals.

4. July 1999: RWF 100 = US$0.3.

5. The DHS was conducted by the ONAPO in collaboration with Macro International and USAID in 2000–01. Households for the DHS were selected as primary sample units from sample cells identified for the Living Conditions Monitoring Survey (LCMS), conducted by the Ministry of Finance in collaboration with UNDP in 2000–01.

6. Note this study was actually designed to look at two community-based insurance schemes, SEWA and the Tribhuvandas Foundation, and a total of 1,120 households were actually interviewed. However, TF households and their controls are not included in this analysis.

7. This model is similar to the two-part demand model developed as part of the Rand Health Insurance experiment to estimate demand for health care services (see Duan and others 1982; Manning and others 1987). For a recent application of the model that analyzes the access impact of school health insurance in Egypt, see Yip and Berman (2001).

REFERENCES

Arhin, D. 1994. "The Health Card Insurance Scheme in Burundi: A Social Asset or a Non-Viable Venture?" *Social Science and Medicine* 39(6): 861–70.

Atim, C. 1998. *Contribution of Mutual Health Organizations to Financing, Delivery, and Access to Health Care: Synthesis of Research in Nine West and Central African Countries.* Technical Report 18. Partnerships for Health Reform Project, Abt Associates Inc., Bethesda, Md.

Atim, C., and M. Sock. 2000. *An External Evaluation of the Nkoranza Community Financing Health Insurance Scheme, Ghana.* Technical Report 50. Partnerships for Health Reform Project, Abt Associates Inc., Bethesda, Md.

Carrin, G., R. Aviva, H. Yang, H. Wang, T. Zhang, L. Zhang, S. Zhang, Y. Ye, J. Chen, Q. Jiang, Z. Zhang, J. Yu, and L. Xi. 1999. "The Reform of the Rural Cooperative Medical System in the People's Republic of China: Interim Experience in 14 Pilot Counties." *Social Science and Medicine* 48: 961–72.

CLAISS (Latin American Center for Health Research). 1999. "Synthesis of Micro-Insurance and Other Forms of Extending Social Protection in Health in Latin America and the Caribbean." Under the supervision and guidance of the ILO and PAHO counterparts, for the ILO-PAHO initiative of extending social protection in health in Latin America. Presented to the Mexico City tripartite meeting of the International Labour Organization (ILO) with the collaboration of the Pan American Health Organzation (PAHO), Mexico City.

Criel, B., P. Van der Stuyft, and W. Van Lerberghe. 1999. "The Bwamanda Hospital Insurance Scheme: Effective for Whom? A Study of Its Impact on Hospitalization Utilization Patterns." *Social Science and Medicine* 48: 897–911

Desmet, A., A. Q. Chowdhury, and K. Islam. 1999. "The Potential for Social Mobilization in Bangladesh: The Organization and Functioning of Two Health Insurance Schemes." *Social Science and Medicine* 48: 925–38.

DeRoeck, D., J. Knowles, T. Wittenberg, L. Raney, and P. Cordova. 1996. *Rural Health Services at Seguridad Social Campesino Facilities: Analyses of Facility and Household Surveys.* Technical Report 13. Health Financing and Sustainability Project, Abt Associates Inc., Bethesda, Md.

Diop, F., and P. Schneider. 2001. *Household Survey in 5 Rwandan Districts.* Technical Report. Partnerships for Health Reform Project, Abt Associates Inc., Bethesda, Md.

Diop, F., A. Yazbeck, and R. Bitran. 1995. "The Impact of Alternative Cost Recovery Schemes on Access and Equity in Niger." *Health Policy and Planning* 10(3): 223–40

Dror, D., and C. Jacquier. 1999. "Micro-Insurance: Extending Health Insurance to the Excluded." *International Social Security Review* 52(1): 71–97.

Duan, N., W. G. Manning Jr., C. M. Morris, and J. P. Newhouse. 1982. *A Comparison of Alternative Models for the Demand for Medical Care.* Report R-2754-HHS. The Rand Corporation, Santa Monica, Calif.

Gilson, L., D. Kalyalya, F. Kuchler, S. Lake, H. Oranga, and M. Ouendo. 2000. "The Equity Impacts of Community Financing Activities in Three African Countries." *International Journal of Health Planning and Management* 15: 291–317.

Gumber, A., and V. Kulkarni. 2000. "Health Insurance for the Informal Sector: Case Study of Gujarat." *Economic and Political Weekly*, September 30, 3607–13.

Hsiao, W. C. 2001. "Unmet Health Needs of Two Billion: Is Community Financing a Solution?" Draft paper for the WHO Commission on Macroeconomics and Health. World Bank, Washington, D.C.

Jakab, M., and C. Krishnan. 2001. "Community Involvement in Health Care Financing: Impact, Strengths and Weaknesses: A Survey of the Literature" Draft Paper for the WHO Commission on Macroeconomics and Health. World Bank, Washington, D.C.

Jütting, J. 2002. *The Impact of Community-Based Health Financing on Financial Protection: Case Study Senegal.* HNP Discussion Paper, World Bank. Washington, D.C.

Liu, Y., S. Hu, W. Fu, and W. C. Hsiao. 1996. "Is Community Financing Necessary and Feasible for Rural China?" *Health Policy* 31: 155–71.

Manning, W. G., J. Newhouse, N. Duan, E. Keeler, A. Leibowitz, and M. Marquis. 1987. "Health Insurance and the Demand for Medical Care: Evidence from a Randomized Experiment." *American Economic Review* 77(3): 251–77.

McPake, B., K. Hanson, and A. Mills. 1993. "Community Financing of Health Care in Africa: An Evaluation of the Bamako Initiative." *Social Science and Medicine* 3(11): 1383–95.

Narayan, D. 1999. "Bonds and Bridges: Social Capital and Poverty." Policy Research Working Paper 2167. World Bank, Poverty Reduction and Economic Management Network, Washington, D.C.

Preker, A., and M. Jakab. 2001. "The Role of Communities in Providing Financial Protection against Illness." In D. Dror and A. Preker, eds., *Social Reinsurance: Improved Risk Sharing for Low-Income and Excluded Populations.* Forthcoming.

Schneider, P., A. K. Nandakumar, D. Porignon, M. Bhawalkar, D. Butera, and C. Barnett. 2000. *Rwandan National Health Accounts 1998.* Technical Report 53. Partnerships for Health Reform Project, Abt Associates Inc., Bethesda, Md.

SEWA brochures. 2000.

Supakankunti, S. 1998. *Comparative Analysis of Various Community Cost Sharing Implemented in Myanmar.* Paper presented to the Workshop of Community Cost Sharing in Myanmar, November 26–28.

Toonen, J. 1995. *Community Financing for Health Care: A Case Study from Bolivia.* Bulletin 337. Amsterdam: Royal Tropical Institute.

Wiesmann, D., and J. Jütting. 2001. "Determinants of Viable Health Insurance Schemes in Rural Sub-Sahara Africa." *Quarterly Journal of International Agriculture* 50(4): 361–78.

World Bank. 2000. *World Development Report 2000: Attacking Poverty.* Washington, D.C.

WHO (World Health Organization). 2000. *World Health Report 2000: Health Systems—Improving Performance.* Geneva.

Yip, W., and P. Berman. 2001. "Targeted Health Insurance in a Low-Income Country and Its Impact on Access and Equity in Access: Egypt's School Health Insurance." *Health Economics* 10(2): 207–20.

Ziemek, S., and J. Jütting. 2000. *Mutual Insurance Schemes and Social Protection.* Bonn: Center for Development Research (ZEF).

CHAPTER 6

Financial Protection and Access to Health Care in Rural Areas of Senegal

Johannes Paul Jütting

Abstract: Community-based health insurance schemes are becoming increasingly recognized as an instrument to finance health care in developing countries. Taking the example of *les mutuelles de santés* (mutual health organization) in rural Senegal, this chapter analyzes whether members in a mutual health insurance scheme have better access to health care than nonmembers. A binary probit model is estimated for the determinants of participation in a mutual and a logit/log linear model is used to measure the impact on health care utilization and financial protection. The results show that, while the health insurance schemes reach otherwise excluded people, the very poorest in the communities are not covered. Regarding the impact on the access to health care, members have a higher probability of using hospitalization services than nonmembers and pay substantially less when they need care. Given the results of this study, community-financing schemes have the potential to improve the risk-management capacity of rural households. To reduce identified limitations of the schemes, an enlargement of the risk pool and a scaling up or linking of the schemes is, however, a prerequisite. Appropriate instruments to be further tested should include reinsurance policies, subsidies for the poorest, and developing linkages to the private sector via the promotion of group insurance policies. All these instruments call for a stronger role for public health policy.

Health insurance schemes are an increasingly recognized tool for financing health care provision in low-income countries (WHO 2000). Given the high latent demand for good quality health care services and the extreme underutilization of health services in several countries, it has been argued that social health insurance may improve access to acceptable quality health care. Many authors have criticized other forms of health care financing and cost-recovery strategies, such as user fees (see, for example, Gilson 1998); insurance seems to be a promising alternative as it offers the opportunity to pool risks, thereby transferring unforeseeable health care costs to fixed premiums (Griffin 1992). However, there is some evidence that neither purely statutory social health insurance nor commercial insurance schemes alone can significantly contribute to an increase in coverage rates and thereby broaden access to health care. Especially in rural and remote areas, unit-transaction cost of contracts are too high, which often leads to a state and market failure (Jütting 2000). Recently, mainly in Sub-Saharan Africa but also in a variety of other countries, nonprofit mutual, community-based health insurance schemes[1] have emerged (Bennett, Creese, and Monasch 1998; Wiesmann and Jütting 2001; Jakab and Krishnan 2001).[2] These schemes are characterized by an ethic of mutual aid, solidarity, and collective pooling of health risks

(Atim 1998). In several countries, these schemes operate in conjunction with health care providers, mainly hospitals in the area.

Proponents argue that these schemes have the potential to increase access to health care (see, for example, Dror and Jacquier 1999). The authors of the few studies so far available, however, are less optimistic (for example, Bennett, Creese, and Monasch 1998; Criel 1998; Atim 1998). They argue that often the risk pool is too small, adverse selection problems arise, the schemes are heavily dependent on subsidies, financial and managerial difficulties arise, and overall sustainability does not seem to be ensured. However, while these studies are important contributions to our knowledge about the schemes' general strengths and weaknesses, not enough attention has been given to the context in which these schemes have been introduced and the objectives of the schemes themselves. Furthermore, the potential social benefit of the schemes, that is, their impact on health care access, labor productivity, and households' risk-management capacity, has been largely ignored.

Against this background, this chapter analyzes whether mutual health insurance schemes improve access to health care in rural Senegal. We tackle two principal questions: What are the important socioeconomic determinants that explain membership in a voluntary health insurance scheme? (We thereby identify important factors influencing the demand for health insurance.) What is the schemes' impact on the utilization of health care by, and the level of financial protection for, members as opposed to nonmembers?

To answer these questions, we use a binary probit model for estimating marginal coefficients for the determinants of participation and a logit/log-linear model to analyze the impact on health care utilization by, and financial protection for, members as opposed to nonmembers. By applying this methodology, we go beyond most of the available studies on the impact of community-financing schemes, which have either relied on secondary literature (for example, Bennett, Creese, and Monasch 1998) or restricted their data analysis to qualitative interpretations (for example, Atim 1998).

We have chosen the case of Senegal because we find here a relatively long (10 years) experience with mutual health insurance schemes and an innovative institutional setting (Tine 2000). There is a contract between a nonprofit health care provider, a Catholic-run hospital, and the mutuals, which allows the latter to receive health care at a lower rate.

The outline of the chapter is as follows. First the chapter gives a quick overview of health insurance schemes in rural Sub-Saharan Africa and presents the specific situation in Senegal. Next it describes the research design and the methodology used. The results of the estimations are then discussed and conclusions presented.

HEALTH INSURANCE IN RURAL SUB-SAHARAN AFRICA

Wiesmann and Jütting (2001) present a detailed overview of health insurance schemes outside formal sector employment in Sub-Saharan Africa, which is

FIGURE 6.1   Urban and Rural Health Insurance Schemes in Sub-Saharan Africa,
Year of Inception and Size

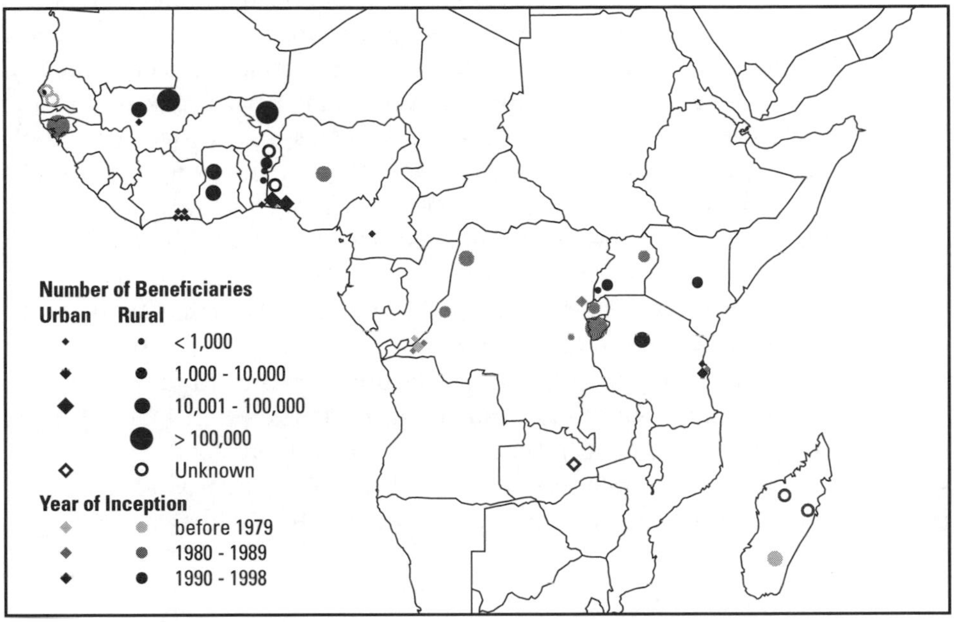

Note: For some schemes, the location is only approximately indicated due to lack of exact data or space problems.

Source: Wiesmann and Jütting (2001).

based on extensive research done in the past few years (Bennett, Creese, and Monasch 1998; Atim 1998; Musau 1999). Most of the schemes were set up in the 1990s. The reasons that promote and foster the development of mutual health insurance schemes have not been analyzed in depth so far, but some trends are obvious (Wiesmann and Jütting 2001). First, people have been forced to think about alternative solutions as health care is no longer offered for free at the public facilities and the introduction of user fees has had negative effects, especially for the poor. Second, in the context of decentralization, more power has been delegated to the communities, which allows them to also assume more responsibilities in the provision of local public goods. Third, the quite positive experience with credit and financing institutions is leading to a discussion about whether the mutuals should enlarge their portfolios to include insurance products. Finally, the debate in the literature over the cost of illness has shown that health shocks often force households into high-cost risk-coping strategies. Access to insurance could reduce these costs substantially (Weinberger and Jütting 2000; Asfaw and others 2001).

The map in figure 6.1 gives a view of health insurance schemes outside the formal employment sector in Sub-Saharan Africa (the following section draws on

Wiesmann and Jütting 2001). The map clearly shows that, thus far, community-based health insurance is more common in West Africa than in Central or East Africa. In some countries, these new schemes are mainly an urban phenomenon—such as those in Côte d'Ivoire and Tanzania—whereas in such states as Uganda, Ghana, and Benin, they predominantly cover people in rural areas.

Some of the schemes are confined to a local cooperative of craftsmen or traders, and therefore the schemes are often very small, perhaps fewer than 100 beneficiaries (Kiwara 1997). Other insurance schemes extend over the whole country and many communities and include up to 1 million or more beneficiaries (Bennett, Creese, and Monasch 1998). The number of beneficiaries can change rapidly and neither reveals the financial balance of the schemes nor says much about the scheme's sustainability. Indeed, a few schemes had to be terminated after some years (Criel 1998; Bennett, Creese, and Monasch 1998), while others have been in operation for decades.

Senegal has a relatively long tradition of mutual health insurance. The first experience began in the village of Fandène in the Thiès region in 1990. From the beginning, the movement in Senegal has been supported by a local health care provider, the nonprofit St. Jean de Dieu Hospital. Today, 16 mutual health insurance schemes operate in the area of Thiès. The main features of the schemes:

- They are community based.

- Ninety percent of them operate in rural areas.

- With the exception of one mutual—Ngaye Ngaye—the schemes cover only hospitalization.

- The mutuals have a contract with St. Jean de Dieu Hospital, where they get a reduction of up to 50 percent for treatment.

- In general, the household is a member of a mutual, which participates in decisions. The member has a membership card on which he or she can list all or selected family members (beneficiaries). The membership fee is per person insured.

Table 6.1 shows that a member has to pay a minimum amount of 3,000 F CFA for a treatment. For surgery, he pays 50 percent of the total costs for the operation. The daily cost of hospitalization, including laboratory analysis, consultation, and some radiography, is paid by the mutual, which receives a reduction of 50 percent. A mutual pays 3,750 F CFA per day for each member hospitalized; nonmembers pay 7,500 F CFA per day. In case of hospitalization, the member has to bring with him a letter of guarantee from the mutual's manager, which is issued if the member has paid the insurance premium regularly. A hospital stay of between 10 and 15 days is entirely paid by the mutual. If the hospitalization exceeds this limit, the mutual pays the hospital the entire invoiced amount because it guaranteed that it would do so. Afterward the member reimburses the

TABLE 6.1   Hospitalization Fees for Members and Nonmembers at St. Jean de Dieu Hospital

		Hospitalization	
	Ticket for consultation	Daily cost	Operation (surgery)
Members	3,000 F CFA	3,750 F CFA mutual	750 F CFA/unit
Nonmembers	6,000 F CFA	7,500 F CFA	1,500 F CFA/unit

Source: ZEF-ISED survey (2000).

mutual in installments. To receive the described benefits, a mutual member has to pay a monthly premium of between 100 and 200 F CFA, and the head of household has to buy a membership card for 1,000 F CFA, a one-time fee.

RESEARCH DESIGN AND METHODOLOGY

Research Design

A household survey was carried out by the Institute for Health and Development (ISED) in Dakar in cooperation with the Center for Development Research in Bonn. The survey began with a pretest in March 2000; the final stage of the survey took place in May 2000. The participation rate in the interviews was very high—more than 95 percent.

For the survey, we chose a two-stage sampling procedure. First, we selected 4 villages out of the 16 villages in which mutuals operate. Each of the selected villages—Fandène, Sanghé, Ngaye Ngaye, and Mont Rolland—has only one mutual, which has the same name as the village. Table 6.2 summarizes the major differences between the analyzed schemes:

In a second step, we randomly selected households for the interviews. In all four villages, members and nonmembers were interviewed. To get a random sample from the four villages, we used household lists of all inhabitants (members and nonmembers) of the four villages to calculate the percentage distribution between members and nonmembers and their respective weight in the

TABLE 6.2   Selection Criteria for Mutual to Be Included in the Survey

Name of mutual/ village	Years of operation	Distance from hospital	Percent of member households in villages	Services
Fandène	10	6 km	90.3	Hospitalization
Mont Rolland	4	15 km	62.6	Hospitalization
Ngaye Ngaye	6	30 km	81.5	Primary health care
Sanghé	3	8 km	37.4	Hospitalization

Source: ZEF-ISED survey (2000).

sample. We interviewed 346 households, 70 percent members and 30 percent nonmembers. The data set contains information on roughly 2,900 persons, 60 percent members and 40 percent nonmembers. This means that some household heads have not insured all of their family.

The data were entered immediately after completing the survey using SPSS Windows. In addition to the household survey, we interviewed key persons (leaders of the mutuals) to get complementary information about the mutuals' functioning, problems, and success.

Methodology

The modeling of mutual health insurance schemes' impact on health care use and expenditure faces the important challenge of dealing with the problem of "endogenity" and "self-selection." This problem is currently receiving a great deal of attention in different areas of development economics, including measuring the impact of microfinance institutions (see Coleman 1999; Nada 1999), estimating the returns of education (see Bedi and Gaston 1999), and analyzing the impact of health insurance on various outcomes, such as health demand and financial protection (see Waters 1999; Yip and Berman 2001). In each of these cases, the evaluation of a policy intervention or institutional innovation involves the problem of assigning individuals randomly to nonprogram control groups and others to program treatment groups. Thus the identification of an adequate control group is the first, and even the most important, step in trying to control for self-selection.

With respect to the impact of health insurance on health care use, Waters (1999) names the potential endogenity of the choice of insurance as the main problem, leading to potential selection bias. Individuals who self-select into the insurance program have unobservable characteristics—related to preference or health status (adverse selection)—that might make them more likely than others to join the program and also might influence their decision to use health care services. An observed association between health insurance affiliation and health care use and expenditure may therefore be due not to the insurance but to the underlying unobservable characteristics. To control for this effect, in the Senegal study an omitted variable version of the Hausman test (Hausman 1978) is applied. This test is based on two steps: estimating the reduced form of the participation equation, and adding the fitted values to the health care demand equation as a regressor. A significantly nonzero coefficient for the predicted value term is an indication that the suspected endogenous variable is in fact endogenous (Waters 1999).[3] To specifically control for self-selection into the program, proxies for the health status and health risks have been included in all of the studies. Finally, village or district dummies are included to control for unobservable characteristics of communities, such as social values and solidarity, to see if they influence individual choice to enroll in a community-financing scheme.

To control for a sample selection bias in the demand equation for health care, the total sample is included, that is, those sick and those not sick as well as those who are members and nonmembers. Finally, the models are checked for stability and robustness by adding and subtracting key variables and by applying the F-test.

To estimate the determinants of participation in a mutual health organization, we follow an approach applied by Weinberger and Jütting (2000). In that approach, participation in a local organization is dependent on the rational choice of an individual weighting costs and benefits of membership. It is assumed that participation of a household (p) in a mutual depends on the current income of the household (y), characteristics of the household head (H), who decides if the household joins or not, household characteristics (Z), community characteristics (C), and the error term u, who is uncovariant with the other regressors.

The following equation describes our model:

(6.1) $p_i = f(y_i, Z_i, H_i, C)$.

To estimate the probability of participation we use a binary probit model:

(6.2) $p_i^* = \beta y_i + \phi Z_i + \alpha H_i + \delta C + u_i,$

$p_i = 1$ if $p^* > 0$, meaning the household $_i$ is a member of the insurance scheme, $p_i = 0$ otherwise.

To assess the impact of mutual health organization on financial protection of members, two aspects have to be taken into account: the probability of visiting a health care provider, and the out-of-pocket expenditure borne by the individuals. The strong disadvantage of using health care expenditure alone as a predictor of financial protection is that this would allow to capture the lack of financial protection for those who choose not to seek health care because they cannot afford it. The first part of the model assesses the determinants of utilization, and we can thereby analyze whether membership in a mutual reduces barriers to assess health care services. We use a two-part model developed as part of the Rand Health Insurance Experiment in the United States (Manning and others 1987)[4]:

a logit model that assesses the probability of visiting a health care provider

(6.3)   Prob (visit > 0) = $X_\beta + M_\alpha + u$, where X stands as a vector for individual, household, and community characteristics (including membership); and

a log-linear model that estimates the incurred level of out-of-pocket expenditures, conditioned on positive use of health care services:

Log(out-of pocket expenditure / visit > 0) = $X_y + M_\chi + e$.

X again represents a set of independent variables that are hypothesized to affect individual patterns of utilization, M represents a dummy variable for membership in a mutual health organization, and u and e represent terms of interference. The independent variables determining the demand for health care and expenditure in the case of illness are—among others—age, gender, education, health status, and income.

As noted above, the modeling of a mutual health insurance scheme's impact faces the important challenge of dealing with the problem of endogenity and self-selection.[5] To control for self-selection, the potential sources have to be identified. With respect to the impact of health insurance on health care use, Waters (1999) names the potential endogenity of the choice of insurance for health care use as the main problem, leading to potential selection bias. To control for this source of self-selection, we estimate the demand for health insurance taking the entire sample instead of only those insured. This also helps us control for potential selection bias due to the potential endogenity of illness and health care use in a reduced sample of sick persons.

To further reduce potential sources of self-selection by bias, each of the four selected villages, as outlined above, has a treatment group (members in a mutual) and a randomly assigned control group (nonmembers). In addition, in the models we have explicitly included a proxy for the health status of individuals as an exogenous variable for health care use and expenditure. Selection bias due to village effects and health status is therefore controlled for. Furthermore, within a single household there are members and nonmembers, which reduces the potential bias related to systematically different preferences between member and nonmember households for health care use and expenditure.

RESULTS

Determinants of Membership in a Health Insurance Scheme

Table 6.3 gives an overview of the variables included in the analysis of the determinants of participation. As outlined above, the decision of a household to participate in a mutual health organization is supposed to be influenced by individual, household, and community characteristics. The variables representing individual characteristics of the household head involve age, education, gender, and membership in another organization. With respect to age, we hypothesize that younger household heads are more open to innovations (age group 1: positive coefficient) and that with increasing age people tend to participate less (age group 3: negative coefficient). Furthermore, we expect that better educated people and male-headed households tend to join a mutual more often than people with less education and female-headed households. The following characteristics of the household are supposed to influence membership in a mutual: income, ethnic group, religion, and the illness ratio (see table 6.3).

The most important variable to be looked at in the context of our research question is income and its effect on the decision to participate or not. In our study, we have measured "income" as calculated by household expenditure per year and member.[6] We assume that income has a positive influence on the decision to participate and that the poorer strata of the population will not participate because of difficulties in paying the premium. In addition, it will be interesting to analyze whether the richer part of the population participates, as

TABLE 6.3   Overview of Variables Used

Variable	Description	Exp. sign for participation decision
Individual and household characteristics		
Age group 1	Age between 21 and 40 years	+
Age group 3	Age between 61 and 90 years	−
Literacy (dummy)	Ability to read/read and write (1 = yes)	+
Sex	Male (1 = yes)	+
Other organization (dummy)	Membership in another group (1 = yes)	+
Relationship (dummy)[a]	Relation to household head (1 = self, spouse, parents, children, and 0 otherwise)	+
Income	Log income/household member in F CFA	+
Income terziles	Lower terzile	−
	Middle terzile	+/−
	Upper terzile	−
Self-wealth	Self-classification of household (poor, average, rich)	−; +/−; +
Wolof (dummy)	Household belonging to ethnic group of Wolof (1 = yes)	+
Religion (dummy)	Christian household (1 = yes)	+
Illness ratio	Number of cases of illness per household in the last six months divided by number of household members	+
Frequency of illness[a]	Number of cases of illness of an individual in the last six months	
Community characteristics		
Fandène (dummy)	Household belonging to Fandène community (1 = yes)	+
Sanghé (dummy)	Household belonging to Sanghé community (1 = yes)	?
Ngaye Ngaye (dummy)	Household belonging to Ngaye Ngaye community (1 = yes)	?
Mont Rolland (dummy)	Household belonging to Mont Rolland community (1 = yes)	?
Solidarity (dummy)	Perceived solidarity in the village (1 = yes)	+

a. These variables are only used in the equation of determinants of participation on the individual level (see table 6.5).

this is important for risk-pooling reasons. Hence we include in the regression analysis income terziles, that is, we divided our sample into three subgroups—rich, average, and poor. Added to the quantitative measures of wealth was relative wealth. Households were asked to classify themselves according to relative

TABLE 6.4   Marginal Coefficients for Determinants of Participation in Mutual Health Insurance (household level). Dependent Variable: Membership in a Mutual (1 if the household is a member and 0 otherwise).

Variable	Model 1	Model 2	Model 3
Constant	−2.048[a]	−0.223	0.064
	(0.541)	(0.155)	(0.147)
Individual characteristics of household head			
Sex (1 = male)	0.054	0.071	−0.001
	(0.083)	(0.083)	(0.083)
Age group 1 (age 21–40)	0.088	0.085	0.079
	(0.092)	(0.092)	(0.091)
Age group 3 (age > 60)	0.087	0.079)	0.101
	(0.061)	(0.061)	(0.062)
Literacy (can read/read and write, 1 = yes)	0.059	0.062	0.043
	(0.063)	(0.063)	(0.063)
Other organization (membership in other group, 1 = yes)	0.180[a]	0.183[a]	0.120[c]
	(0.066)	(0.066)	(0.065)
Household characteristics			
Wolof (household belonging to ethnic group of Wolof, 1 = yes)	0.249[c]	0.284[b]	0.229[c]
	(0.135)	(0.137)	(0.133)
Religion (1 = Christian)	0.370[a]	0.369[a]	0.347[a]
	(0.085)	(0.085)	(0.083)
Income (expenditures per household member log)	0.167[a]		
	(0.046)		
Income terzile: lower		−0.110[c]	
		(0.063)	
Income terzile: upper		0.165[b]	
		(0.073)	
Self-wealth (self-classification of household): Poor			−0.254[a]
			(0.058)
Self-wealth: rich			0.018
			(0.113)
Illness ratio (number of cases of illness per household divided by number of household members)	0.002	0.007	0.037
	(0.088)	(0.088)	(0.086)

(continued)

wealth within the community on a rank from one (poorer than the average) to three (wealthier than the average). We expect the same findings in tendency for the relative measures as for the quantitative measures.

We have included a dummy variable "Wolof" to measure the influence of belonging to a specific ethnic group. The Wolof are known for their openness to institutional innovations in the Senegalese context (Diallo 2000). The variable "religion" is included to take into account that the mutuals have an exclusive contract with the Catholic-owned St. Jean de Dieu Hospital. Moreover, the mutu-

TABLE 6.4 Continued

Variable	Model 1	Model 2	Model 3
Community characteristics			
Fandène (household belonging to Fandène community, 1 = yes)	−0.029	−0.011	−0.119
	(0.151)	(0.152)	(0.150)
Sanghé (household belonging to Sanghé community, 1 = yes)	−0.277[b]	−0.261[c]	−0.383[a]
	(0.132)	(0.134)	(0.130)
Mont Rolland (household belonging to Mont Rolland community, 1 = yes)	−0.225	−0.202	−0.308[b]
	(0.139)	(0.141)	(0.137)
Solidarity (perceived solidarity in the village, 1 = yes)	0.103	0.100	0.104[c]
	(0.066)	(0.067)	(0.065)
Number of observations	338	338	341
Pseudo R	0.567	0.569	0.568
Chi	120.32	121.39	127.96
Prob > Chi	0.000	0.000	0.000
Frequencies of actual/predicted outcomes	80%	80%	80%

a. Significant at 0.01 level.

b. Significant at 0.05 level.

c. Significant at 0.1 level.

Source: Author's estimation based on ZEF-ISED survey data.

als get active support from the diocese of Thiès. Hence we expect that more Christians will enroll than Muslims. We also assume a positive relationship between membership in a mutual and membership in other organizations. People who already have experience participating in local organizations are more willing to join a mutual insurance group than people who have no experience participating. To control for adverse selection, we integrate the illness ratio of the household as a proxy for the health status. The variable describes the number of cases of illness of household members in relation to the overall household size. It is assumed that less healthy households tend to join mutuals more than healthier ones, leading to adverse selection problems.

Finally, we include dummy variables capturing village characteristics: acknowledgement of solidarity in the village (solidarity) and village factors. We assume that people acknowledging a high value of solidarity in their village tend to participate more. With respect to the village effects, we want to control for the type of insurance—whether it covers hospitalization or only primary health care (Ngaye Ngaye)—as well as for the specific local setting—the cultural environment in the specific village and specific characteristics of the mutual, such as distance to the hospital and the functioning of the mutual.

The results presented in table 6.4 show the marginal effects of the probit analysis. Three different models were evaluated, differing in their definition of the income variable. In the first model, income is defined as a metric variable so as to analyze whether income has an influence on membership in a mutual. In the second model, income groups are established to determine effects between different income groups. In the third model, income groups were also formed, but in contrast to model 2 they were not based on expenditure but on self-assessment by the people surveyed.[7]

Table 6.4 shows that all three methods used are highly significant. Income has the anticipated positive influence on membership. Models 2 and 3 show furthermore that the lower income groups in the villages are significantly less represented in the mutuals. That means that the wealthy people in the communities are more likely to (be able to) participate in the insurance schemes. At the household level, religion and ethnic identity also play an important role. The higher participation by Christians—the probability increases by nearly 40 percentage points compared with that for non-Christians—was to be expected because of the Catholic Church's intensive promotion of the mutuals.

While household characteristics do have an influence on the membership decision, this is obviously not the case for the individual characteristics of the head of the household, such as education, gender, and age. None of these three characteristics is significant. Membership in other organizations, however, is a positive factor. People who have already experienced the advantages and disadvantages of being associated with local groups are obviously more disposed toward membership in a health insurance scheme.

The village effects that were discovered are also interesting. Different model variations show, for example, that the inhabitants of the villages of Sanghé and Mont Rolland have a significantly lower probability of membership than people from the villages of Ngaye Ngaye and Fandène. These results indicate that the different type of health insurance provided—primary health care in Ngaye Ngaye and inpatient care in the other three mutuals—had no significant influence on the decision to participate. Instead, specific village factors, such as the management of the mutual, seemed to play a role. The mutual of Sanghé has faced several financial and managerial difficulties that led to a suspension of operations for some time. As a consequence, several people left the mutual. Efforts to reestablish the mutual have been successful, and today it is functioning again, but with a lower participation rate than before.

Thus far the results have shown that the main factors influencing the demand for health insurance in rural Senegal are religion, income, belonging to a certain ethnic group, access to a social network, and village effects. These results are largely confirmed by looking at the determinants of participation at the individual level. Regarding the individual level, it is interesting to analyze which type of household members are insured. From a theoretical perspective, one would assume that individuals more prone to the risk of illness are insured. As table 6.5 shows, this is largely confirmed as the probability for women and older people is higher than for men and younger persons in the household. It is reasonable to assume that women of child-bearing age and older people do need hospitalization care more often than other household members.

TABLE 6.5   Marginal Coefficients for Determinants of Participation in Mutual Health Insurance (individual level). Dependent Variable: Membership in a Mutual

Variable	Model 2
Constant	−0.100[c]
	(0.056)
Individual and household characteristics	
Sex (1 = male)	−0.042[b]
	(0.021)
Age group 1 (age < 26)	0.000
	(0.027)
Age group 3 (age > 50)	0.077[b]
	(0.035)
Literacy (can read/read and write, 1 = yes)	0.109[a]
	(0.022)
Other organization (membership in other group, 1 = yes)	0.070[b]
	(0.028)
Relationship (self, spouse, parents, children, 1 = yes)	0.115[a]
	(0.022)
Health status (number of cases illness in last 6 months)	−0.011
	(0.020)
Wolof (household belonging to ethnic group of Wolof, 1 = yes)	0.182[a]
	(0.049)
Religion (1 = Christian)	0.386[a]
	(0.033)
Income terzile: lower	−0.047[b]
	(0.024)
Income terzile: upper	0.219[a]
	(0.028)
Community characteristics	
Fandène (household belonging to Fandène community, 1 = yes)	−0.058
	(0.058)
Sanghé (household belonging to Sanghé community, 1 = yes)	−0.358[a]
	(0.050)
Mont Rolland (household belonging to Mont Rolland community, 1 = yes)	−0.332[a]
	(0.055)
Number of observations	2.855
Pseudo R	0.549
Chi	989.02
Prob > Chi	0.000
Frequencies of actual/predicted outcomes	77%

a. Significant at 0.01 level.

b. Significant at 0.05 level.

c. Significant at 0.1 level.

Source: Author's estimation based on ZEF-ISED survey data.

TABLE 6.6   Probability of Hospitalization and Determinants of Expenditure in Case of Hospitalization

Variable	Model 1[a] (hospital)	Model 1[b] (hospital)	Model 2[a] (expend.)	Model 2[b] (expend.)
Constant	−0.301[a] (0.065)	−0.137[a] (0.021)	4.611[a] (2.016)	9.445[a] (0.642)
Individual and household characteristics				
Sex (1 = male)	−0.014[b] (0.007)	−0.014[b] (0.006)	0.370 (0.214)	0.401 (0.21)
Age group 1 (age < 26)	−0.016[b] (0.008)	−0.016[b] (0.008)	−0.495[a] (0.258)	−0.520[a] (0.210)
Age group 3 (age > 50)	0.022[b] (0.009)	0.022[b] (0.009)	−0.008 (0.323)	−0.141 (0.327)
Literacy (can read/read and write, 1 = yes)	−0.107 (0.007)	−0.010 (0.007)	0.07 (0.243)	0.035 (0.239)
Membership (in health insurance without Ngaye Ngaye, 1 = yes)	0.020[b] (0.009)	0.020[b] (0.009)	−0.452[b] (0.287)	−0.514[b] (0.291)
Frequency of illness	0.009 (0.006)	0.008 (0.006)	−0.02 (0.16)	−0.03 (0.157)
Type of illness (complications during pregnancy/childbirth, 1 = yes)			1.273[b] (0.303)	1.125[b] (0.299)
Severity of illness (number of days hospitalized)				0.015[a] (0.005)
Wolof (household belonging to ethnic group of Wolof, 1 = yes)	−0.007 (0.020)	−0.005 (0.019)	−0.002 (0.576)	−0.033 (0.582)
Religion (1 = Christian household)	−0.005 (0.012)	−0.004 (0.012)	0.089 (0.324)	0.142 (0.323)
Income (expenditures per household member log)	0.015[a] (0.005)		0.441[b] (0.174)	
Income terzile: lower		−0.008 (0.008)		−0.120 (0.273)
Income terzile: upper		0.016[b] (0.008)		0.67[a] (0.238)

(continued)

Whereas the coefficient for both variables is significant, the marginal effect with less than 0.1 percentage points is rather low, which makes it too difficult to diagnose severe adverse selection problems.

Impact of Membership on Access to Modern Health Care Services

In this section, we test the hypothesis that members of a mutual have better access to modern health care facilities than nonmembers. We measure access in two respects: the probability of frequentation of a health care facility, in this case a hospital, and the out-of-pocket expenditure at point of use. Our primary vari-

TABLE 6.6   Continued

Variable	Model 1[a] (hospital)	Model 1[b] (hospital)	Model 2[a] (expend.)	Model 2[b] (expend.)
Community characteristics				
Fandène (household belonging to Fandène community, 1 = yes)	0.046[b] (0.022)	0.046[b] (0.022)	0.550 (0.67)	0.568 (0.676)
Sanghé (household belonging to Sanghé community, 1 = yes)	0.017 (0.020)	0.018 (0.020)	1.573 (0.643)	1.588 (0.643)
Mont Rolland (household belonging to Mont Rolland community, 1 = yes)	0.027 (0.022)	0.027 (0.021)	1.986[c] (0.636)	1.779 (0.629)
Number of observations	2,855	2,855	118	118
Chi/F value	103.00	103.96	3.990	4.176
Corrected r squared			0.264	0.289
Prob > Chi/F value	0.000	0.000	0.000	0.000
Frequencies of actual/predicted outcomes	94.7 %	94.7 %		

a. Significant at 0.01 level.

b. Significant at 0.05 level.

c. Significant at 0.1 level.

Source: Author's estimation based on ZEF-ISED survey data.

able of interest is membership in a mutual. We hypothesize that the probability of members' frequenting a hospital is higher, while at the same time they pay less for their treatment in comparison to nonmembers after controlling for individual, household, and community characteristics. This would mean that membership has a positive coefficient for health care demand and a negative one for the effect on expenditure. Besides membership, the other key variable is income as we want to see how much of demand health care utilization and out-of-pocket expenditure is due to the income level and the ability to pay.

As control variables we include age, gender, education, and frequency of illness, which capture the need for health care and the health status of an individual. Household characteristics are included to control for health preferences due to factors such as religion and belonging to an ethnic group. Finally, village effects are taken into account for differences in the cost of seeking health care as well as in the specific design of the mutuals. One assumption here is that inhabitants from the village in Fandène have better access to health care because of their relatively short distance from the hospital as well as the fact that the mutual reportedly functions well. The results of the estimates for the determinants of demand for health care services and costs in the case of illness are presented in table 6.6.

Both models are highly significant. Of the 2,856 people, 151 have been in the hospital within the past two years.[8] The findings of the estimates for both models suggest that the members of a mutual have better access to health care services than nonmembers. The probability of making use of hospitalization increases by 2 percentage points with membership, and expenditure in case of need is reduced by about 50 percent compared with nonmembers. Regarding individual characteristics, in addition to membership, age and gender play a role. Moreover, the results suggest that younger people make less use of the hospital than the elderly, and they pay less on average if they do fall ill. Furthermore, women use the hospital more than men. Women go to the hospital especially when they have problems during pregnancy or childbirth.

As far as the variables at the household level are concerned, it turns out that income has an impact on the demand for health care services and expenditure. The relatively better-off people in a community make more use of services and spend more money in the event of hospitalization. This is in line with findings on demand for health care in other developing countries (Gertler and van der Gaag 1990).

With respect to village effects, people living in Fandène have a higher effective demand for hospitalization than people in the other three communities.[9] A possible explanation is the fact that Fandène is the oldest mutual, and according to our interview partners, it is well-organized and functions well. It is also the closest mutual to St. Jean de Dieu Hospital.

To sum up, it can be said that members are (can be) hospitalized more often and pay considerably less for treatment than nonmembers. Other important factors are age, type of illness, gender, income, and village effects.

The case study on the community-based health insurance schemes in Senegal shows that the formation of a health insurance scheme for households in rural areas is possible and can result in better access to health care for otherwise excluded people. Especially in places where local institutions have already developed forms of mutual help, possibilities seem to exist for developing the schemes into more formalized approaches. From the Senegalese case study, in addition to an existing local network, the existence of a viable health care provider is of tremendous importance. Without the financial support of the hospital as well as a perception that the care provided is of good quality—the hospital is well known for its good quality in service provision—it is difficult to imagine that the mutuals would still exist. Hence subsidies seem to be necessary if one wants to set up an insurance scheme for poor people.

Finally, individual and household characteristics also play a role in the viability of rural health insurance schemes. In areas with widespread poverty and a scattered population, setting up a health insurance scheme is much more difficult than in richer and more densely populated areas. As the analysis of the determinants of participation in microinsurance schemes has revealed against the expectations of most donors and policymakers, they do not necessarily reach all population groups in a village. In fact, for the lowest income group the premium to insure the whole family reaches nearly 8 percent of the household's annual income.[10] Support for this group should therefore be secured by the state. This could be done, for example, in the form of subsidized premiums.

CONCLUSIONS

The results of experience with mutual health organizations in Senegal suggest that rural health insurance for the poor is feasible under certain conditions. More important, it could be shown that access to health insurance can have a positive impact on the members' economic and social situation. Further investigation should be devoted to discovering the extent to which health insurance, or its lack, affects labor productivity and investors' willingness to undertake risky, but potentially profitable, investments.

To enlarge access to health care for the poor and the rural population, community-based health insurance schemes can be an important element and a first step. They allow some limited pooling of risks and thereby lead to an improvement in the health care system, since most people otherwise have to pay their health expenditure out-of-pocket. However, the study also points to the persistent problem of social exclusion—that the community's poorest members have no opportunity to participate and not enough resources to pay the required premium. To overcome these limitations of community-based health insurance, broader risk pools are required. In particular, the role of external financial support, such as government subsidies, donor funding, and reinsurance in encouraging social inclusion needs to be further explored. More research is needed on how these schemes can be scaled up, replicated, and linked to other social risk-management instruments such as social funds.

Acknowledgments: The author is grateful to the World Health Organization (WHO) for having provided an opportunity to contribute to the work of the Commission on Macroeconomics and Health and to the World Bank for having published the material in this chapter as an HNP Discussion Paper.

The author would like to thank Hana Ohly for her valuable research assistance. Financing from the ILO-STEP project is gratefully acknowledged. The findings, interpretations, and conclusions expressed in the chapter are entirely those of the author and do not necessarily represent the views of the World Bank, its Executive Directors, or the countries they represent.

NOTES

1. The terms *community-based health insurance* and *mutual health insurance* are used interchangeably throughout this chapter.

2. For a more detailed typology see Jakab and Krishnan (2001).

3. The test of endogenity of the membership variable in health care use and expenditure had to be rejected, that is, we supposed that membership is exogenous.

4. For a recent application see Yip and Berman (2001).

5. The problem of self-selection is not relevant for our first research question on determinants of participation. But it is relevant for the second research question, which looks at the demand for health care and the amount of expenditure, with "health insurance membership" as an exogenous variable.

6. Alternatively, we have also measured income as calculated by the revenue from on-farm and off-farm activities as well as remittances. It turned out, however, that there was some estimation bias in the data because some of the people interviewed were unwilling to report their true income.

7. Estimating the income of households in developing countries is difficult. Since many of the people surveyed are reluctant to reveal their real income, income is generally measured by using expenditure. This method of measuring can be supplemented by asking the protagonists to do a self-assessment, comparing themselves with other households in the neighbourhood.

8. A certain percentage of the hospitalized persons had to be excluded from the "expenditure" analysis as they were not aware of the costs they had to pay because other family members made the payments.

9. This effect clearly pops up when the Fandène mutual is left outside and the remaining mutuals get a significant negative coefficient.

10. An individual household has to weigh these costs against the probability of being hospitalized and the average cost for treatment. The direct average financial costs for one hospitalization of a household member is already above 20 percent of the annual income of the household.

REFERENCES

Asfaw, A., A. Admassie, J. von Braun, and J. Jütting. 2001. "New Dimensions in Measuring Economic Costs of Illness: The Case of Rural Ethiopia." Submitted to *Social Science and Medicine*.

Atim, C. 1998. *Contribution of Mutual Health to Financing, Delivery, and Access to Health Care: Synthesis of Research in Nine West and Central African Countries*. Technical Report 18. Partnerships for Health Reform Project. Abt Associates Inc., Bethesda, Md.

Bedi, A. and N. Gaston. 1999. "Using Variation in Schooling Availability to Estimate Educational Returns for Honduras." *Economics of Educational Review* 18: 107–16.

Bennett S., A. Creese, and R. Monasch. 1998. *Health Insurance Schemes for People Outside Formal Sector Employment*. ARA Paper 16. WHO, Geneva.

Coleman, B. 1999. "The Impact of Group Lending in Northeast Thailand." *Journal of Development Economics* 60: 105–41.

Criel, B. 1998. "District-Based Health Insurance in Sub-Saharan Africa. Part II: Case-Studies." *Studies in Health Services Organisation and Policy* (Antwerp) 10.

Diallo, I. 2000. "Impact des mutuelles de santé sur l'accessibilite des populations aux soins de santé modernes dans la région de Thiès au Sénègal." Institute for Health and Development, Dakar.

Dror, D., and C. Jacquier. 1999. "Microinsurance: Extending Health Insurance to the Excluded." *International Social Security Review* 52(1): 71–97.

Gertler, P., and J. van der Gaag. 1990. *The Willingness to Pay for Medical Care*. Baltimore: World Bank, Johns Hopkins University Press.

Gilson, L. 1998. "The Lessons of User Fee Experience in Africa." In A. Beattie, J. Doherty, L. Gilson, E. Lambo, and P. Shaw, eds., *Sustainable Health Care Financing in Southern*

Africa: Papers from an EDI Health Policy Seminar Held in Johannesburg, South Africa, June 1996. Washington, D.C.: EDI Learning Resources Series.

Griffin, C. 1992. *Health Care in Asia: A Comparative Study of Cost and Financing.* World Bank Regional and Sectoral Studies. Washington, D.C.

Heckman, J. 1979. "Sample Bias as a Specification Error." *Econometrica* 47(1): 153–61

Jakab, M., and C. Krishnan. 2001. "Community Involvement in Health Care Financing: Impact, Strengths and Weaknesses: A Synthesis of the Literature." Background paper prepared for Working Group 3 of the Commission on Macroeconomics and Health of the WHO. World Bank, Washington, D.C.

Jütting, J. 2000. "Social Security Systems in Low Income Countries: Concepts, Constraints, and the Need for Cooperation." *International Social Security Review* 53(4): 3–25.

——. 2001. "Health Insurance for the Poor?" In *Development and Cooperation* 6: 4–5.

Kiwara, A. 1997. "Mutual Society for Health Care in the Informal Sector (UMASIDA) Backup Report—January to August 1997." Dar es Salaam.

Manning, W., J. Newhouse, N. Duan, E. Keeler, A. Leibowitz, and M. Marquis. 1987. "Health Insurance and the Demand for Medical Care: Evidence from a Randomized Experiment." *American Economic Review* 77: 251–77.

Musau, S. 1999. *Community-Based Health Insurance: Experiences and Lessons Learned from East and Southern Africa.* Technical Report 34. Partnerships for Health Reform Project, Abt Associates, Inc., Bethesda, Md.

Nada, P. 1999. "Women's Participation in Rural Credit Programmes in Bangladesh and Their Demand for Formal Health Care: Is There a Positive Impact?" *Health Economics and Econometrics* 8: 415–28.

Tine, J. 2000. *Les mutuelles de santé rurales de la région de Thiès au Sénegal: Des initiatives communautaires pour améliorer l'accès aux soins de santé.* ILO/ZEF Project Report 4. Center for Development Research, Bonn.

Waters, H. 1999. "Measuring the Impact of Health Insurance with a Correction for Selection Bias: A Case Study of Ecuador." *Health Economics and Econometrics* 8: 473–83.

Weinberger, K., and J. Jütting. 2000. "The Role of Local Organizations in Risk Management: Some Evidence from Rural Chad." *Quarterly Journal of International Agriculture* 39(3): 281–99.

——. 2001. "Women's Participation in Local Organizations: Conditions and Constraints." *World Development* 29(8): 1391–404.

WHO (World Health Organization). 2000: *World Health Report 2000: Health Systems—Measuring Performance.* Geneva.

Wiesmann, D., and J. Jütting. 2001. "Determinants of Viable Health Insurance Schemes in Rural Sub-Saharan Africa." *Quarterly Journal of International Agriculture* 50(4): 361–78.

Yip, W., and P. Berman. 2001. "Targeted Health Insurance in a Low-Income Country and Its Impact on Access and Equity in Access: Egypt's School Health Insurance." *Health Economics* 10: 207–20.

ZEF-ISED. 2000. Survey info.

CHAPTER 7

Community-Based Health Insurance in Rwanda

Pia Schneider and François Diop

Abstract: This chapter evaluates the impact of prepayment schemes on access to health care for poor households, based on household survey data. Rwanda is one of the poorest countries in the world. After the genocide in 1994, public health care services were provided free to patients, financed by donors and the government. In 1996, the Ministry of Health reintroduced prewar level user charges. By 1999, utilization of primary health care services had dropped from 0.3 in 1997 to a national average of 0.2 annual consultations per capita. This sharp drop in health service use, combined with growing concerns about rising poverty, poor health outcome indicators, and a worrisome HIV prevalence among all population groups, motivated the Rwandan government to develop community-based health insurance to assure access to the modern health system for the poor. In early 1999, the Rwandan Ministry of Health, in collaboration with the local communities and with the technical support of the USAID-funded Partnerships for Health Reform (PHR) project, began the process to pilot test 54 prepayment schemes in three districts. At the end of their first operational year, the 54 schemes comprised more than 88,000 members. The findings presented in this chapter reveal that insurance enrollment is determined by household characteristics such as the health district of household residence, education level of household head, family size, distance to the health facility, and radio ownership; health and economic indicators did not influence enrollment. Insurance members report up to five times higher health service use than nonmembers. The analysis confirms findings reported by PHR based on provider data: health insurance has significantly improved equity in health service use for members while out-of-pocket spending per episode of illness has decreased.

In response to declining health service utilization after the reintroduction of user fees for services and drugs in public health facilities in 1996, the Rwandan Ministry of Health (MOH) decided to pilot test alternative health care financing and provider payment methods. During the first six months of 1999, the MOH developed an ongoing collaboration with the local communities involving 54 community-based health insurance (CBHI) plans—each of them partnering with a health center. The MOH selected three pilot districts, Kabutare, Byumba, and Kabgayi, to pilot test these prepayment schemes (PPS). The three districts were chosen based on the extent of their health infrastructure, the repeated demand for technical assistance from the population in developing and implementing CBHI, and the districts' political will to participate in the health insurance pilot experience. By July 1, 1999, all 54 health centers, which had collaborated in the set up of their CBHI in the three pilot districts, signed a contract with their partnering health insurance scheme. Thereafter, the district population began to enroll in the schemes, which are

TABLE 7.1   Community-Based Health Insurance in Rwanda, First Year Performance (July 1999–June 2000)

| | Pilot districts with CBHI | | | |
Indicators	Byumba	Kabgayi	Kabutare	All 3 districts
All prepayment schemes (status on 6/30/2000)				
Total number of PPS	21	17	16	54
Total target population in districts	459,329	368,020	288,160	1,115,509
Total population enrolled	48,837	21,903	17,563	88,303
Average number of members per PPS	2,326	1,288	1,098	1,635
First year average PPS enrollment rate	10.6%	6.0%	6.1%	7.9%

Source: Schneider and others (2001).

democratically managed by their members as mutual health associations. At the end of the first year, membership in the 54 health insurance plans rose to 88,303 individuals, corresponding to 8 percent of the total population of the three districts (see table 7.1). Technical and financial assistance for the entire design, development, implementation, and evaluation phase was provided to the Rwandan government by Partnerships for Health Reform (PHR), a project funded by USAID and administered by Abt Associates. (For detailed information on the development and implementation of prepayment schemes in Rwanda, see Schneider, Diop, and Bucyana 2000.)

The objective of this chapter is to respond to two questions about the prepayment schemes' impact: What are the population groups that enroll in community-based health insurance schemes? Does health insurance membership improve financial accessibility to care without increasing the burden of out-of-pocket health expenditures? These questions are addressed by presenting a synopsis of the findings from the household survey conducted by PHR in the three health districts. The impact of prepayment schemes on insurance and providers' utilization, cost, and finances has been analyzed from monthly routine data collected from providers and health insurance schemes over a two-year period in the three districts. Findings of this detailed analysis on the financial sustainability of CBHI plans and their impact on health care providers are presented in the PHR Technical Report No. 61 (Schneider and others 2001). This chapter will therefore respond to the question about the insurance impact on households' financial accessibility to the modern health care system by focusing on information collected in the household survey.

The next section provides a brief summary of the design, development, and implementation of prepayment schemes in Rwanda, which took place from January 1999 until September 2000. The third section introduces the method used to address the research questions and presents the household survey data and variables used. Results are presented in the fourth section; and the fifth section has a discussion and conclusion.

BACKGROUND

In January 1999, the Rwandan MOH initiated the design and development phase of prepayment plans by creating a strategic steering committee, which was headed by the director of health care and included representatives and stakeholders from the central and regional levels. The design and implementation of health insurance modalities and management features were discussed and agreed upon during 28 district-level workshops attended by community and health care representatives and in a series of community gatherings with the local populations. Proposals stemming from these district and community meetings were shared with the central steering committee, which provided feedback and advice to the communities. As a result of this ongoing discussion between the central and local levels, the scheme features were designed, the legal, contractual, and financial tools were developed, and workshop participants were trained and prepared to manage the 54 prepayment schemes, each entering into partnership with a health center on July 1, 1999.

Under Rwandan law, the schemes are deemed mutual health associations, headed by an executive bureau with four volunteers, elected by and among the scheme members during a CBHI general assembly. At the district level, the schemes have formed a federation. Six members have been elected by and among all PPS executive bureau representatives in their general assembly to constitute the district federation of prepayment schemes. The federation is the partner to the district hospital as well as to the health district and other authorities. Each prepayment bureau has signed a contract with the affiliated health center, and each federation with the district hospital, defining in 17 articles the rules of collaboration between the insurer and the provider. According to the schemes' bylaws, members are invited at least once a year to attend the prepayment scheme general assembly.

Individuals and households who would like to be insured pay, at the time of enrollment, an annual premium of 2,500 francs per family, for up to seven persons (July 1999: RWF 2,500 = US$7.50). The premium is paid to the CBHI affiliated with their "preferred" health center.[1] In case of sickness, members first contact their preferred health center, which is usually the nearest public or church-owned facility. Health centers play a gatekeeper function; hospital services are covered for members only if the preferred health center has referred them. This is done to dissuade members and providers from frivolous use of more expensive hospital services. PPS membership entitles members—after a one-month waiting period—to a basic health care package covering all services and drugs provided in their preferred health center, including ambulance transfer to the district public or church-owned hospital, where a limited package is covered.[2] Members pay a 100 francs copayment for each health center visit (July 1999: RWF 100 = US$0.30).

The MOH was concerned that the availability of health insurance to a population group with an accumulated demand for health services could lead to adverse selection and moral hazard, causing health care costs to rise. Therefore, the MOH recommended to the district workshop participants that they incorporate into the design of the prepayment schemes a provider-payment mechanism that would set the necessary incentives for providers to improve their productivity while controlling for unnecessary use of health services. After several discussions between providers and future scheme managers, the workshop participants selected capitation provider payment to the health center as a measure for controlling cost escalations caused by supply-side induced increases in demand for health care. Each prepayment bureau disburses monthly one-twelfth of its accumulated premium fund, 5 percent of which is withheld to cover the scheme's administrative costs, 10 percent is paid to the district's prepayment federation, and the rest is paid as capitation payment to the partnering health center. The federation reimburses the district hospital for covered services provided to members, paying per episode of illness (for caesarean sections, malaria, and pediatrics), and by service for overnight stays and physician consultations for all other illnesses. Thus insurance members share their hospital costs on a district level and health center costs on a health center catchment-area level. (For a detailed analysis of PPS impact on utilization, cost, and finances in health centers, see Schneider and others 2001.)

DATA SOURCES AND METHODOLOGY

The analysis presented in this chapter is based on data collected in the prepayment scheme household survey, conducted by PHR in collaboration with the Rwandan National Population Office (ONAPO). Data collection took place during 40 days in October–November 2000. The household survey includes 2,518 households that were successfully interviewed in the three pilot districts, and number 11,583 individuals. The sample was designed to provide information on the impact of prepayment schemes on households' enrollment and health care seeking behavior, as well as on the related financial implications. The sample was based on the same sampling frame as the Rwandan Demographic and Health Survey (DHS) 2000, covering 11 health regions in Rwanda.[3] Households for the prepayment household survey in the three districts were sampled at random from a list of primary households from sample cells identified in the national DHS sample, rendering the household survey sample representative to the district level.

The prepayment household survey used three structured questionnaires for data collection: a socioeconomic household questionnaire, a curative questionnaire, and a preventive care questionnaire. The household questionnaire collected information on households' and individuals' sociodemographic and economic characteristics, including household expenditures for consumer goods, health, and education, and participation in CBHI. The curative care questionnaire was addressed to household members who were sick two weeks prior to the interview, and the preventive care questionnaire was used to interview women of childbearing age who had delivered a child in the past five years or who were pregnant during the year preceding the interview (Diop, Schneider, and Butera 2001).

The three pilot districts (Byumba, Kabgayi, Kabutare) are similar in their socioeconomic situation. There is little urban activity, and the populations are mainly active in agriculture and animal husbandry. Households are assumed to be equally poor, with few of them owning cattle, a sign of wealth. For the analysis, the sample population is divided into two groups: CBHI members in pilot districts, and CBHI nonmembers in pilot districts.

Three models are used in this chapter to estimate first, the probability of buying health insurance for specific population groups in the three pilot districts; second, the probability of access to basic health care services for the insured and uninsured population groups in the pilot districts; and third, the estimated out-of-pocket health expenditures per episode of illness for all sick individuals and for those who sought professional care, based on a set of explanatory variables. For each categorical variable used in the three models, one category has been selected as a reference category. Odds ratios are estimated in the logit regression models for each category to estimate the factor that measures the magnitude of the difference in relation to the reference category. Interaction effects were tested for significance.

Model 1: Demand for Health Insurance

The following model estimates the probability of CBHI enrollment for households in pilot districts. The objective is to determine if the poorest buy basic health insurance, and if the poor benefit from a redistribution from richer members of the financial pool. The willingness to join CBHI is a discrete choice—to join or to not join. A logit regression model is used to determine households' CBHI enrollment probability and the extent to which this decision is influenced by specific sociodemographic and economic characteristics. The hypothesis to be tested is that the CBHI member and nonmember households do not differ in their socioeconomic characteristics. In a logit regression, the dependent variable "demand for insurance" (D_i) will equal 1 if individuals buy insurance or 0 otherwise. Formally, the logit model can be written as a linear function of the explanatory variables:

(7.1) $L_i = b_1 + b_2 X_{2i} + \ldots + b_k X_{ki}$

and

P_i (D for CBHI membership) $= 1/(1 + 1/e^{L_i})$.

The second equation shows that the conditional probability of buying insurance P_i is a nonlinear function of the explanatory variables X_i, which represents a series of attributes assumed to have caused a household to buy health insurance membership in the three pilot districts. We will estimate the unknown coefficients b_i, which are the weights assigned to each of the households' sociodemographic and economic characteristics in the probability that $D_i = 1$ for given X_i. Insurance was an option only for households within the pilot districts. Therefore,

TABLE 7.2   Summary Statistics: Independent Variables Used to Determine Probability of CBHI

Independent variables	Mean	Std. dev.	N (Households)
Kabgayi District	0.41	0.492	2,518
Byumba District	0.22	0.411	2,518
Kabutare District	0.37	0.482	2,518
Male HH head	0.66	0.474	2,518
Average age HH head	44.33	15.789	2,512
HH head 40 years and older	0.83	0.377	2,518
HH head attended school	0.54	0.498	2,515
HH with child < 5	0.07	0.249	2,518
HH with pregnancy in past year	0.03	0.167	2,518
HH with cattle	0.18	0.386	2,503
HH with radio	0.34	0.475	2,505
HH with 5 or more members	0.45	0.498	2,518
HH size	4.57	2.255	2,518
Less than 30 minutes from HH cell to health facility	0.38	0.487	2,518
Income quartiles			
1	0.26	0.437	2,518
2	0.25	0.431	2,518
3	0.25	0.435	2,518
4	0.24	0.430	2,518

the logit regression was performed with weighted household survey data from pilot districts, based on household heads as the unit of analysis.

Description of Variables Included in Model 1

The response to enroll in CBHI is the dependent variable in this model and is made primarily by the head of household, based on a set of independent variables X. These explanatory variables are classified into demographic, socioeconomic, and health attributes of the household. Table 7.2 presents their sample size, mean, and standard deviation.

Model 2: Access to the Modern Health Care System

Patients' health-seeking behavior was measured based on weighted data for individuals who reported sickness during the two weeks preceding the interview in the household survey and who responded to the curative care questionnaire. As in the first model, the second model applies a logit regression model to estimate the probability of entering (or not entering) the modern health care system for the insured and uninsured in the pilot districts. Access probabilities are estimated based on spe-

TABLE 7.3   Summary Statistics of Explanatory Variables for Probability of Professional Visit

Independent variable	Mean	Standard deviation	N (Sick individuals)
Kabgayi District	0.23	0.421	3,130
Byumba District	0.37	0.482	3,130
Kabutare District	0.40	0.491	3,130
Prepayment member in pilot district	0.06	0.236	3,130
Male patient	0.42	0.494	3,130
Average age patient	24.60	21.003	3,127
Patient age 0–5 years	0.23	0.423	3,127
Patient with pregnancy in past year	0.07	0.251	3,130
Patient spent 4 or more days in bed	0.56	0.497	1,599
HH with 5 or more members	0.57	0.495	3,130
HH head attended school	0.56	0.496	3,130
HH with cattle	0.21	0.404	3,130
HH with radio	0.36	0.481	3,130
Less than 30 minutes from HH cell to health facility	0.39	0.488	3,130
Income quartiles			
1	0.23	0.421	3,130
2	0.26	0.441	3,130
3	0.26	0.439	3,130
4	0.24	0.430	3,130

cific sociodemographic and economic household characteristics that determine a sick individual's care-seeking behavior. The hypothesis is tested that the sick who access health care do not significantly differ in their sociodemographic, economic, and health characteristics. Therefore, the logit regression was performed with weighted curative survey data from the pilot districts, based on sick individuals as the unit of analysis. The logit model, based on equation 7.1 presented in the first model, leads to the following definition of the probability of accessing modern health care:

(7.2) P_i (access to professional care) $= 1/(1 + 1/e^{Li})$,

where X represents a set of explanatory variables that are assumed to have caused a sick person to seek care with a professional provider at a health center or district hospital during the two weeks prior to the interview.

Description of Variables Included in Model 2

The decision to seek professional care is influenced by households' socioeconomic conditions, insurance status, and the sick individuals' health status. These explanatory variables are summarized in table 7.3, showing for each attribute the sample size, mean, and standard deviation.

Model 3: Financial Impact of Household Out-of-Pocket Health Expenditures

The third model is a log-linear regression that serves to estimate first, that sick individuals' total average out-of-pocket spending per episode of illness and second, that total out-of-pocket spending conditioned on the positive use of health care services (Manning and others 1987; Yip and Berman 2001). The model is a linear regression for the logarithm of total health-related spending per episode of illness of the sick and for the logarithm of total health-related spending for the sick who reported at least one visit. The logarithmic transformation of health expenditures per episode of illness eliminates skewness in the distribution of health expenses among users, yielding roughly normal error distributions. The model can be written as follows:

(7.3)   Log (total illness related out-of-pocket spending) = a + b X + e

and

Log (total illness related out-of-pocket spending | visit > 0) = a + b X + e,

where X represents a set of continuous and dummy attributes assumed to influence patients' health expenditures. Detailed health expenditures are reported by episode of illness, which includes spending before and during a professional care visit, and will show to what extent patients rely on alternative sources of care outside the formal health sector. The regressions were performed with weighted curative survey data from the pilot districts, based on sick individuals as the unit of analysis. It is assumed that the amount spent on nonprofessional medicine will be higher for patients whose access to professional care is limited by financial barriers.

Description of Variables Included in Model 3

Model 3 uses the same variables as in the second model and adds the variable professional care visit to estimate out-of-pocket health expenditures for those individuals who were sick and for those who sought professional care. Table 7.4 presents sample size, mean, and standard deviation for each explanatory variable.

RESULTS

Description of the Sample Group

Tables 7.5 and 7.6 describe sociodemographic and economic characteristics for the sample population included in the household survey conducted in the three pilot districts. Males head about 82 percent of PPS member households. One-third of the heads of member households have five or more years of schooling, 41 percent of the household heads are in the 40–59 age group and belong to households in higher expenditure quartiles as compared with the nonmember households in the same districts. Distance to the health facility also seems to be

TABLE 7.4   Summary Statistics of Explanatory Variables for Estimated Out-of-Pocket Spending per Episode of Illness

Independent variable	Mean	Standard deviation	N (Sick individuals)
All sick with 1+ professional care visits	0.16	0.371	3,130
Kabgayi District	0.23	0.421	3,130
Byumba District	0.37	0.482	3,130
Kabutare District	0.40	0.491	3,130
Prepayment member in pilot district	0.06	0.236	3,130
Male patient	0.42	0.494	3,130
Average age patient	24.60	21.003	3,127
Patient age 0–5 years	0.23	0.423	3,127
Patient with pregnancy in past year	0.07	0.251	3,130
Patient spent 4 or more days in bed	0.56	0.497	1,599
HH with 5 or more members	0.57	0.495	3,130
HH head attended school	0.56	0.496	3,130
HH with cattle	0.21	0.404	3,130
HH with radio	0.36	0.481	3,130
Less than 30 minutes from HH cell to health facility	0.39	0.488	3,130
Income quartiles			
1	0.23	0.421	3,130
2	0.26	0.441	3,130
3	0.26	0.439	3,130
4	0.24	0.430	3,130

an important criterion as almost 50 percent of the member households live within 15 minutes of the health facility. Membership begins to taper off as the distance to the health facility increases.

Almost 61 percent of insured households interviewed in the survey said all individuals living in the household had been enrolled. In the remaining households, individuals not enrolled were usually young adults above the age of 18, who are supposed to enroll either in a group category or as individuals.[4] Table 7.6 presents households' monthly average per capita monetary expenditures for each expenditure quartile, as well as the average household size for insured and uninsured households. Independent means tests were performed to compare differences. Households' monetary expenditures were used as proxy to classify households in income quartiles. Insured households number on average significantly more individuals than uninsured ones in the pilot districts. The possibility of signing up in a CBHI plan as a family of up to seven members for the same annual premium might have been an incentive for larger households to enroll with all their family members. Each of the two groups shows a decreasing average household size with higher expenditure quartiles.

TABLE 7.5   Descriptive Sample Characteristics (Column Percentages Sum to 100 Within Each Category)

	Pilot districts		
	Nonmembers (N 2,337)	PPS members (N 181)	Total (N 2,518)
Characteristics of head of household			
Gender			
Female	35.4%	17.8%	34.1%
Male	64.6%	82.2%	65.9%
Level of schooling			
Never	47.0%	28.4%	45.7%
Primary < 5	22.6%	22.5%	22.6%
Primary = or > 5	24.2%	33.3%	24.9%
Above primary	6.2%	15.9%	6.9%
Age group			
< 30	17.1%	17.6%	17.2%
30–39	25.2%	27.2%	25.4%
40–59	36.3%	41.2%	36.7%
60 & +	21.3%	14.0%	20.8%
Characteristics of household			
Income quartiles			
1	26.1%	19.8%	25.6%
2	24.7%	24.2%	24.6%
3	25.0%	29.9%	25.3%
4	24.3%	26.1%	24.4%
Time distance (minutes) to health facility			
15	37.6%	48.6%	38.4%
45	14.6%	20.8%	15.1%
75	25.6%	24.2%	25.5%
105	22.1%	6.4%	21.0%

Smaller households in higher expenditure quartiles pay the same premium per household as larger families in the lowest expenditure quartiles. Depending on members' service use and financial contribution to health for uncovered services, this negative relationship between household size and income status can lead to cross-subsidies from the smaller, predominantly richer to the larger, poorer families in the prepayment health insurance pool.

Table 7.7 presents the summary statistics for monthly per capita monetary expenditures for households living in the pilot districts. Figure 7.1 shows that the monetary expenditure data are very right-skewed, confirming that this is an equally poor population with very few households reporting high monetary expenditures: the 90th percentile amount is 5,975 francs compared with the maximum amount of 192,950 francs.

The figure shows that Rwandan households living in these rural districts are poor. They live mostly from subsistence farming in areas with a high-density

TABLE 7.6   Household Characteristics, by Income Quartile

Household characteristics	Nonmembers	PPS members	Total
Monthly average per capita expenditure (RWF)			
Quartile 1	333	347	334
Quartile 2	1,050	1,007	1,047
Quartile 3	2,241	2,056	2,225
Quartile 4	8,154	9,367	8,247
In all 4 quartiles	**2,884**	**3,370**	**2,919**
Average household size, number of individuals			
Quartile 1	4.6	5.5	4.7
Quartile 2	4.7	5.6	4.8
Quartile 3	4.6	5.8	4.7
Quartile 4	4.1	4.8	4.1
In all 4 quartiles	**4.5**	**5.5[a]**	**4.6**

Note: t-tests were performed to compare the average values of the insured with the uninsured sample.

a. Significant at 1 percent level of significance.

TABLE 7.7   Summary Statistics on Distribution of Monthly Monetary Expenditures per Capita

Monetary expenditures		Households
N		2,518
Mean	RWF	2,919.1
Standard Error of Mean		126.798
Median		1,475.5
Standard Deviation		6,362.787
Minimum		0
Maximum		192,950
Percentiles	10	267.0
	25	624.5
	50	1,475.5
	75	3,190.0
	90	5,975.0

population. Rwanda is recovering from the recent civil war, and an estimated 10 percent of the male population is still missing. Muller (1997) found in a household survey conducted in 1983 that the average land area farmed by Rwandan households is very small at 1.24 hectares, and households produced agricultural product worth an average of US$51 per capita per year, 90 percent of which is

FIGURE 7.1   Monthly Monetary Expenditure per Capita

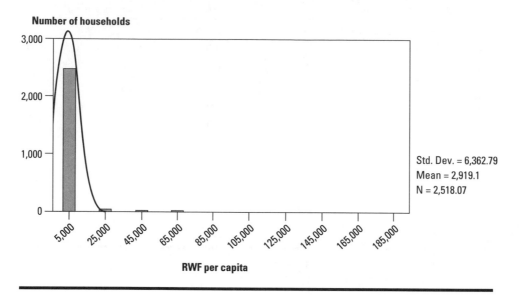

used for consumption. Findings in our household survey, conducted 17 years later, estimated annual monetary expenditure is approximately US$100 per capita for these rural households. The Rwandan Ministry of Finance is conducting a living standard survey in Rwanda, which will provide more insight into the socioeconomic conditions of Rwandan households.

Model 1: Who Demands Health Insurance?

The means comparison in tables 7.1 and 7.2 has shown that, compared with the uninsured, insured households are more likely to be headed by a male individual who has attended some schooling. In addition, proportionally more CBHI member households are likely to come from higher income quartiles and from larger households.

The logit regression results presented in table 7.8 show that the household head's level of education, family size, district of residence, distance to the health facility, and radio ownership are the major determining factors in whether to join a health insurance plan. Households' health and economic indicators did not influence demand for health insurance. Radio ownership is indicative of a household's ability to access information and exposure to advertising about the CBHI. It may also be seen to a certain extent as an economic indicator for these very poor households.

Households in Kabgayi are more than twice as likely, and those in Byumba about 15 times as likely, to buy health insurance as households in Kabutare. Household heads who attended school are 103 percent more likely to enroll in health insurance than the illiterate. Households with five and more members are

TABLE 7.8   Logit Regression Results for Households' Probability to Demand Community-Based Health Insurance (Prepayment Schemes)

Explanatory variable	Reference category variable	Insurance membership in pilot districts		
		Odds ratio	S.E.	Sign
Kabgayi District	Kabutare District	3.51[a]	0.362	0.001
Byumba District		15.80[a]	0.268	0.000
Male HH head	Female HH head	1.55	0.253	0.084
HH head, age 40+	HH head, younger than 40	1.13	0.239	0.598
HH head, attended school	HH head, illiterate	2.03[a]	0.196	0.000
Large HH size, 5+	Small HH size, fewer than 5	1.60[a]	0.189	0.013
HH with child < 5	No child < 5	0.87	0.488	0.768
HH with pregnancy in past year	No pregnancy in past year	1.23	0.674	0.761
Less than 30 minutes to health facility	More than 30 minutes to health facility	3.96[a]	0.187	0.000
HH with cattle	No cattle	1.28	0.210	0.237
HH with radio	No radio	1.47[a]	0.184	0.038
Quartile 1	Quartile 4	1.19	0.264	0.513
Quartile 2		1.21	0.244	0.437
Quartile 3		1.15	0.228	0.535
	Ancillary statistics			
	N (households)	2,474		
	– 2 Log likelihood	1,054.901		
	Goodness fit (chi-squared test)	236.998		
	Degree of freedom	14		
	Nagelkerke R Square	22%		

Note: HH = Household. Z-tests were performed to test the probability of enrollment for each characteristic in a logit model.

a. Significant at 1 percent level of significance.

60 percent more likely to buy insurance than smaller households. This is probably because, irrespective of the family size (up to seven members), households pay a 2,500 francs membership fee per year.[5] Therefore, larger families effectively pay less per household member. Households who live within 30 minutes of their health facility have a 296 percent higher probability of joining than those who live farther away. This latter result might have been influenced by health centers' and prepayment schemes' awareness campaigns, which could have been more intense in the vicinity of a health facility. Households who own a radio are 47 percent more likely to enroll than those without a radio, another result that might have been caused by the regular awareness campaigns transmitted by radio. Although male-headed households are 55 percent more likely to join than female-headed, and households with pregnant women are 23 percent more

likely to join, these results are not significant. Other economic attributes, such as household cattle ownership and different income quartiles were not significant in the demand for health insurance. Households in the lowest and lower income quartiles were as likely to enroll as those in the fourth income quartile.

The findings from the first model respond to the question, Who enrolls in CBHI? Households living in Byumba and Kabgayi, who number five and more individuals, whose household head attended school, who live in the vicinity of a health center, and who own a radio appear to be more likely to buy insurance.

Other important factors also influence households' probability of enrolling, such as their risk aversion and their exposure to effective information campaigns on prepayment schemes, as well as their trust in the scheme management, which is related to households' willingness to see CBHI as an investment and which supports the argument that enrollment in health insurance is not necessarily driven by economic conditions such as household income. The following reasons were identified in different surveys (focus group, household, and patient exit interview) to be important in households' enrollment decisions:

- Both Byumba and Kabgayi had intensive awareness and information campaigns on PPS during the first year, supported by the district authorities and prepayment federation, which resulted in steady monthly enrollment increases.

- The prepayment schemes' features, including benefit package, premium level, enrollment categories, copayments, and waiting period, were designed, discussed, and agreed upon (by voting) in a series of about 30 workshops in the three districts. These workshops were attended by the local populations. As a result, the health insurance schemes were "tailored" as desired by, and in response to, the needs of the local people.

- The main determinant of PPS participation is trust, which might be captured by the time variable. People living near the facilities are more likely to enroll because they know the health center personnel, as well as the prepayment scheme management team, and have been exposed to regular information campaigns on prepayment.

- The participatory approach and the democratic management of PPS lead to sentiments of "ownership" and increased trust among the poor, which are basic conditions for poor households to engage in any investment.

- Households that do not have the 2,500 francs (about US$8) to pay the one-year PPS enrollment fee join a "tontine." Over a five-week period, each tontine household pays 500 francs per week to the "tontine-caisse" as an installment toward the 2,500 francs total fee. Households are enrolled as full members once they have contributed 2,500 francs.

- Local initiatives (churches and members who attended the PPS general assemblies) have helped to pay enrollment fees for indigents, widows, orphans, and poor high-risk patients such as HIV-positive individuals.

This shows that poor households will enroll in well-designed health insurance schemes that improve access to health care. At the same time, these solidarity groups contribute to positive social capital in a society that is recovering from a civil war. Therefore, community-based health insurance becomes a form of social cohesion and provides a link between the poor and the health facilities.

The following section answers the second question, Does health insurance membership improve financial accessibility to care without increasing members' financial burden?

Model 2: Equity in Financial Accessibility to Professional Care[6]

Evaluation of the first year of prepayment schemes in Rwanda has been based on extensive data collection. The analysis of monthly health service utilization data in health centers and hospitals has revealed that the overall use of curative services for adults and children, and preventive health services for children and women, was up to five times higher for PPS members than for nonmembers (Schneider and others 2001).[7]

Results in table 7.9 reveal that the insured report considerably better access to the modern health care system with a visit probability of 0.45, compared with a 0.15 visit probability for the uninsured in the pilot districts. Given the relatively moderate visit probability for sick PPS members of 0.45, it can be assumed that prepayment enrollment was not driven by adverse selection, and there was no frivolous use of health care caused by members' moral hazard behavior.

Probability of visit by members does not vary by patients' gender, age, and income quartile; it is determined by patients' geographic access to the health facility (time distance) and health status, with the sick and very sick being three times more likely to seek care than healthier individuals. Interestingly, CBHI members who said they were not very sick or were sick reported higher visit likelihood (0.22 and 0.64, respectively) than the average nonmember (0.05 and 0.15), indicating that CBHI membership causes sick individuals to seek care at the onset of illness. Access to professional care is lowest for the uninsured in the lowest income quartile, who are about four times less likely to seek care than the insured in the same income group.

The logit regression results presented in table 7.10 estimate the probability of a professional health care visit for members and nonmembers and controls for skewness in the data distribution that could have influenced the access. The logit regression coefficient estimates were translated into odds ratios to facilitate interpretation.

Findings show that health insurance has tremendously improved the financial accessibility of its members to the modern health care system, particularly for women, children, and the poor. Access to care is determined by prepayment membership, patient age, pregnancy, patients' health status, distance to the health facility, and households' income group. Most important, prepayment members are 559 percent more likely than nonmembers to enter the modern

TABLE 7.9   Probability of Using a Professional Provider by Insurance Status

	Pilot districts	
Probability of visit	*Members (N 376)*	*Nonmembers (N 3,459)*
Sick individuals (N 3,835)	0.45[a]	0.15
Patient gender		
Female	0.42	0.14
Male	0.50	0.16
Patient age		
6 years and older	0.45	0.13
0–5 years	0.46	0.19
Time from household to health facility		
More than 30 minutes	0.33	0.12
Less than 30 minutes	0.60	0.19
Income (expenditure) groups		
Quartile 1	0.40	0.06
Quartile 2	0.35	0.13
Quartile 3	0.49	0.14
Quartile 4	0.54	0.26
Self-perceived health status		
Not very sick	0.22	0.05
Sick	0.64	0.15
Very sick	0.61	0.30

Note: Probability of sick individuals with at least one visit with a professional provider during the two weeks prior to the interview. T-tests were performed to compare the rates of the insured with the uninsured in the pilot districts.

a. Significant at 1 percent level of significance.

health care system when sick. Health-related indicators significantly influenced health-seeking behavior, with children under five years of age being 92 percent more likely to report a visit than older patients. In addition, pregnant women report 65 percent higher probability than nonpregnant women for seeking care, and the sick individuals who spent four or more days in bed were 96 percent more likely to go to a modern health care provider than people who were not sick in bed as long. People who live close to the health facility are significantly more likely to seek care (61 percent) than those who live farther away. Patients in the lowest income quartile are far less likely to seek care than those in the highest income quartile. This means that while the prepayment scheme has significantly increased access to health care for members, including those who are poor, the impact at the district level in increased access to health care for the poor remains an issue. The solution is to find mechanisms to increase enrollment of the poor households in the prepayment schemes.

TABLE 7.10   Logit Regression Results for Probability of at Least One Professional Provider Visit for Members and Nonmembers

Explanatory variable	Reference category variable	Probability of visit		
		Odds ratio	S.E.	Sign
Prepayment members	Nonmembers	6.59[a]	0.263	0.000
Male patient	Female patient	1.21	0.140	0.170
Patient age 0–5 years	Patient age 6 years and older	1.92[a]	0.158	0.000
Pregnant in past year	No pregnancy in past year	1.65[a]	0.248	0.043
Patient spent 4 or more days in bed	Less than 4 days in bed	1.96[a]	0.139	0.000
Less than 30 minutes to health facility	More than 30 minutes to health facility	1.61[a]	0.137	0.000
HH with 5 or more members	HH with fewer than 5 members	1.17	0.142	0.277
HH head attended school	HH head illiterate	0.91	0.141	0.519
HH with cattle	No cattle	1.26	0.162	0.162
HH with radio	No radio	1.33	0.143	0.050
First income quartile	Fourth income quartile	0.18[a]	0.230	0.000
Second income quartile		0.44[a]	0.174	0.000
Third income quartile		0.46[a]	0.172	0.000
	Ancillary statistics			
	N	1,502		
	− 2 Log likelihood	1,434.941		
	Goodness fit (chi-squared test)	211.744		
	Degree of freedom	13		
	R Square	19.3%		

Note: Z-tests were performed to test the probability of enrollment for each characteristic in a logit model.

a. Significant at 1 percent level of significance.

Model 3: Average Out-of-Pocket Health Expenditures per Episode of Illness[8]

Based on detailed provider and insurance data, the evaluation of the prepayment pilot phase has shown that health insurance has a substantial impact on members' financial contribution to health care as well as on the providers' cost and financial situation (Schneider and others 2001). Findings in PHR report no. 61 have shown that the PPS members' annual per capita contributions to the modern health care system are up to five times higher than those of nonmembers (see Schneider and others 2001, table 3.14).[9] However, the out-of-pocket expenditures per episode of illness are significantly lower for members as compared with those for nonmembers. This means that by paying insurance, scheme

TABLE 7.11   Average Health Expenditure (RWFᵃ) per Sick Individual with or without a Visit to a Professional Provider, by Health Insurance Status and Expenditure Quartile, in Pilot Districts

Out-of-pocket spending RWF	Income quartile	Pilot districts					
		Nonmembers			Members		
		No prof. visit	1+ prof. visit	Total	No prof. visit	1+ prof. visit	Total
Home and other care	1	90	85	90	276	0	165
	2	124	178	131	68	23	53
	3	171	230	180	28	20	24
	4	277	322	288	79	133	108
	Total	**160**	**245**	**172**	**93**	**52**	**74**
First professional provider	1	11	693	49	10	112	51
	2	10	1,356	180	20	178	75
	3	43	1,445	246	9	220	112
	4	36	2,228	600	105	966	572
	Total	**24**	**1,693**	**269**	**32**	**418**	**207**
Other professional providers	1	0	262	15	0	0	0
	2	0	27	3	0	0	0
	3	1	42	7	0	1	1
	4	9	22	13	0	91	50
	Total	**2**	**50**	**9**	**0**	**28**	**12**
Total illness-related expenditure	1	101	1,041	154	286	112	216
	2	134	1,561	314	88	201	128
	3	215	1,717	433	37	242	137
	4	322	2,573	901	184	1,190	730
	Total	**186**	**1,987**	**450**	**126**	**497**	**294**

Source: National Bank of Rwanda.

a. Nominal Exchange Rate: US$1 = RWF 370 (official period average in 2000).

members face lower fees at the time of illness and have greater access at times of need. Furthermore, in Rwanda, with very low per capita use rates, the higher utilization by members should not be interpreted as an effect of moral hazard but rather as improved access to essential basic health services.

The third model in this chapter documents insured and uninsured patients' out-of-pocket health expenditures per episode of illness. This information is first shown for all sick, independent of their care-seeking behavior, and second for those who reported at least one health facility visit.

Table 7.11 presents total health-related out-of-pocket expenditures paid for each of the different health-related services during an episode of illness, which includes care received before visiting a provider, out-of-pocket spending at the first professional visit, and out-of-pocket spending for other professional providers. This total health expenditure information is shown for the insured and uninsured sick in the pilot districts and is further broken down for each group by "with and without a professional provider visit." Within these categories, the different health expenditures are shown by patients' income quartiles. It is found that per episode of illness, sick members pay on average 294 francs for all health-related expenditures. This amount is higher for nonmembers in the pilot districts (450 francs). The differences are even stronger when comparing only the sick insured and uninsured with a professional care visit. Sick members with a professional visit pay 497 francs for the full episode of illness, whereas nonmembers' out-of-pocket health expenditures per episode of illness with a professional visit amount to 1,987 francs in the pilot districts.

Insurance membership has significantly decreased out-of-pocket spending for a full episode of illness for sick members with and without a visit and at the same time has substantially improved members' access to the modern health care system. In addition, health insurance has changed patients' health care–seeking behavior. A comparison of members' and nonmembers' average out-of-pocket spending for home and other care in table 7.11 shows that the uninsured spend almost two and a half times more on home care and traditional remedies than the insured, who are more likely to seek quality care in the modern health system. Thus not only have prepayment schemes reduced financial barriers in accessing better quality care and thus equity in accessing care, but insurance membership has shifted the demand for health care toward more efficient care as well.

Members who seek care pay a 100 francs copayment per episode of illness at the health center. Sick individuals from richer households spend more on home care and on professional care compared with lower income groups, and this holds for the insured and the uninsured. The fact that the richer insured pay up to 10 times more per episode of illness than the poorest CBHI members supports the assumption made in the previous model. That is, prepayment schemes favor cross-subsidies from richer to poorer members if there is a uniform premium per family, if poorer families number more individuals than richer families, and if members' care-seeking behavior is independent of their income status. Thus far this argument holds. However, the richer insured may still pay more because they are willing to pay additional amounts for care not covered by the insurance scheme, such as drugs excluded from the MOH essential drug list.

The following log-linear regression (table 7.12) estimates sick individuals' average health expenditures for the insured and uninsured in the pilot districts. Findings show that prepayment schemes have significantly decreased out-of-pocket spending for the entire episode of illness for sick individuals who are members. Individuals' out-of-pocket health expenditures are positively influenced by the patient's gender, with men paying more than women, by household size, and by use of professional care. Patients classified in the three lower income quartiles report significantly lower out-of-pocket spending for an episode of illness, with or without a visit, than those in the fourth income quartile. In addition, out-of-pocket spending per episode of illness is significantly influenced negatively if patients live in the health center's vicinity and if they own cattle (which can be interpreted as a sign of wealth).

TABLE 7.12   Log-Linear Regression Results: Estimated Total Health-Related Expenditures per Episode of Illness for Sick Individuals with and without a Visit

Explanatory variable	Reference category variable	Out-of-pocket all sick		
		Coeff.	S.E.	P > t
Sick insured members	Sick uninsured in pilot districts	−0.604[a]	0.141	0.000
Male patient	Female patient	0.056[a]	0.061	0.000
Patient age 0–5 years	Patient age 6 years and older	−0.006	0.075	0.362
Pregnant in past year	No pregnancy in past year	−0.227	0.120	0.933
Patient spent 4 or more days in bed	Less than 4 days in bed	0.228	0.060	0.057
Less than 30 minutes to health facility	More than 30 minutes to health facility	−0.125[a]	0.062	0.000
HH with 5 or more members	HH with fewer than 5 members	0.111[a]	0.063	0.045
HH head attended school	HH head illiterate	0.262	0.061	0.075
HH with cattle	No cattle	−0.090[a]	0.075	0.000
HH with radio	No radio	0.258	0.067	0.234
First income quartile	Fourth income quartile	−0.544[a]	0.091	0.000
Second income quartile		−0.290[a]	0.085	0.000
Third income quartile		−0.183[a]	0.085	0.001
All sick w/ 1+ professional care visit	All sick without visit	1.645[a]	0.077	0.030
(Constant)		1.048[a]	0.101	0.000
Ancillary statistics				
N		1,596		
F		52.686		
Degree of freedom		(141,582)		
Prob > F		0.000		
R square		0.318		

Note: Includes total health related out-of-pocket spending for sick with and without visit. T-tests were performed to test significant difference for each characteristic.

a. Significant at 1 percent level of significance.

Table 7.13 presents log-linear regression results on out-of-pocket spending per episode of illness for the 336 patients who reported a professional health care visit. As can be expected, CBHI membership has significantly decreased health care costs for the sick members with a visit. Patients classified in the first income quartile report significantly lower out-of-pocket spending per episode of illness if they had a visit than do patients in the fourth income quartile. However, those in the second and third quartiles report lower out-of-pocket spending per

TABLE 7.13   Log-Linear Regression Results: Estimated Out-of-Pocket Health Expenditures per Episode of Illness for Sick Individuals Who Reported a Professional Visit in Past 2 Weeks

		Log of total health expenditures with a visit	Out-of-pocket with a visit		
Explanatory variable	_Reference category variable_		_Coeff._	_S.E._	_P > t_
Sick insured members	Sick uninsured in pilot districts		−0.808[a]	0.145	0.000
Male patient	Female patient		0.274[a]	0.099	0.006
Patient age 0–5 years	Patient age 6 years or older		0.068	0.107	0.523
Pregnant in past year	No pregnancy in past year		−0.127	0.172	0.460
Patient spent 4 or more days in bed	Less than 4 days in bed		0.088	0.101	0.386
Less than 30 minutes to health facility	More than 30 minutes to health facility		−0.121	0.098	0.215
HH with 5 or more members	HH with fewer than 5 members		0.061	0.103	0.556
HH head attended school	HH head illiterate		0.133	0.106	0.213
HH with cattle	No cattle		−0.068	0.112	0.547
HH with radio	No radio		0.007	0.103	0.948
First income quartile	Fourth income quartile		−0.464[a]	0.181	0.011
Second income quartile			−0.152	0.124	0.221
Third income quartile			−0.143	0.124	0.250
(Constant)			2.850[a]	0.155	0.000
Ancillary statistics					
N			336		
F			5.286		
Degree of freedom			(13 323)		
Prob > F			0.000		
R square			0.175		

Note: Includes total health-related out-of-pocket spending for the full episode of illness for those who were sick and went to seek professional care. T-tests were performed to test significant difference for each characteristic.

a. Significant at 1 percent level of significance.

episode but are not statistically significant. Male patients with visits spend significantly more per episode of illness than female patients.

Combining these findings with the results presented in the first and second model show that community-based health insurance in Rwanda has been successfully used as a tool to improve financial accessibility to care for the poor who enroll in the scheme while, at the same time, their out-of-pocket health care expenditures could be reduced per episode of illness.

DISCUSSION AND CONCLUSION

Findings confirm that prepayment schemes in Rwanda successfully target the rural poor, with their members having an annual average per capita income of approximately US$100. Logit regression results have shown that the probability of enrolling in prepayment schemes is equal among all income groups and is determined by factors such as households' distance from the health center, exposure to radio awareness campaigns, age, gender, and education status of the household head. Other factors have influenced enrollment, such as precautionary behavior for one's family's health, foresight, and the possibility of seeing the insurance premium as a trustworthy investment. Survey findings also allude to the fact that social capital such as trust and sentiments of ownership are important determinants of participation in prepayment schemes. Prepayment schemes are forms of solidarity and social cohesion that help strengthen the link between the poor and the health facilities where the local people would like to seek care.

Health insurance has significantly improved equity in financial accessibility to care for members by increasing their probability of a visit while at the same time possibly reducing the financial burden per episode of illness. This argument holds for all income groups in the insurance pool, although richer members still pay up to 10 times more out-of-pocket, supporting the argument of possible cross-subsidies to poorer patients. Health insurance has helped to eliminate financial barriers in access to care for the poorest among the insured members, whereas the uninsured in the lowest expenditure quartiles continue to report significantly worse access to care than the richer insureds. In addition to improved access, faster access to care of the insured patients has contributed to a shift in demand for care from the traditional to the modern health sector and has improved the efficient use of limited medical resources such as drugs and staff in district health facilities.

The analysis of the financial impact of prepayment schemes on health care providers has shown that community-managed health plans, combined with provider capitation payment, have built up expertise and capacity among insurance members about their rights and obligations and, as a result, have empowered consumers in discussions for better quality care with health center managers during the schemes' general assemblies.

Although data collection during the pilot phase was extensive and included patient exit interviews and focus group information as well as routine provider insurance and household data, it is too early to conclude that better access to care due to prepayment membership has caused members' health to improve. However, findings from different sources suggest that conclusion.

Still, about 90 percent of the population in the three districts has not enrolled with prepayment schemes and continues to report dismal health care utilization patterns. Although the large majority of nonmembers interviewed in the household survey said they would like to become members, three-fourths of them had serious doubts that they would have the 2,500 francs available to pay the annual fee for their family, raising concerns about how successful the schemes are in improving equity of access to care. During the pilot year, church groups facilitated enrollment by financing membership for widows, orphans, indigents, and poor HIV-infected individuals. This targeted demand-side subsidy contributed to a welfare gain if they benefited the indigents' insurance enrollment without decreasing benefits for patients who did not enroll. The church groups' experience with financing health insurance membership has caused prepayment to become a promising tool to subsidize targeted access to care for the vulnerable.

Acknowledgments: The authors are grateful to the World Health Organization (WHO) for having provided an opportunity to contribute to the work of the Commission on Macroeconomics and Health and to the World Bank for having published the material in this chapter as an HNP Discussion Paper. This analysis is supported by the Partnerships for Health Reform Project, which is administered by Abt Associates Inc. and funded by the United States Agency for International Development (USAID). Helpful comments on this analysis were received from Charlotte Leighton, A. K. Nandakumar, and Manjiri Bhawalkar.

NOTES

1. Premium rates were set by taking into account existing user fees and by assuming that utilization rates would increase by 25 percent compared with baseline levels. See Schneider, Diop, and Bucyana (2000), chap. 3.1.1.

2. The Kabgayi PPS covers full episodes of caesarean sections, malaria, and nonsurgical pediatrics at the hospital, whereas the Kabutare and Byumba PPSs cover full episode C-sections, as well as each physician consultation and overnight stay at the district hospitals.

3. The DHS was conducted by the ONAPO in collaboration with Macro International and USAID in 2000–01. Households for the DHS were selected as primary sample units from sample cells identified for the Living Condition Monitoring Survey (LCMS), conducted by the Ministry of Finance in collaboration with UNDP in 2000–01.

4. The enrollment category "household" includes two adults and all children up to the age of 18 living in the same household. Other household members need to enroll in a group or individual category.

5. Households with up to seven members pay 2,500 francs per household per year. Individual enrollment costs 2,000 francs per year, and enrollment in a group for eight and more individuals costs 530 francs per person per year. Premiums are slightly higher in Kabgayi due to the larger hospital coverage (household—2,600 francs, individual—2,200 francs, and group enrollment per person—550 francs).

6. Professional care means public- and church-owned health centers, district hospitals, and dispensaries. This excludes sick individuals who sought care at traditional healers and others (for example, drug vendors, pharmacies).

7. District averages are 1.5 curative consultations per member per year in Kabutare and Kabgayi, and 1.1 curative consultations per member in Byumba, whereas nonmembers' curative care consultation level scores around 0.2 consultation per nonmember per year.

8. See note 6 above.

9. Members in Byumba reported 580 francs annual per capita contributions to health centers, whereas this amount is only 104 francs per capita per year for nonmembers, due to their lower health service use.

REFERENCES

Diop, F., P. Schneider, and D. Butera. 2001. *Summary of Results: Prepayment Schemes in the Rwandan Districts of Kabgayi, Byumba, and Kabutare.* Technical Report No. 59. Partnerships for Health Reform Project, Abt Associates Inc. Bethesda, Md.

Manning, W., J. Newhouse, N. Duan, E. Keeler, A. Leibowitz, and M. Marquis. 1987. "Health Insurance and the Demand for Medical Care: Evidence from a Randomized Experiment." *American Economic Review* 77(3): 251–77.

Muller, C. 1997. "Transient Seasonal and Chronic Poverty of Peasants: Evidence from Rwanda." WPS/97–8. Centre for the Study of African Economics, Institute of Economics and Statistics, University of Oxford, Oxford.

Schneider, P., F. Diop, and S. Bucyana. 2000. *Development and Implementation of Prepayment Schemes in Rwanda.* Technical Report No. 45. Partnerships for Health Reform Project, Abt Associates Inc. Bethesda, Md.

Schneider, P., F. Diop, D. Maceira, and D. Butera. 2001. *Utilization, Cost and Financing of District Health Services in Rwanda.* Technical Report No. 61. Partnerships for Health Reform Project, Abt Associates Inc. Bethesda, Md.

Yip, W., and P. Berman. 2001. "Targeted Health Insurance in a Low-Income Country and Its Impact on Access and Equity in Access: Egypt's School Health Insurance." *Health Economics* 10(2): 207–20.

CHAPTER 8

The SEWA Medical Insurance Fund in India

M. Kent Ranson

Abstract: This chapter assesses the impact of the Self-Employed Women's Association's (SEWA's) Medical Insurance Fund, Gujarat, in terms of inclusion of the poor, hospital utilization, and expenditure. Age-matched insured and uninsured women were compared using survey data (2000). We found that wealth was not a determinant of membership in the Fund; that is, the poor were not excluded. Of 28 hospitalizations among Fund members over one year, only 5 were reimbursed. Membership in SEWA was not significantly associated with increased frequency of hospitalization, but there was a significant association with lower costs of hospitalization, net of reimbursement. Unlike many other CBHI schemes, the Fund has overcome barriers that exclude the poorest. This is due in part to nesting of the Fund within a larger development organization. Utilization of the Fund, and thus impact on hospital utilization and expenditure was minimal. This may relate to a lack of awareness of benefits among Fund members or costs and difficulties associated with submitting an insurance claim.

Community-based health insurance (CBHI) schemes—also referred to as micro-insurance units and mutual health insurance—are mechanisms wherein people prepay for some component of health care and there is some pooling of revenues and risks, with the healthy cross-subsidizing health care for the sick. Policymakers generally see CBHI as a means of improving access to effective health care, particularly among the poor, and preventing indebtedness and impoverishment as a result of trying to access such care (WHO 2000).

A few studies have investigated the impact of CBHI schemes in developing countries. In general, these studies suggest that it is difficult to include the poorest individuals and households in a CBHI scheme but that a well-designed and well-managed scheme can increase demand for, and utilization of, health care while protecting members from catastrophic costs.

There are many reasons why the poorest in a population might not join a CBHI scheme, including lack of information about the scheme, lack of solidarity within the population, limited participation in planning or managing the scheme, unaffordable premiums, and priorities that are more important or immediate than health and medical insurance (for example, food and shelter). In their review of 83 health insurance schemes for the informal sector, Bennett, Creese, and Monasch (1998) found that most of them relied on flat-rate premiums and that for several schemes unaffordable premiums were a major deterrent to participation. For example, a study conducted in rural Senegal found the average income of members of four CBHI schemes to be three times as high as that of randomly selected nonmembers; the authors attributed this difference to premiums that were unaffordable to the poorer part of the population (Jütting 2001). Despite problems of affordability, very few schemes have adopted sliding scales or exemptions for people who could not afford to pay (Bennett, Creese, and Monasch 1998).

Numerous studies have found that CBHI schemes increase utilization while (or as a result of) decreasing costs to the consumer. Schemes that cover hospital inpatient care have resulted in increased rates of utilization in such diverse settings as China (Bogg and others 1996), the Democratic Republic of Congo (Criel and Kegels 1997), Ghana (Atim 1999), and Kenya (Musau 1999). In Bwamanda District, Democratic Republic of Congo, Criel and Kegels found that rates of hospital utilization by members of a voluntary insurance scheme for hospital care were twice as high as those for the uninsured (49 versus 24.9 per thousand per year). The Nkoranza Community Financing Scheme in Ghana (Atim 1999) covers 100 percent of the costs of hospitalization. Members of the scheme were consistently more likely to be admitted to the hospital (4.6 to 6.3 percent admitted per year) than nonmembers (1.5 to 2.6 percent per year). We make the assumption in this study that increasing utilization rates among the poor in developing countries is a "good thing," at least from the perspective of scheme members. However, the inefficient overutilization of services (moral hazard) and the escalation of costs borne by the insurer or provider have been problematic, particularly in schemes that cover hospital inpatient care (Bennett, Creese, and Monasch 1998).

The Integrated Social Security Scheme of the Self-Employed Women's Association (SEWA) was initiated in 1992. This scheme provides life insurance, medical insurance, and asset insurance. Those who pay the annual Social Security Scheme premium of 72.5 rupees—30 rupees of which is earmarked for the Medical Insurance Fund (herein referred to as the Fund)—are covered to a maximum of 1,200 rupees yearly in case of hospitalization in any registered (private or public) facility. Only women between the ages of 18 and 58 are eligible for membership in the Fund. Women also have the option of becoming lifetime members of the Social Security Scheme by making a fixed deposit of 700 rupees. Interest on this is used to pay the annual premium, and the deposit is returned to the woman when she turns 58. Upon discharge from the hospital, members must first pay for the hospitalization out of pocket. They submit receipts and doctors' certificates to the Fund, and if the insurance claim is approved, they are reimbursed by check. Excluded from coverage under the Fund are certain chronic diseases (for example, chronic tuberculosis, certain cancers, diabetes, hypertension, piles) and "disease caused by addiction" (SEWA brochures 2000). Throughout the 10 districts of Gujarat where it operates, the Fund had approximately 23,000 members in 1999–2000. This compares with roughly 150,000 women covered under the broader SEWA trade union statewide.

The purpose of this chapter is to assess the impact of the Fund. The data for this analysis were collected from households in the Anand and Kheda Districts using an interview-administered questionnaire. We will look at impact in terms of (a) population reach of the Fund, particularly inclusion of the poor; (b) hospital utilization during the one-year period preceding the survey; and (c) annual cost of hospitalizations, conditional on reporting one or more hospitalizations.

We hypothesize that the Fund will do the following. First, it will include the very poor. The broader SEWA trade union organizes poor women working in the informal sector and seems to target quite effectively. By restricting membership in the Social Security Scheme (and hence the Fund) to members of the SEWA trade union, the Fund is likely to include women who are, on average, poorer than the general population.

Second, it will increase the frequency of hospitalization among the insured by removing some component (that is, the maximum 1,200 rupees) of the financial barrier to seeking inpatient care. Note that the impact on utilization is likely to be lessened by the fact that women must first pay out of pocket—which often means borrowing money, selling valuables, or performing extra work—before seeking reimbursement from SEWA.

Third, it will decrease the total annual hospital costs per person hospitalized. This basically assumes that (a) among insured women, some hospitalizations will be caused by conditions that are covered by the Fund, (b) women will actually seek reimbursement when they have been hospitalized for a covered condition, and (c) the Fund will reimburse women for some portion of the claims that are submitted.

METHODS

Data Collection and Analysis

This was a cross-sectional cohort study; respondents were interviewed at only one point in time, and we fixed in advance the number of SEWA and uninsured households (the two "cohorts"). Two-stage, random cluster sampling was used. The primary sampling units (PSUs) were villages. Twenty villages were selected randomly (using random-number tables); the probability of selection was equal for all villages regardless of size. The secondary sampling units were households. Within each village, the insured were randomly selected from lists compiled by SEWA, and the uninsured were randomly selected from census or voting lists. In 10 villages, 14 SEWA households and 14 uninsured households were sampled, and in 10 villages, 14 SEWA households and 28 uninsured households were sampled (20 villages × 14 SEWA households = 280 SEWA households; 10 villages × 14 controls + 10 villages × 28 controls = 420 controls; therefore, 700 households are included in this analysis).[1] The household questionnaire was administered between February 14, 2000, and May 6, 2000. An attempt was made to interview the female head of household.

Data were double entered into a Microsoft Access Database. Analysis was conducted using Stata. Special statistical tools (the "svy function" in Stata) have been used to correct for clustering and stratification. This means that all measures of central tendency, association, and variance have been weighted or adjusted to account for the different probability of a household's being selected in each of the primary sampling units.

The survey estimators are based on maximum likelihood estimation. We present adjusted Wald tests for all models; this is equivalent to the F-test of the significance of the regression. A p-value of 5 percent or less was used as criterion for significant association.

The analyses in this chapter are restricted to women of ages 18 to 58 years, as only they are eligible for participation in SEWA's Medical Insurance Fund.

Models

What was the population reach of the Fund? The model for looking at sociodemographic determinants of membership is a logit model, written as follows:

(8.1) $\ln(p/(1-p)) = X\beta + \varepsilon$

where p is the probability of being a member in the Fund, given female gender and age 18 to 58 years, and X represents a set of independent variables that are hypothesized to affect membership in community-based schemes.

Did the Fund affect hospital utilization over the past year? The model is a logit model. It estimates the probability of an individual's being hospitalized during the one-year period preceding the interview. It can be written as follows:

(8.2) $\ln(p/(1-p)) = X\beta + \varepsilon$

where p is the probability of hospitalization, given female gender and age 18 to 58 years, and X represents a set of independent variables that are hypothesized to affect individual patterns of hospital utilization.

Did the Fund affect net annual hospital costs per person hospitalized? The model is a log-linear model that estimates the net costs incurred for all hospitalizations (over one year), conditioned on positive hospitalization. Costs were net of reimbursement by insurance schemes, including the Fund. The model can be written as follows:

(8.3) $\ln Y = X\beta + \varepsilon$

where Y is the net annual hospital costs per person, given female gender, age 18 to 58 years, and one or more hospitalizations over one year, and X represents a set of independent variables hypothesized to affect individual patterns of hospital expenditure.[2]

Equations 8.2 and 8.3 are equivalent to the "two-part" (utilization and expenditure) model developed as part of the Rand Health Insurance Experiment and used more recently by Yip and Berman (2001) in their study of the impact of Egypt's School Health Insurance Programme.

Dependent Variables

Table 8.1 describes the independent variables included in the analyses. We include a number of household-level demand-side factors. Independent of insurance,

TABLE 8.1   Independent Variables Included in the Regression Analyses

Variables	Model 1	Model 2	Model 3
Characteristics of the household			
ESI1 to ESI5 = quintiles of economic status index, this is an approximation of HH wealth based on assets, ESI1 being the poorest and ESI5 the wealthiest. (These variables are exhaustive, ESI1 is left out of the models.)	✔	✔	✔
HINDU = 1 if Hindu religion, 0 if Muslim or Christian	✔	✔	✔
BKWDCASTE = 1 if scheduled caste, scheduled tribe, and other "backward caste," 0 if castes that have *not* been identified by government as "backward" (Bhakshipanch, Brahmin, Patel, Shah, etc.).	✔	✔	✔
HHSIZE1 = 1 if 1 to 2 people in HH HHSIZE2 = 1 if 3 to 4 people in HH HHSIZE3 = 1 if 5 to 9 people in HH HHSIZE4 = 1 if > 10 people in HH (These variables are exhaustive, HHSIZE1 is left out of the models.)	✔	✔	✔
Characteristics of the individual	✔	✔	✔
NON-INS = 1 if not insured by SEWA and not living with someone who is insured by SEWA SEWA-INS = 1 if covered by SEWA's Social Security Scheme SEWA-FAM = 1 if uninsured but living in the same household as someone insured by SEWA (These variables are exhaustive, NON-INS is left out of the models.)		✔	✔
AGE1 = 1 if 18 to 29 years of age AGE2 = 1 if 30 to 39 years of age AGE3 = 1 if 40 years of age or older (These variables are exhaustive, AGE1 is left out of the models.)	✔	✔	✔
LITERATE = 1 if person can read and write a simple letter, 0 if not	✔	✔	✔
MARRIED = 1 if married, 0 if never married, widowed, divorced, separated, or other	✔	✔	✔
DAILYWAGE = 1 if unskilled worker being paid daily wage (agricultural or factory worker) DOMESTIC = 1 if primary occupation is domestic work or housework OTHERWORK = 1 if other than unskilled daily wages or domestic work (These variables are exhaustive, OTHERWORK is left out of the models.)	✔	✔	✔
NUMBACUTE = number of acute illness episodes reported during the past 30 days (ranged from 0 to 3), intended to control for general level of health. We include this variable as a proxy, based on the hypothesis that those who are more sickly will have experienced illness episodes within the past month. This variable was included only in model 1 as it was collinear with SEWA-INS, the independent variable of interest in models 2 and 3.	✔		
Characteristics of the hospitalization			
PUBLIC = 1 if government or ESIS hospital PRIVATE = 1 if private for-profit hospital NONPROF = 1 if "trust" or charitable hospital (These variables are exhaustive, PUBLIC is left out of the models.)			✔
SHORT = 1 if 0 to 3 days hospitalized MEDIUM = 1 if 4 to 7 days hospitalized LONG = 1 if 8 days or more hospitalized (These variables are exhaustive, SHORT is left out of the models.)			✔
OB/GYN = 1 if cause of hospitalization was pregnancy, delivery, or family planning, 0 if other			✔

wealth is hypothesized to be positively associated with rates of hospitalization and with net costs of hospitalization. As a proxy for wealth, we construct an economic status index (ESI) based on household assets, allowing the weights of these assets to be determined by the statistical procedure of principal components (Filmer and Pritchett 2001). The other household-level variables controlled for are religion, caste, and number of people living in the household.

A number of individual-level, demand-side variables are controlled for. In all models, we control for age, literacy, marital status, and primary occupation. For models 2 and 3, individuals are classified as SEWA insured, uninsured but living in a household with at least one other insured person, and uninsured and not living with someone who is insured by SEWA. It was not uncommon for some adult women in a household to join the scheme while others abstained. We hypothesize that uninsured women living in the same households may also have increased rates of utilization, due to the information and education provided by SEWA and the positive wealth effect of having insured people in the household. In model 1, we control for the number of acute illness episodes reported during the past 30 days as a proxy for general level of health (unfortunately, we did not collect information on whether or not individuals had chronic diseases). We hypothesize that those in poorer health are more likely to join the Fund.

In model 3 only, we control for characteristics of the hospitalization. We hypothesize that use of private for-profit and private nonprofit hospitals (generally perceived to be of higher quality) will be associated with higher net costs of hospitalization than use of government facilities. Women who report longer episodes of hospitalization are expected to have experienced higher net costs. Finally, we anticipate that women hospitalized for pregnancy, delivery, and family planning will generally have experienced an uncomplicated hospitalization without major surgical procedures and for this reason will have lower net costs.

RESULTS

In total, 242 SEWA households and 381 control households were included in the analyses (some households were dropped from the analyses due to misclassification). In the 242 SEWA households, there were 270 members and 125 women ages 18 to 58 who were nonmembers. In the 381 control households, there were 607 women ages 18 to 58.

The demographic data (before controlling for any potential confounders) suggest that the SEWA-insured were of lower socioeconomic status than the uninsured in control households (see table 8.2). They ranked lower on the ESI. They were almost twice as likely as the uninsured to be of a "backward caste" and tended to be from smaller households. They were older (mean 40.1 versus 35.0 years), less likely to be literate, more likely to report primary occupation as unskilled labor for daily wages, and almost 60 percent more likely to have reported illness within the past 30 days (our proxy for frequency of chronic disease).

TABLE 8.2   Sample Characteristics

Variable	SEWA-INS	SEWA-FAM	NON-INS
Number of households	242		381
Number of individuals	270	125	607
Mean ESI	0.29		0.84
Cat: Quintiles of ESI			
% in 1st quintile	13.1		15.8
% in 2nd quintile	23.9		13.8
% in 3rd quintile	30.1		22.0
% in 4th quintile	13.8		18.9
% in 5th quintile	19.1		29.5
Religion			
% Hindu	80.7		79.3
% Muslim	7.4		18.5
% Christian	12.0		2.1
% ST, SC, or other "backward" caste	54.0		29.4
Mean number of household members	5.8		7.0
Cat: Number of HH members			
% 1–2	6.1		3.5
% 3–4	30.4		20.8
% 5–9	53.0		52.6
% >10	10.5		23.1
Mean age	40.1	26.3	35.0
Cat: Age			
% 10–<20	0.1	12.1	6.3
% 20–<30	15.9	61.4	34.0
% 30–<40	29.7	18.2	21.2
% 40+	54.3	8.3	38.4
% Literate	41.5	55.5	51.6
% Married	79.3	74.5	79.8
% Working for daily wages	25.0	11.4	16.9
% Doing domestic work	56.7	70.2	71.5

In the SEWA households interviewed, more than two-thirds of women ages 18 to 58 were enrolled in the Fund (see table 8.2). The SEWA-insured, in comparison to the uninsured living with SEWA members, were older (mean 40.1 versus 26.3 years), less likely to be literate, more than twice as likely to report that primary occupation was unskilled labor for daily wages, and more than four times as likely to have reported illness within the past 30 days.

TABLE 8.3   Hospital Utilization and Expenditure per Hospitalization by SEWA Coverage

	SEWA-INS (n = 270)		SEWA-FAM (n = 125)		NON-INS (n = 607)
Hospital utilization					
Total hospitalizations reported	28		12		56
Women with > 0 hospitalizations, 1 year	26		12		51
Probability of hospitalization	0.095	NS	0.105	NS	0.063
Hospital costs					
Total hospitalizations reimbursed	5		0		0
Women with > 0 reimbursement	5		0		0
Mean total hospital costs, 1 year	2,425	NS	3,532	NS	4,977

US$1 is approximately equal to 44 Rs.

Note: T-tests were performed to compare rates and expenditures of the SEWA-INS with NON-INS, and the SEWA-FAM with NON-INS.

Among the SEWA-insured who experienced hospitalizations during the one-year recall period, the frequency of reimbursement by SEWA was low (see table 8.3). There were 28 hospitalizations among Fund members; only 5 of these hospitalizations (18 percent) were reimbursed by SEWA. For the five members who were reimbursed, the costs before reimbursement were 4,431 rupees and after reimbursement 3,434 rupees.

Before controlling for sociodemographic variables, SEWA-insured were 1.5 times more likely than uninsured women in control households to have been hospitalized (0.095 versus 0.063). Among those hospitalized, the net annual hospital costs for the SEWA-insured were less than half those for the uninsured women in control households. (Clearly, this difference cannot be attributed to the Fund, given that even among the very few people reimbursed, the mean reimbursement amounted to less than one-quarter.)

Regression Analyses

Controlling for other sociodemographic variables, only older age and higher frequency of illness episodes within the past month were significantly associated with membership in the Fund (see table 8.4). Results were the same for the "full" and "best fit" models. Wealth, proxied by quintiles of ESI, was not significantly associated with membership in the Fund; there was a trend suggestive of higher levels of membership among the second and third income quintiles (compared with the first, or poorest, quintile), but this did not reach significance at the 95 percent level. Women of ages 30 years and above were 3.4 times as likely to join the Fund as those ages 18 to 20 (full model). Each additional illness reported within the past month (acute illnesses as well as exacerbations of chronic disease) was associated with a 70 percent (full model) to 80 percent (best fit) increase in the probability of joining the Fund.

TABLE 8.4   Regression Results for Equation 1, the Odds of Being SEWA-INS Based on Sociodemographic Variables: Logit Model (N = 987)

	Odds ratios (t-statistics)		*Odds ratios (t-statistics)*
	Full model		*Best fit model*
ESI2	1.906[a]	ESI2	1.837[a]
	(2.060)		(1.880)
ESI3	1.922	ESI3	1.793
	(1.280)		(1.090)
ESI4	0.961	ESI4	0.988
	(−0.150)		(−0.030)
ESI5	1.300	ESI5	1.287
	(0.700)		(0.650)
HINDU	0.720	HINDU	—
	(−0.550)		—
BKWDCASTE	2.450[a]	BKWDCASTE	2.563[a]
	(2.000)		(1.910)
HHSIZE2	0.821	HHSIZE (cont.)	0.940
	(−0.320)		(−1.220)
HHSIZE3	0.631		
	(−1.120)		
HHSIZE4	0.454		
	(−1.100)		
AGE2	3.356[c]	AGE (cont.)	1.040[c]
	(4.840)		(6.220)
AGE3	3.423[c]		
	(4.930)		
LITERATE	1.166	LITERATE	1.166
	(0.410)		(0.470)
MARRIED	0.970	MARRIED	—
	(−0.160)		—
DAILYWAGE	0.672	DAILYWAGE	0.888
	(−1.720)		(−0.470)
DOMESTIC	0.601	DOMESTIC	0.675
	(−1.640)		(−1.390)
NUMBACUTE	1.695[b]	NUMBACUTE	1.799[c]
	(2.690)		(3.090)
Adjusted Wald Test, F =	55		97
P-value =	0.003		0.000
Percent of predictions correct =	72.8%		72.9%

a. 10% (borderline) significance level.

b. 5% significance level.

c. 1% significance level.

TABLE 8.5   Regression Results for Equation 2, the Probability of Being Hospitalized within the Last Year: Logit Model (N = 987)

	Odds ratios (t-statistics)	Odds ratios (t-statistics)
	Full model	Best fit model
SEWA-INS	2.042	1.668
	(1.220)	(0.960)
SEWA-FAM	1.639	1.999
	(1.000)	(1.640)
ESI2	0.564	0.522
	(−1.370)	(−1.540)
ESI3	0.801	0.762
	(−0.460)	(−0.540)
ESI4	0.798	0.690
	(−0.540)	(−0.890)
ESI5	0.275[a]	0.253[a]
	(−1.960)	(−1.940)
HINDU	1.578	1.638
	(1.100)	(1.100)
BKWDCASTE	0.785	—
	(−0.700)	—
HHSIZE2	2.328	2.729
	(1.020)	(1.200)
HHSIZE3	1.687	2.307
	(0.680)	(1.010)
HHSIZE4	0.846	1.233
	(−0.190)	(0.240)
AGE2	0.450	—
	(−1.270)	—
AGE3	0.386[a]	—
	(−1.990)	—
LITERATE	0.585	0.766
	(−1.190)	(−0.620)
MARRIED	1.522	1.453
	(0.670)	(0.750)
DAILYWAGE	0.733	0.719
	(−0.470)	(−0.520)
DOMESTIC	1.254	1.499
	(0.390)	(0.690)
Adjusted Wald Test, F =	36	21
P-value =	0.027	0.002
Percent of predictions correct =	91.6%	91.6%

a. 10% (borderline) significance level.

Neither membership in the Fund nor any of the sociodemographic variables tested were significantly associated with the probability of having been hospitalized (see table 8.5). Again, results were similar for the full and best fit models. There was a trend suggestive of higher rates of hospitalization among Fund members (and even women living in the same households as Fund members), but this association was not significant. There were also trends toward lower frequency of hospitalization among higher ESI quintiles and lower frequency of hospitalization with increasing age, but again these were not significant at the 95 percent level.

Results of the model of annual hospital costs per person hospitalized varied somewhat with changes in the variables included and the removal of outliers (see table 8.6). In some models, hospital expenditures were significantly lower among the SEWA insured (models 3B, 3C, and 3D). Interestingly, this finding *was not* sensitive to removal from the model of the five cases of hospitalization that were reimbursed; in model 3D, being insured by SEWA was associated with a decrease in hospital expenditures of 54 percent (β = –0.789) even though the five reimbursed hospitalizations were removed from the calculations. Consistent in the various iterations of model 3 were the findings that hospital expenditures varied directly (and significantly) with quintiles of ESI, were significantly higher for private than for public hospitalizations, and were significantly lower for pregnancy, delivery, or family planning than for other causes.

DISCUSSION

Strengths and Limitations of the Study

Perhaps the greatest limitation of this study was its small sample size. The study shows trends toward higher rates of utilization and lower spending per episode of hospitalization among SEWA members (significant in some models). Had the study been larger, these associations might have been statistically significant (or in the case of spending, consistently statistically significant). Insufficient sample size arose in part because there were fewer Fund members in "insured" households than had been expected and because of the problem of misclassification of households—that is, households were identified as including a Fund member when in fact they did not. Such households were dropped from the analysis without replacement.

It is difficult to say how accurately the economic status index reflected household "wealth." A very similar index developed for Indian survey data (Filmer and Pritchett 2001) was closely correlated with state domestic product (SDP) and poverty rates data. Using data from Indonesia, Nepal, and Pakistan, they also showed their asset index to be consistent with consumption expenditures. Comparison of our asset index with the interviewers' assessments of wealth and with daily household expenditures on food suggested strong correlation (data not presented here). Nonetheless, it is possible that some of the "negative results" in this study were due to insufficiently controlling for wealth. For example, if, as

TABLE 8.6   Regression Results for Equation 3

	Odds ratios (t-statistics)			
	3A full model N = 77	3B best fit N = 81	3C outliers removed N = 74	3D reimbursed removed N = 70
SEWA-INS	−0.630 (−1.190)	−1.744[b] (−2.350)	−0.812[b] (−2.290)	−0.789[b] (−2.140)
SEWA-FAM	0.560 (0.900)	0.289 (0.300)	0.000 (0.000)	−0.048 (−0.100)
ESI2	1.662[b] (2.270)	1.908[c] (2.930)	1.356[c] (4.000)	1.353[c] (3.960)
ESI3	1.779[b] (2.800)	1.237[c] (2.900)	0.550[a] (1.740)	0.551 (1.690)
ESI4	2.171[b] (2.810)	1.273[c] (3.180)	1.235[b] (2.640)	1.234[b] (2.630)
ESI5	2.443[b] (2.7Z0)	2.356[b] (2.580)	1.266[b] (2.480)	1.345[b] (2.620)
HINDU	3.630[c] (3.300)	— —	— —	— —
BKWDCASTE	0.465 (1.700)	1.103[b] (2.120)	0.270 (1.560)	0.268 (1.450)
HHSIZE2	−1.301[c] (−3.440)	— —	— —	— —
HHSIZE3	−1.610[c] (−3.500)	— —	— —	— —
HHSIZE4	−0.581 (−1.490)	— —	— —	— —
AGE2	−0.246 (−0.570)	— —	— —	— —
AGE3	0.403 (1.090)	— —	— —	— —

(continued)

hypothesized, SEWA membership was inversely associated with wealth, and wealth was directly associated with hospital spending, then failure to fully control for wealth could result in an observed estimate of effect diluted toward the null. Though not presented in this chapter, all of the models were run using two other indicators of wealth (interviewers' assessments and daily per capita food consumption) with no major changes in the results.

Several questions were not included in the household questionnaire that, in retrospect, should have been included. For example, it is common in such analyses to control for the presence of "chronic diseases," but these data were not available from our questionnaire. It would have been both interesting and informative to know, among the SEWA-insured women who had undergone hospitalization, the number who had submitted claims but were still awaiting a response

TABLE 8.6   Continued

	Odds ratios (t-statistics)			
	3A full model N = 77	3B best fit N = 81	3C outliers removed N = 74	3D reimbursed removed N = 70
LITERATE	0.152 (0.420)	— —	— —	— —
MARRIED	2.861[b] (2.620)	0.659 (0.560)	−0.019 (−0.020)	−0.004 (0.000)
DAILYWAGE	0.885 (0.950)	0.412 (0.430)	−0.223 (−0.450)	−0.247 (−0.510)
DOMESTIC	0.793 (0.980)	0.674 (0.830)	0.325 (0.510)	0.345 (0.540)
PRIVATE	4.306[c] (10.710)	4.453[c] (5.140)	2.600[c] (8.220)	2.601[c] (8.300)
NONPROF	3.115[a] (2.080)	3.058[a] (2.080)	1.763[b] (2.290)	1.737 (2.070)
MEDIUM (4 to 7 days)	0.206 (0.420)	1.092[a] (1.810)	0.249 (0.740)	0.242 (0.690)
LONG (> 7 days)	0.716 (1.370)	1.433[a] (1.750)	1.445[c] (4.800)	1.453[c] (4.640)
OB/GYN	−1.379[b] (−2.430)	−1.357[c] (−4.170)	−1.312[c] (−4.190)	−1.334[c] (−3.940)
Adjusted Wald Test, F =	95	47	8	7
P-value =	0.081	0.001	0.031	0.069
R-squared =	79.32%	66.19%	67.24%	67.76%

a. 10% (borderline) significance level.

b. 5% significance level.

c. 1% significance level.

or had been unsuccessful in their claims. Finally, for purposes of triangulation (that is, verifying the ESI), we could have collected data on household expenditures on a small number of items, as a proxy for total household expenditures (Morris and others 2000).

It is possible, though unlikely, that observation bias affected the study results. Interviewer bias may have occurred if investigators elicited or interpreted information differently among the insured and the uninsured. It was impossible to blind interviewers to the insurance status of the household. Certainly, the interviewers came to make generalizations about households (for example, that SEWA households tended to be very poor). Thus there may have been some bias in the way they recorded household asset information. It is also possible that the interviewers probed more carefully into health care seeking and spending among poorer households. Study subjects may also have reported events in a noncomparable manner (recall bias). For example, SEWA members may be likelier to recall episodes of hospitalization or to remember how much they have paid for hospitalization as they have been sensitized to the subject by the information, education, and communication from SEWA (or they have spent months collecting and processing the related paperwork). Perhaps the lower hospital expenditures reported by the SEWA insured is a function of more accurate recall (that is, a lower probability of accidentally inflating the figures).

Unlike many other CBHI schemes, SEWA has not excluded the very poor. What design factors have facilitated inclusion of the poor in the SEWA scheme? The fact that the SEWA Integrated Social Security Scheme is nested within the larger development organization (the SEWA workers union) has undoubtedly been an important factor. Bennett, Creese, and Monasch (1998, p. 20) hypothesize that "communities may be more willing to participate actively in health insurance schemes (initiated by NGOs involved in broad community development activities) since they consider that their priority needs—for a stable income, for instance—are also being addressed." Other factors that are likely to have facilitated inclusion of the poor include an affordable premium, village-level representatives who are themselves poor, self-employed women, and efforts to serve geographically isolated villages.

The positive associations between older age and higher frequency of illness and membership in SEWA's insurance scheme suggest that adverse selection may be occurring. Bennett, Creese, and Monasch (1998), in their review of community-based health insurance schemes, found that adverse selection affected schemes covering hospital inpatient care, in particular. The fact that membership in the SEWA scheme is voluntary and individual may enable adverse selection. However, the waiting period after joining and the exclusion of preexisting or chronic diseases are meant to limit adverse selection. It is likely that adverse selection is to some extent encouraged by scheme functionaries, insofar as poor households with limited expendable income may be encouraged to insure the household member most likely to fall ill. Furthermore, the scheme does fall somewhere on the spectrum between health insurer (strictly defined) and "social service" in that the scheme does aim to improve access to hospital care among the poor and to protect the poor from the costs of hospitalization. As such, adverse selection may be viewed in a positive light. If it is decided to try to deter adverse selection under the scheme, additional methods that could be used include (a) making the household, or even the village, the unit of membership and enforcing this rule strictly; (b) stipulating that if a village is to be allowed to enter a scheme a certain proportion of households in the village must join; and (c) making the scheme compulsory (Bennett, Creese, and Monasch 1998, p. 56).

We found no significant association between membership in SEWA's Medical Insurance Fund and frequency of hospitalization, although there was a non-significant trend toward higher rates of hospitalization among SEWA members. Table 8.7 summarizes the results of other studies that have examined the impact

TABLE 8.7   Summary of Studies Looking at the Impact of CBHI Schemes on Utilization and Out-of-Pocket Expenditures

Study	Description of study	Utilization	Expenditure
Rwanda (Schneider and Diop 2001)	Fifty-four prepayment schemes in 3 districts covering some outpatient and inpatient costs. What does the scheme cover? Sample size of 11,583 (2,518 HH). Data collection, yr. 2000.	Increased probability (6.6 times) of "at least one visit to professional health care provider."	Decreased (by approx. 60%) "total out-of-pocket payment per illness episode."
Senegal (Jütting 2001)	Three Mutual Health Insurance Schemes that cover part of the costs of hospitalization. Sample size of 2,987 (346 HH). Data collection, yr. 2000.	Increased "proportion of sample with at least one hospitalization."	Decreased "out-of-pocket spending on hospitalization" (48%).
India (Gumber 2001)	Self-Employed Women's Association (SEWA); covers hospital costs only, to 1,200 rupees. Sample size 1,200 HH in nonrandomly selected clusters. Data collection, yr. 1998–99.	Decreased likelihood (down by 63%) of seeking ambulatory care in case of illness. (Perhaps women are "jumping the queue"?)	No change in "total annual cost (direct and indirect) of health care use." Neither ambulatory nor inpatient.
Democratic Republic of Congo (Criel and Kegels 1997)	District-level scheme that covers 80% of hospitalization costs at referral hospital. Routinely collected hospitalization data.	Rates of hospitalization were consistently higher (1.5 to 2 times) among the insured.	—
Ghana (Atim 1999)	Nkoranza community-financing scheme. Covers 100% of hospital costs for referred patients. Hospital data from 1992 to 1994.	Members are consistently more likely (2.3 to 4 times) to be admitted to a hospital than nonmembers.	—
China (Bogg and others 1996)	Comprehensive health insurance system in Jintan County. Partial reimbursement for drugs, outpatient and inpatient visits. Data from 1986 to 1994.	Evidence for increased utilization of inpatient care.	—
Niger (Diop and others 1995)	Boboye district. Mandatory taxation. Coverage of "pharmaceutical products." Longitudinal data.	The number of initial visits (outpatient) increased by nearly 40% during the year following implementation.	Total illness-related expenditure dropped by 48%.

Note: HH = household.

Source: Format adapted from Jakab and others (2001).

of CBHI schemes on rates of hospitalization. Almost all other studies found that community-based insurance covering the costs of hospitalization increases hospital utilization.[3] This may reflect a publication bias, wherein the most successful schemes are the ones most likely to have been studied and reported on. If we accept these findings as valid, then a question arises: Why has the SEWA scheme not resulted in significantly increased rates of utilization? The scheme's failure to affect hospital utilization is attributable to the factors that have prevented women from using the Fund (that is, the factors that have prevented women from submitting insurance claims). Data from qualitative interviews (Ranson 2001) suggested that members of the Fund are sometimes unaware of their membership or the benefits of the scheme. Furthermore, among those who do know about the scheme, rates of reimbursement may be considered low by members (as the Fund does not cover, for example, transportation or bribes), while the costs of submitting a claim (for example, transportation to the SEWA office, opportunity cost of missed work, bribes paid to doctors for hospital certificates) are potentially quite high.

There were significant (but not consistently so) associations between SEWA membership and lower costs of hospitalization. Very few other studies have looked at whether CBHI has actually resulted in decreased out-of-pocket expenditures (see table 8.7). In a small study of four mutuals in Senegal (carried out in 2000), Jütting (2001) found that "being a member reduces the expenditure for hospitalization by 48 percent in comparison to nonmembers holding all other variables constant." Other studies (Schneider and Diop 2001; Diop, Yazbeck, and Bitran 1995) have found decreased spending (both outpatient and inpatient) per illness episode. Interestingly, in our study the association between membership in SEWA's Fund and decreased hospital spending was not due to reimbursement by the scheme, as the associations remained even after we removed the five reimbursed hospitalizations from the sample. The difference then may result from methodological problems, such as failure to adequately control for wealth or other potential confounders (most important, severity of illness resulting in hospitalization). Alternatively, it may be that the scheme confers protection from hospital costs in some other way. For example, doctors may charge SEWA members less as the doctors know the scheme is restricted to the poor, self-employed (unlikely, given that providers are usually unaware of SEWA, far less a woman's membership status in the organization or insurance scheme). It may also be that SEWA members are more sensitive to the costs of hospitalization and as a result are more likely, or better able, to seek out low-cost hospital care.

Conclusions and Policy Recommendations

Members of the Fund were similar to the general population in terms of wealth. The Fund's success at including the poor was probably due to its being nested within a development organization committed to serving poor, self-employed women. Members of the Fund were older and sicker than the general population, suggestive either of adverse selection or effective targeting of those most in need of inpatient care. In either case, the Fund can facilitate risk pooling by broadening its membership to include younger and healthier individuals, by requiring, for example, enrollment of all eligible women in a household.

Relatively few of those who were members of the Fund and were hospitalized were reimbursed through the scheme. This suggests that either women are not submitting claims even when they might be eligible for reimbursement or that the claims are not eligible for reimbursement (for example, if the hospitalization resulted from certain chronic illnesses). Given the low rate of utilization of the Fund by those who are members, it is not surprising that the Fund had no discernable affect in terms of health care utilization. Rates of Fund utilization may be increased by providing members with information and education about their membership in the Fund and its benefits, and by making the process of claims submission easier, faster, and less expensive.

Acknowledgments: The author of this report is grateful to the World Health Organization (WHO) for having provided an opportunity to contribute to the work of the Commission on Macroeconomics and Health and to the World Bank for having published the material in this chapter as an HNP Discussion Paper.

This research was supported by the British Department for International Development (DfID). The author wishes to thank members of the Self-Employed Women's Association for their support and Anne Mills and Kara Hanson for stimulating review comments. The findings, interpretations, and conclusions expressed in the chapter are entirely those of the author and do not necessarily represent the views of the World Bank, its Executive Directors, or the countries they represent.

NOTES

1. Note that this study was actually designed to look at *two* community-based insurance schemes, SEWA and the Tribhuvandas Foundation (TF), and a total of 1,120 households were actually interviewed. However, TF households and their controls are not included in this analysis.

2. In the log-linear model, the coefficient β for a *continuous* independent variable gives the relative change in the mean value of Y for a unit change in X. To obtain the relative change in mean Y for a *dummy variable,* one must take the antilog (to base e) of the estimated dummy coefficient and subtract it from 1 (Gujarati 1995, p. 525).

3. Note that the other study of the SEWA scheme, by Gumber (2001), has not examined the impact of the scheme on hospital utilization

REFERENCES

Atim, C. 1999. "Social Movements and Health Insurance: A Critical Evaluation of Voluntary, Nonprofit Insurance Schemes with Case Studies from Ghana and Cameroon." *Social Science and Medicine* 48(7): 881–96.

Bennett, S., A. Creese, and R. Monasch. 1998. *Health Insurance Schemes for People Outside Formal Sector Employment.* Geneva: World Health Organization.

Bogg, L., D. Hengjin, W. Keli, C. Wenwei, and V. Diwan. 1996. "The Cost of Coverage: Rural Health Insurance in China." *Health Policy and Planning* 11(3): 238–52.

Criel, B., and G. Kegels. 1997. "A Health Insurance Scheme for Hospital Care in Bwamanda District, Zaire: Lessons and Questions after 10 Years of Functioning." *Tropical Medicine and International Health* 2(7): 654–72.

Diop, F., A. Yazbeck, and R. Bitran. 1995. "The Impact of Alternative Cost Recovery Schemes on Access and Equity in Niger." *Health Policy and Planning* 10(3): 223–40.

Filmer, D., and L. H. Pritchett. 2001. "Estimating Wealth Effects Without Expenditure Data—or Tears: An Application to Educational Enrollments in States of India." *Demography* 38(1): 115–32.

Gujarati, D. 1995. *Basic Econometrics,* 3d ed. London: McGraw-Hill.

Gumber, A. 2001. *Hedging the Health of the Poor: The Case for Community Financing in India.* HNP Discussion Paper. Washington, D.C.: World Bank.

Jakab, M., A. S. Preker, C. Krishnan, P. Schneider, F. Diop, J. Jütting, A. Gumber, K. Ranson, and S. Supakankunti. 2001. *Social Inclusion and Financial Protection through Community Financing: Initial Results from Five Household Surveys.* Report submitted to Working Group 3 of the Commission on Macroeconomics and Health, Jeffrey D. Sachs (Chairman). WHO, Geneva.

Jütting, J. 2001. *The Impact of Community-Based Health Financing on Financial Protection: Case Study Senegal.* HNP Discussion Paper. Washington, D.C.: World Bank.

Morris, S., C. Carletto, J. Hoddinott, and L. Christiaensen. 2000. "Validity of Rapid Estimates of Household Wealth and Income for Health Surveys in Rural Africa." *Journal of Epidemiology and Community Health* (London) 54: 381–87.

Musau, S. 1999. *Community-Based Health Insurance: Experiences and Lessons Learned from East and Southern Africa.* Technical Report No. 34. Partnerships for Health Reform Project, Abt Associates, Inc., Bethesda, Md.

Ranson, M. K. 2001. "The Consequences of Health Insurance for the Informal Sector: Two Non-Governmental, Nonprofit Schemes in Gujarat." Ph.D. thesis in progress. London School of Hygiene and Tropical Medicine.

Schneider P., and F. Diop. 2001. *Synopsis of Results on the Impact of Community-Based Health Insurance (CBHI) on Financial Accessibility to Health Care in Rwanda.* HNP Discussion Paper. Washington, D.C.: World Bank.

WHO (World Health Organization). 2000. *The World Health Report 2000: Health Systems: Improving Performance.* Geneva.

Yip, W, and P. Berman. 2001. "Targeted Health Insurance in a Low Income Country and Its Impact on Access and Equity in Access: Egypt's School Health Insurance." *Health Economics* 10(2): 207–20.

CHAPTER 9

The Potential Role of Community Financing in India

Anil Gumber

Abstract: This chapter reviews the existing community-based and self-financing health insurance schemes in India that cater to the general population and address the needs of the society's poor and vulnerable section. It discusses critical issues of accessibility and use of health care services, out-of-pocket expenditure on treatment, and the need for health insurance for poor rural and urban households pursuing varied occupations. The chapter examines in detail the determinants of enrollment in the community-based financing scheme, using the household-level data from the pilot study undertaken in Gujarat. It also investigates the issue of how much health insurance mitigates the households' burden of health care expenditure. The findings suggest that the community plan fairly addresses equity in enrollment but that, in terms of providing financial protection, social insurance coverage is much more successful.

More than 90 percent of India's population and almost all its poor have no health insurance coverage. They primarily meet health care needs through direct out-of-pocket expenditure on services provided by the public and private sectors. Furthermore, various health care services studies show that the poor and other disadvantaged groups (scheduled castes and scheduled tribes) are forced to spend a higher proportion of their income on health care than better-off groups. For the disadvantaged, the burden of treatment, especially inpatient care, is disproportionately heavy (Visaria and Gumber 1994). In addition, this group suffers a high incidence of morbidity, which adversely affects their household budgets in two ways: in the large amounts of money and resources they have to spend on medical care, and in the earnings they have to forgo during periods of illness. Thus they often have to borrow funds at very high interest rates to meet both medical expenses and other household consumption needs. One possible consequence of this is that these families could be pushed into a zone of permanent poverty.

There are also concerns about problems in accessibility and the use of subsidized public health facilities. Most poor households, especially rural ones, reside in backward, hilly, and remote regions, where neither government facilities nor private medical practitioners are available. These households have to depend heavily on poor quality services provided by local, often unqualified, practitioners and faith healers. Wherever accessibility is not a constraint, the primary health centers are generally found to be either dysfunctional or providers of low-quality services. The government's claim to provide free secondary and tertiary care does not stand up; in reality, patients are charged for various services (Gumber 1997).

Estimates based on a large-scale health care utilization survey of 1993 suggest that, overall, about 6 percent of household income is spent on curative care, which amounts to Rs. 250 per capita per year (Shariff and others 1999). However, the burden of expenditure on health care is unduly heavy on households in the informal sector, indicating the potential for voluntary comprehensive health insurance schemes for these segments of society.

Overall, health insurance coverage is low. Only 9 percent of the Indian workforce is covered by some form of health insurance (through the Central Government Health Scheme [CGHS], the Employees' State Insurance Scheme [ESIS], and Mediclaim), and most of those insured belong to the organized sector (Gumber 1998). Health insurance coverage is so sparse because government policy has been to provide free health services through public hospitals, dispensaries, and clinics. As noted above, however, public sector providers charge patients for various services, and outreach is also poor. According to estimates based on the National Sample Survey (NSS) 1986–87, nationally 42 percent of inpatients and 30 percent of outpatients using public sector facilities had paid for various services; the percentages varied substantially between rural and urban areas and among states (Gumber 1997). Furthermore, health care costs have increased enormously. A comparison of NSS data for 1986–87 and 1995–96 suggests that the cost of inpatient care and outpatient care grew annually at 26–31 percent and 15–16 percent, respectively, putting severe strains on efforts to achieve equity in health care (Gumber 2001).

Nongovernmental organizations (NGOs) and charitable institutions (not-for-profit) have played an important role in the delivery of affordable health services to the poor, but their coverage has always been small. The issue is how to reach the unreached and how to ensure that the uninsured receive at least a minimum of affordable quality services.

The public insurance companies so far have paid very little attention to voluntary medical insurance because of low profitability, high risk, and lack of demand. From the consumer point of view, insurance coverage is low because consumers lack information about the private insurance plans, and the mechanisms used by the health insurance providers are not suitable for consumers. Furthermore, compared with ESIS and with the community-based schemes, the private plans offer a modicum of benefits (table 9.1), that is, only hospitalization and that with many exclusions (such as preexisting conditions). One analysis suggests that the existing voluntary health insurance plans cover only between 55 and 67 percent of total hospitalization costs and, on average, only 10 to 20 percent of the total annual out-of-pocket expenditure on health care (Gumber 2000a).

Gender bias in use of health care persists. For various socioeconomic and cultural reasons, men have better access than women. Poor women are most vulnerable to diseases and ill health because they live in unhygienic conditions, carry a heavy childbearing burden, place little emphasis on their own health

TABLE 9.1   Type of Health Care Burden on Households Covered by Health Insurance Schemes

	Type of care or cost	ESIS	SEWA	Mediclaim
Inpatient	Medical	✔	✔	✔
	Transport and other direct cost	✗	✗	✗
	Loss of earnings	✔	✗	✗
Outpatient	Medical	✔	✗	✗
	Transport and other direct cost	✗	✗	✗
	Loss of earnings	✔	✗	✗
Preventive and promotive	Immunization	✔	✗	✗
	Prenatal and postnatal care	✔	✗	✗
	Maternity care	✔	✔	✗
	Family planning	✗	✗	✗

Note: Self-Employed Women's Association (SEWA) and Mediclaim are reimbursement plans (subject to the sum assured) while ESIS is a facility-based plan.

care needs, and encounter severe constraints in seeking health care for themselves. Thus far institutional arrangements to correct these gender differentials have been lacking. A pioneering study undertaken by Gumber and Kulkarni (2000) looked into issues related to the availability and needs of health insurance coverage for the poor, especially women, and the scope and likely problems in extending current health insurance benefits to workers in the informal sector.

This chapter attempts to review existing community-based and self-financing health insurance schemes in India that serve the general population and address the needs of the poor and vulnerable. It discusses some critical issues concerning accessibility and use of health care services, out-of-pocket expenditure on health care, and the need for health insurance for poor rural and urban households pursuing varied occupations. The chapter examines in detail the determinants of enrollment in the community-based financing scheme, using household-level data from the pilot study. It also investigates the issue of how much health insurance mitigates the households' burden of health care expenditure.

COMMUNITY FINANCING IN INDIA AND THE SEWA PROGRAM

Community and self-generated financing programs are usually run by NGOs or nonprofit organizations. These organizations rely on financing from various sources, including government, donor agencies, and community and self-generated sources. Among the many innovative methods being used to finance health care services are progressive premium scales, community-based prepayment and insurance schemes, and income-generating schemes. These organizations' target populations for health care services are primarily workers and families outside the formal sector. Program revenue comes from the following sources:

- User fees, defined as the payment made by the beneficiaries directly to the health care provider (for example, fees for services or prices paid for drugs and immunizations). This mode of financing is not common.

- Prepayment-insurance schemes, including payment by members for drugs at either subsidized rates or cost.

- Commercial for-profit schemes actively run by health care finance organizations.

- Fund-raising activities by organizations to pay for health care services. This type of revenue represents more than 5 percent of some organizations' total funding.

- Contributions in-kind (for example, rice, sorghum, community labor). Because this method is hard to manage, it is not very popular.

Other sources of community-based and self-financing include the Tribhuvandas Foundation, which provides health care through village milk cooperatives, and Amul Union (the milk cooperative organization), which puts a tax on milk collection to pay for health care.

Tables 9.2 and 9.3 describe select schemes. Most of the successful case studies (Dave 1991) happen to be in the states of Assam, Gujarat, Maharashtra, Nadu, Orissa, Tamil, and West Bengal. The experience of such schemes could be useful for understanding their merits and disadvantages and their potential for replication in other states. The most pertinent points about these schemes are that they are rurally oriented and have the ability to mobilize resources in a village community. However, most of these schemes have served only a small segment of the population, and their health coverage has been restricted to elementary, preventive, and maternal and child health (MCH) care.

Microcredit Linked Health Insurance Schemes

To break the vicious circle of poverty, malnutrition, disease, low productivity, and low income, several NGOs and governments in developing countries have started microcredit schemes for vulnerable groups. Microcredit is considered not only an effective tool for reducing poverty but also an instrument for empowering the poor, especially women. This operation generates income for the poor by extending small credits for self-employment and other economic activities. However, loan repayments by these groups fell far below the expected level. The experience suggested that ill health, expenditures on treatment, and associated consumption needs were the prime reasons for defaults. To stop the erosion of borrowers' income by health care needs, some NGOs (such as Grameen Bank in Bangladesh and the Self-Employed Women's Association [SEWA] in India) have introduced health insurance schemes for their members. The Grameen Bank Health Program was started in 1994 to adopt disease-prevention measures, to arrange for minimum-cost treatment, and to build a nonprofit primary health care system. Under this scheme, the borrowers were asked to pay a fixed annual amount of 60 taka per family as a premium and a small sum at the time of use. A 2000 study found that the scheme had met the desired objectives (Rahman 2000).

TABLE 9.2 Salient Characteristics of Selected NGO-Managed Health Insurance Schemes

Voluntary organizations/ location	Date started	Service provided	Health service delivery/ organization	Population served	Total annual cost (Rs.)
Sevagram/ Wardha, Maharashtra	Hospital—1945 Community health program—1972	500-bed hospital Outreach community health program	Trained male VHW provides basic curative, preventive, and promotive health care. Mobile with doctor and ANM provides care every 2 months.	— 19,457	— 69,459
Bombay Mother and Child Welfare Society (BMCWS)/ Chawla, Bombay	1947	Health activities: two maternity hospitals (40 beds each) with child welfare centers Nonhealth activities: day care centers, convalescent home	Outpatient and inpatient maternity care Outpatient pediatric care, including immunization	—	120,175 (health and nonhealth combined)
Raigarh Ambikapur Health Association (RAHA)/Raigarh, Madhya Pradesh	Hospital—1969 Community health services—started 1974	Federation of 3 referral hospitals and 65 independent health centers with outreach community care	RAHA functions include management of insurance scheme, training, and support for health centers. Health centers staffed by nurse provide outpatient care, run MCH clinic. VHWs provide community-based care.	400,000	30,000–50,000 (cost range of individual health centers of which there are 65)
Christian Hospital/ Bissamaucuttak, Orissa	Hospital—1954 Outreach community care—1980	120 bed hospital Community project currently not operational	Outpatient/inpatient care, specialties include obstetrics, gynecology, surgery, ophthalmology	—	1,911,740 (hospital only)
UPASI/ Coocnoor, Tamil Nadu	19th century CLWS—1971	Association of tea growers runs comprehensive labor welfare scheme (CLWS)	CLWS provides training and management support to health programs of individual tea estates. Tea estates have small cottage hospital and outreach care provided by local workers.	250,000	300,000
Goalpur Co-operative Health Society/ Shanthiniketan, West Bengal	1964	Dispensary, periodic community health services	Doctor provides outpatient care twice weekly	1,247	32,000

(continued)

TABLE 9.2 Continued

Voluntary organizations/ location	Date started	Service provided	Health service delivery/ organization	Population served	Total annual cost (Rs.)
Students Health Home/ West Bengal	1955	Polyclinic plus 28 regional clinics	Polyclinic has 20 beds, provides outpatient and inpatient care. Regional clinics provide outpatient care only, health education campaigns, and blood donation camps.	550,000	2,950,745
Saheed Shabsankar Saba Samithi (SSSS)/ Burdwan, West Bengal	1978	Dispensary, occupational health activities, rural health program, school health program, and fair-price medicine shop	Doctors provide outpatient care weekly at MCH clinic.	—	87,780
Arvind Eye Hospital/ Madurai, Tanil Nadu	1976	2 urban hospitals (100 beds), 2 rural hospitals (500 beds), and outreach program	Outpatient and inpatient eye care provided. Regular eye camps organized.	—	10,987,700
Tribhuvandas Foundation/ Anand, Gujarat	1980	Community-based health program linked with milk cooperatives, regional rehabilitation centers, and Balwadis women's income-generating scheme.	CHWs provide basic curative, preventive, and promotive care. Field supervisors provide support to CHWs, milk society building used as base for coordinating health services.	300,000	1,080,000 (health and nonhealth combined)
SEWA/ Ahemadabad, Gujarat	Union—1972 Health program—1984	Union of self-employed women helps organize women into cooperatives of various traders and provides credit facilities. It provides health care as a support that stocks rational generic drugs.	Health centers established in urban slums and rural villages. CHWs provide basic care; doctors provide support twice weekly.	63,000	391,850 (health program only)
CINI/Daulatpur, West Bengal	1975	Community-based health programs, dispensary, and outreach rehabilitation center. Other activities: income-generating schemes, farm, health training, research	CHWs provide MCH care through Mahila Mandals. Doctors run daily OPD, weekly MCH clinic, supplementary feeding.	70,000 (community health project)	1,900,000

Notes: — not available; ANM, auxiliary nurse and midwife; MCH, maternal and child health; VHW, village health worker.
Source: Dave (1991).

TABLE 9.3 Prepayment and Insurance Mechanisms in Selected NGO-Managed Health Insurance Schemes

Features	Sevagram	RAHA	Tribhuvandas Foundation	Goalpur	Students Health Home	SSSS
Coverage provided	Household	Individual	Household	Household	Institutional and individual	Individual
Annual subscription fee	8 payali sorghum (landless) and 2 payali sorghum per acre extra (landholders), or equivalent cash	Rs. 5 or Rs. 2 rice	Rs. 10	Rs. 18 in cash or in kind (rice or labor)	Rs. 2— institutions Rs. 6—individuals	Rs. 2 or Rs. 5
Number of members	At least 75% of households (23 villages covered). Total insured: 14,390	75,000	Approximately 1/5 to 1/6 of all households in villages, (319 villages covered)	150 out of 175 households in village	630 institutes; total 350,000 students covered	6,800
Member entitlement	Community care: free CHW services, drugs, and mobile (doctor + ANM) services. Hospital: free care for unphased illness episodes; 25% subsidy for anticipated illness episodes, such as pregnancy and chronic ailments	Community care: free CHW services and drugs. Free health center services, including MCH clinic. Hospital: free care after paying entrance fee up to ceiling of Rs. 1000	Community care: free services, subsidized drugs. Hospital: 50% subsidy	Dispensary: free doctor consultations and drugs at cost; free periodic public health activities	Polyclinic/regional clinics: free consultations, drugs, diagnostic tests, operations, and bed stay at nominal charges	Outpatient clinic: free consultations, drugs at cost, and free MCH care
Nonmember entitlement	Nonmembers not entitled to use community health services	Nonmembers charged for drugs (over cost), not entitled to attend MCH clinic	Nonmembers have same emoluments to community services as members but not to hospital care	Nonmembers charged for drugs (over cost)	Nonmembers not entitled to avail themselves of services	Nonmembers are not entitled to avail themselves of services
Management of fund	VHW responsible for membership collections. Collections once a year at harvest time. Compulsory that 75% of villages covered.	Individual health centers responsible for membership collections. Collections once a year. New members waiting period 2 months before services entitlements. Rs. 3 retained by center, Rs. 2 to RAHA for referral fund.	VHW services responsible for membership collections. Collected once a year when bonus payments distributed (nonadult society members can also enroll in scheme).	Village health communities— funds collections once a year.	Institutions enrolled once a year. Individuals' enrollment ongoing (no waiting period).	Able to enroll throughout the year. No waiting period between enrollment and service entitlements.

Source: Dave (1991).

In India, SEWA is a trade union of 215,000 female workers in the informal sector. It organizes them at the household level toward the goals of full employment and self-reliance. Full employment includes social security, which in turn incorporates insurance. SEWA's experience revealed that women's efforts to escape from poverty through enhanced employment opportunities and increased income were repeatedly frustrated by crises such as sickness, a breadwinner's death, and accidental damage to, or destruction of, their homes and work equipment. Too often maternity also becomes a crisis for a woman, especially if she is poor, malnourished, and living in a remote area. One SEWA study observed that women identified sickness of themselves or their family members as the major stress events in their lives (Chatterjee and Vyas 1997). Sickness was also a major cause of indebtedness among women.

From the start, the health insurance program was linked to SEWA's primary health care program, which includes occupational health services. Thus insured members also have access to preventive and curative health care with health education. Health insurance accounts for most of the claims and for 50 percent of the premiums paid out to the insurance program by SEWA members. The SEWA Bank introduced the scheme in March 1992, with an initial enrollment of 7,000 women from Ahmedabad City (Chatterjee and Vyas 1997). Later extended to cover rural woman from nine districts of Gujarat, it now has 30,000 women enrolled, half of them rural dwellers.

Health insurance is an integral part of SEWA's insurance program. The main motivation for initiating a women's health insurance scheme was the recognition that maintaining an active, health-seeking behavior is vital for ensuring a good quality life and women tend to place a low priority on their own health care needs.

The SEWA health insurance program includes maternity coverage, hospitalization coverage for a wide range of diseases, and coverage for occupational illnesses and diseases specific to women (table 9.4). It covers diseases not covered by the GIC's Mediclaim plan and also provides life and asset insurance for the woman and for her husband or, in the case of widowhood or separation, for other household members. Administrative procedures under the plan are simplified.

The SEWA health insurance scheme functions in coordination with the Life Insurance Corporation of India (LIC) and the New India Assurance Company (NIAC). SEWA has integrated the schemes of LIC and NIAC into a comprehensive health insurance package to address women's basic needs. The claimants are needy health-benefits seekers, and as the insurance is an additional benefit, the beneficiaries willingly pay the premium. Most of the insurers opt for a fixed deposit of Rs. 500 or Rs. 700 (depending upon the type of coverage) with the SEWA Bank; accrued interest on the deposit goes toward the annual premium. The SEWA Bank's large membership and assets have enabled it to provide this insurance coverage at low premiums.

TABLE 9.4   Coverage under SEWA Scheme

Provider	Description of coverage	Coverage amount (Rs.)	Premium (Rs.)
New India Assurance	Accidental death of the woman member	10,000	3.50
	Loss of assets		
	Accidental death of a member's husband	10,000	3.50
SEWA	Loss during riots, fire, floods, theft, and so forth		8.00
	(a) of work equipment	2,000	
	(b) of the housing unit	3,000	
	Health insurance, including coverage for:	1,200	30.00
	(a) gynecological ailments		(10)
	(b) occupational health-related diseases		(5)
	Maternity benefits	300	—
Life Insurance Corporation of India	Natural death	3,000	15.00
	Accidental death	25,000	

Note: Total premium for the entire package is Rs. 60 plus a service charge of Rs. 5.

RESEARCH DESIGN AND METHODOLOGY

Research Design

This chapter is based on a primary household survey undertaken in Gujarat's Ahmedabad District in 1998–99. The survey covered about 1,200 households from rural and urban areas. The households were stratified into four categories according to health insurance status. About 360 households belonged to a contributory plan known as the Employees' State Insurance Scheme (ESIS) for industrial workers. Another 120 households subscribed to a voluntary plan (Mediclaim), and 360 households belonged to a community-based financing scheme run by an NGO, the Self-Employed Women's Association (SEWA). The remaining 360 households were uninsured and were purchasing health care services directly on the market. This last subsample served as a control group. The idea behind selecting such stratification was to understand the varying health needs, access to health services, treatment pattern, and the types of benefits received by sample households in the different health insurance environments.

The survey was conducted in eight slum-dominated localities in the city of Ahmedabad and six neighboring villages. On average, 60 households per village and 90 households per urban locality were selected. The criterion for selecting a village or an urban locality was that the settlement should have a cluster of households covered by the SEWA and ESIS plans. The sample canvassed from each settlement included about equal numbers of households from the ESIS, SEWA, and uninsured categories (20 each from a village and 30 each from an urban locality). The sample was purposive, and no house listing prior to the survey was carried out. The sample of Mediclaim/Jan Arogya beneficiaries belonging to Ahmedabad city was selected from the list of subscribers obtained from the offices of two companies, United India Insurance and New India Assurance.

Methodology

Determinants of Participation in Mutual Health Organization

(9.1)   Prob (membership > 0) = $X\beta + \varepsilon$,

where X represents a set of independent variables that are hypothesized to affect membership in community-based schemes. These variables include income, gender, age, marker on chronic illness, and disability. β is a vector of coefficient estimates and ε is the error term.

Level of Financial Protection Provided by SEWA

To assess the impact of mutual health organizations on financial protection of members, two aspects have to be taken into account: the probability of visiting a health care provider and the out-of-pocket expenditure borne by the individual. We use a two-part model developed as part of the Rand Health Insurance Experiment:

- a logit model that assesses the probability of visiting a health care provider

(9.2)   Prob (visit > 0) = $X\beta + u$,

where X stands as a vector for individual, household, and community characteristics;

- a log-linear model that estimates the incurred level of out-of-pocket expenditures per episode, conditioning on positive use of health care services:

(9.3)   Log (out-of pocket expenditure / visit > 0) = $X\beta + e$,

where X represents a set of independent variables hypothesized to affect individual patterns of utilization and expenditure on treatment.

Variables Used in the Model

Table 9.5 gives an overview of the variables included in the analysis.

RESULTS

Determinants of Participation

A multinomial logit model is used to identify various determinants of being enrolled in the SEWA health insurance plan among members of SEWA. Out of the total 645 SEWA members above 15 years of age in the sample, 236 (36.6 percent) were enrolled in the plan. Out of 10 variables used in the model, 3 depicted

TABLE 9.5   Overview of Variables Used

Variable	Description
Individual characteristics	
Gender	Male and female
Age	Completed years of age at the time of last birthday; broad age groups are used in the model
Marital status	Never married, currently married, and widowed/divorced/separated
Education level	Years of schooling: broadly classified as illiterate, below primary, primary, middle, secondary, graduate, and above
Activity status	Usual activity status during the past year: broadly classified as nonworker, self-employed in agriculture, casual laborer, home-based production worker, trade or sales worker, salaried worker in organized sector, salaried worker in unorganized sector, and subsidiary status worker
Health characteristics	
Acute morbidity	Episode of illness during past 30 days not involving hospitalization
Chronic morbidity	Prevalence of any chronic disease/ailment
Hospitalization	Any illness resulting in hospitalization during the past 365 days
Childbirth	Childbirth during past two years
Duration of illness	Number of days the person was ill and also categorized into groups
Source of care	Source of treatment; broadly categorized as no treatment, use of public facility, including ESIS, and private facility
Cost of treatment	Cost of treatment includes: direct out-of-pocket payments toward fees, medicines, diagnostic tests, surgery, bed charges, transportation, and special diet. Indirect costs include income or wage loss of the patient and the caring person as well as interest payments on amount borrowed to meet treatment expenses.
Health insurance enrollment	Community-based plan (SEWA), social insurance (ESIS), private plan (Mediclaim), and uninsured
Household characteristics	
Income and expenditure	Annual household income from different sources; categorized into quintile groups. Monthly household expenditure by broad items—but not considered in the model.
Household size	Number of members usually residing in the house and sharing food from the common kitchen
Community characteristics	
Area of residence	Usual place of residence: rural or urban area

health status (whether suffering from any chronic ailment, hospitalized during last 365 days, and had delivery during the past two years), 4 personal characteristics (age, education, marital status, and activity status), 2 household characteristics (household size and income quintile), and 1 community variable (area of residence). The description of these variables is provided in table 9.5. The mean value of the enrollment rate varied across these characteristics. The enrollment rate was higher among women who had reported suffering from any chronic ailment or had been hospitalized in the previous 365 days but not among those who had reported delivery during the past two years. Among personal characteristics, the mean enrollment rate was found to be higher in the middle age groups, 36–45 years and 46–55 years, than the other age groups; it was also higher among currently married women. However, with level of education the mean enrollment rate tended to decline. The rate was found to be much lower among nonworkers or subsidiary status workers than among home-based production or salaried workers. The rate tended to decline with the size of household and did not vary much across income quintiles, except in the top quintile, where it was marginally higher. Overall, the enrollment rate was higher among urban women than rural women, mainly due to better access to information as well as to the SEWA Bank (located in Ahmedabad city), which manages the scheme.

The alternative results of multinomial logit models (interchanging activity status and income variables) are presented in table 9.6. The explanatory power of the model (Pseudo R^2) ranged between 0.185 (without income variable) to 0.218 (with inclusion of both income and activity status variables). The following are the main findings.

There was no adverse selection in terms of whether the member had been suffering from any chronic ailment or had been hospitalized before. However, maternity, a predictable event, had increased the likelihood of enrollment to take advantage of a benefit allowance of Rs. 300 and coverage of the high risk of hospitalization.

Among the personal attributes, the odds of being enrolled were five to seven times higher among middle-age groups than in the 16–25 years age group. For currently married women, the odds were twice as high as for never-married women. Education level turned out to be an insignificant predictor. The type of activity pursued by a SEWA member was found to be a highly significant predictor (the predictive power was much higher than that of the income effects). The odds ratios were much higher for self-employed, home-based, or agricultural workers than for nonworkers. The odds were found to be insignificant for salaried workers in the formal sector.

Household size showed an inverse relationship with enrollment, and the odds ratios tended to decline significantly in medium-size and large households. Income was not found to be a significant predictor. When activity status was not taken into account, women in the top income quintile were twice as likely to enroll as women in the bottom quintile.

There seemed to be an urban bias in enrollment, which may be due to better outreach and accessibility factors. An urban woman was three times more likely to enroll than a rural woman.

Determinants of Financial Protection in Community Financing

A multinomial logit model is used to identify various determinants of utilization of services for ambulatory care, and an attempt is also made to explore predictors for choosing a private facility for ambulatory and inpatient care over a public one. This model uses the cases of illnesses reported by all households, irrespective of health insurance status (SEWA, ESIS, Mediclaim, and uninsured). Out of the total 1,327 illnesses reported by the sample population during the previous 30 days, treatment was sought for 1,271 ailments (96 percent). The first model uses all illnesses (excluding hospitalization) reported during the previous 30 days and predicts the probability of seeking treatment (only for 56 illnesses was the treatment not sought). The second and third models are subsets of the first model (treated in public facility versus no treatment—383 cases—and treated in private facility versus treated in public facility—1,271 cases). The third model shows that of the total treated ambulatory cases, nearly 74 percent relied on the private facility, thus suggesting the dominant role of the private sector in handling the ambulatory care burden. The last model is exclusively for hospitalization cases during previous 365 days (that is, treated in a private hospital versus public hospital—362 cases). Here the inpatient load was almost equally distributed between the private and public sectors (53 percent of inpatients used public hospitals).

Of 11 variables used in the model, 3 depicted health characteristics (whether suffering from any chronic ailment, duration of illness, and type of health insurance coverage), 5 personal characteristics (gender, age, education, marital status, and activity status), 2 household characteristics (household size and income quintile), and 1 community variable (area of residence). The mean value of utilization and the proportion using private health service facilities both for ambulatory and inpatient care varied considerably across these characteristics.

The results of multinomial logit models for utilization and private/public choice for ambulatory care are presented in table 9.7.

The explanatory power of the utilization model (Pseudo R^2) was 0.148. For the other two models, it was 0.372 (treated in a public sector facility versus no treatment) and 0.226 (treated in a private versus a public sector facility). The following are the main findings.

Of 11 variables used for predicting utilization rate, only 3 (illness duration, type of health insurance enrollment, and area of residence) were found to be significant. None of the personal and household attributes exerted significant influence on utilization rate. The odds of being untreated were higher among those enrolled with the community plan (SEWA) as well as among rural residents.

In the case of choosing a private facility over the public facility, including ESIS for ambulatory care, seven variables had a significant impact. The odds of choosing a public facility were higher if the person had a chronic ailment, a salaried work status, or coverage under social insurance. Males, educated graduates and above, and those covered by a private plan (Mediclaim) tended to choose a private facility for ambulatory treatment. Patients from small households in urban areas tended to choose a public facility. The income effect for opting out the private facility was clearly discernable. Members of the SEWA plan also tended to choose the private facility for ambulatory care.

TABLE 9.6   Determinants of Being Enrolled in SEWA Health Insurance Plan among SEWA Members

Variables	Model 1		
	Odds ratio	Coefficient	Significance
Whether chronic ailment	1.155	0.144	0.655
Whether hospitalized	1.602	0.471	0.152
Whether had children in the past 2 years	1.835	0.607	0.047
Urban resident	3.096	1.130	0.000
Activity status (nonworker)			
Agricultural	3.357	1.211	0.011
Casual labor	3.006	1.101	0.001
Home-based worker	4.095	1.410	0.001
Trade or sales worker	2.475	0.906	0.013
Salaried worker—organized	2.257	0.814	0.136
Salaried worker—unorganized	2.753	1.013	0.006
Other worker—subsidiary status	2.016	0.701	0.089
Education level (0)			
1–4 std.	1.400	0.336	0.292
5–7 std.	0.668	−0.404	0.147
8–9 std.	0.540	−0.617	0.122
10–12 std.	0.721	−0.328	0.334
Graduate and above	1.483	0.394	0.530
Age (16–25 years)			
26–35	2.235	0.804	0.008
36–45	5.444	1.694	0.000
46–55	6.729	1.906	0.000
56 and above	4.453	1.494	0.002
Marital status (never married)			
Currently married	2.089	0.737	0.099
Widowed/divorced/separated	1.154	0.143	0.799
Household size (1–4)	−0.375		
5–6	0.687	−0.907	0.170
6–8	0.404	−0.925	0.004
9–10	0.397	−1.391	0.015
11 and above	0.249		0.005
Annual household income quintile (lowest)			
2	0.867	−0.143	0.659
3	1.182	0.167	0.643
4	1.094	0.090	0.785
5 (top)	1.872	0.627	0.098
Constant		−2.929	0.000
Pseudo R^2		0.218	

Model 2			Model 3		
Odds ratio	Coefficient	Significance	Odds ratio	Coefficient	Significance
1.164	0.152	0.630	1.121	0.114	0.719
1.716	0.540	0.087	1.528	0.424	0.193
1.480	0.392	0.184	1.761	0.566	0.063
2.720	1.001	0.000	3.131	1.141	0.000
			3.316	1.199	0.012
			2.777	1.021	0.002
			4.835	1.576	0.000
			2.599	0.955	0.009
			2.328	0.845	0.115
			2.802	1.030	0.004
			1.811	0.594	0.145
1.173	0.160	0.600	1.511	0.413	0.190
0.715	−0.336	0.208	0.701	−0.355	0.196
0.484	−0.725	0.062	0.578	−0.549	0.163
0.599	−0.512	0.111	0.805	−0.217	0.512
1.058	0.056	0.927	1.813	0.595	0.325
2.752	1.012	0.000	2.203	0.790	0.009
6.294	1.840	0.000	5.801	1.758	0.000
6.746	1.909	0.000	6.878	1.928	0.000
3.334	1.204	0.010	4.867	1.582	0.001
2.251	0.811	0.061	1.939	0.662	0.134
1.299	0.262	0.629	1.122	0.116	0.835
0.690	0.359	0.176	0.792	−0.233	0.370
0.455	−0.787	0.009	0.482	−0.729	0.011
0.470	−0.755	0.039	0.497	−0.700	0.044
0.264	−1.333	0.005	0.367	−1.001	0.026
0.885	−0.122	0.699			
1.202	0.184	0.594			
1.203	0.185	0.564			
2.106	0.745	0.041			
	−2.490	0.000		−2.936	0.000
	0.185			0.212	

TABLE 9.7 Determinants of Being Treated and Use of Public or Private Facility for Ambulatory Care (Multinomial Logit Model)

Predictor	Treated vs. untreated		
	Odds ratio	Coefficient	Significance
Illness duration (1–3 days)			
4–7	0.9975	−0.003	0.995
8–14	1.5286	0.424	0.369
15–29	7.6682	2.037	0.057
30 and older	5.4784	1.701	0.095
Whether chronic ailment	0.2392	−1.430	0.154
Whether male	0.8775	−0.131	0.697
Age (0–14 years)			
15–24	2.9836	1.093	0.337
25–34	0.9822	−0.018	0.990
35–44	0.8176	−0.201	0.893
45–54	0.5992	−0.512	0.730
55 and older	0.4542	−0.789	0.588
Marital status (never married)			
Currently married	1.2941	0.258	0.853
Widowed/divorced/separated	1.3710	0.316	0.828
Education level (illiterate)			
1–4 Std.	0.9347	−0.068	0.852
5–7 Std.	1.1325	0.124	0.765
8–9 Std.	1.09E+14	32.323	1.000
10–12 Std.	1.8429	0.611	0.388
Graduate and above	1.0233	0.023	0.984
Activity status (nonworker)			
Agricultural	1.5643	0.447	0.590
Casual labor	1.0278	0.027	0.956
Home-based worker	0.5168	−0.660	0.426
Trade or sales worker	0.7356	−0.307	0.627
Salaried worker—organized	1.23E+14	32.441	1.000
Salaried worker—unorganized	1.34E+14	32.527	1.000
Other worker—subsidiary status	1.1006	0.096	0.905
Health insurance enrollment (uninsured)			
Community plan—SEWA	0.3669	−1.003	0.035
Social insurance—ESIS	1.1657	0.153	0.671
Private plan—Mediclaim	9.50E+13	32.185	1.000
Urban resident	2.0618	0.724	0.019
Household size (1–4)			
5–6	0.8953	−0.111	0.750
7–8	1.6893	0.524	0.293
9–10	1.1413	0.132	0.832
11 or more	1.0451	0.044	0.951
Annual household income quintile (lowest)			
2	1.8603	0.621	0.168
3	0.9483	−0.053	0.902
4	1.8409	0.610	0.227
5 (top)	1.3011	0.263	0.613
Constant		1.915	0.000
Pseudo R^2		0.148	
Number of cases (dependent valued as): 1		1,271	
0		56	

Note: Out of 1,327 illness episodes reported during the past 30 days, 56 were not treated. Of the treated episodes, the public facility, including ESIS, was contacted in 327 cases; in the remaining 944 cases a private facility was contacted. Figures in brackets refer to the reference category of the variable.

Public contact vs. untreated			Private vs. public contact		
Odds ratio	Coefficient	Significance	Odds ratio	Coefficient	Significance
0.6281	−0.465	0.426	0.8946	−0.111	0.661
1.4671	0.383	0.564	0.8339	−0.182	0.492
8.3126	2.118	0.081	0.5712	−0.560	0.065
4.6462	1.536	0.311	1.4982	0.404	0.304
0.5453	−0.606	0.678	0.2108	−1.557	0.000
0.7512	−0.286	0.561	1.4326	0.359	0.046
10.0297	2.306	0.076	0.6249	−0.470	0.151
1.2636	0.234	0.855	0.6186	−0.480	0.329
2.1255	0.754	0.617	0.4862	−0.721	0.148
0.3484	−1.054	0.471	0.6338	−0.456	0.376
0.5865	−0.534	0.707	0.4829	−0.728	0.149
0.8231	−0.195	0.883	1.9124	0.648	0.124
0.9973	−0.003	0.999	1.7128	0.538	0.286
0.6011	−0.509	0.307	0.9139	−0.090	0.696
1.4707	0.386	0.487	0.6471	−0.435	0.052
2.48E+15	35.448	1.000	0.7109	−0.341	0.252
0.9979	−0.002	0.998	0.8000	−0.223	0.432
0.1647	−1.804	0.292	3.2589	1.181	0.036
0.6132	−0.489	0.699	0.8316	−0.184	0.745
3.4850	1.248	0.097	0.6730	−0.396	0.160
1.6128	0.478	0.668	0.9354	−0.067	0.894
2.0847	0.735	0.397	0.5980	−0.514	0.213
5.35E+15	36.217	1.000	0.2761	−1.287	0.000
4.54E+15	36.051	1.000	0.5682	−0.565	0.083
7.4579	2.009	0.080	0.2318	−1.462	0.001
0.0798	−2.529	0.003	2.1073	0.745	0.043
5.9587	1.785	0.000	0.1715	−1.763	0.000
0.40E+15	36.666		4.4984	1.504	0.050
8.1439	2.097	0.000	0.2525	−1.377	0.000
2.0201	0.703	0.166	0.5795	−0.546	0.006
7.4421	2.007	0.004	0.4030	−0.909	0.000
2.0905	0.737	0.386	1.0896	0.086	0.806
4.4154	1.485	0.159	0.5556	−0.588	0.138
0.6607	−0.414	0.513	1.6769	0.517	0.033
0.1623	−1.818	0.008	2.2582	0.815	0.002
0.1336	−2.013	0.016	3.3027	1.195	0.000
0.1134	−2.177	0.007	2.6790	0.985	0.001
	−0.550	0.481		3.116	0.000
	0.372			0.226	
	327			944	
	56			327	

TABLE 9.8   Determinants of Using Private Facility for Inpatient Care (Multinomial Logit Model)

Predictor	Private vs. public hospital		
	Odds ratio	Coefficient	Significance
Illness duration (1–3 days)			
4–7	0.4685	–0.7583	0.026
8–14	0.1998	–1.6105	0.000
15–29	0.1299	–2.0410	0.000
30 or more	0.3191	–1.1423	0.027
Whether male	1.1257	0.1184	0.719
Age (0–14 years)			
15–24	1.2172	0.1966	0.725
25–34	3.6314	1.2896	0.069
35–44	1.5422	0.4332	0.591
45–54	3.2025	1.1639	0.132
55 or more	1.1200	0.1134	0.877
Marital status (never married)			
Currently married	0.5864	–0.5337	0.345
Widowed/divorced/separated	0.7650	–0.2679	0.730
Education level (illiterate)			
1–4 Std.	0.9722	–0.0282	0.947
5–7 Std.	0.5129	–0.6678	0.089
8–9 Std.	0.7450	–0.2944	0.575
10–12 Std.	0.6452	–0.4383	0.336
Graduate and above	2.0286	0.7074	0.419
Activity status (nonworker)			
Agricultural	0.5824	–0.5406	0.537
Casual labor	0.5931	–0.5224	0.259
Home-based worker	0.6837	–0.3802	0.622
Trade or sales worker	2.0432	0.7145	0.382
Salaried worker—organized	1.4176	0.3489	0.553
Salaried worker—unorganized	0.4821	–0.7297	0.158
Other worker—subsidiary status	0.5435	–0.6097	0.443

(continued)

For inpatient care, the results of the multinomial logit model for choosing a public or private hospital are presented in table 9.8. Of the 10 variables used in the model, only 4 (illness duration, type of health insurance enrollment, area of residence, and income) showed a significant influence. The odds of choosing a public hospital for inpatient care were much higher for illnesses requiring a longer stay in a hospital. This is entirely due to price considerations because for longer stays, out-of-pocket expenditure would be huge if treatment were in a private hospital. People covered under social insurance tended to use public and ESIS hospitals much more. Only patients from households in the top quintile, who could afford treatment, chose private hospitals over public for inpatient

TABLE 9.8   Continued

Predictor	Private vs. public hospital		
	Odds ratio	Coefficient	Significance
Health Insurance Enrollment (uninsured)			
Community plan—SEWA	0.7946	−0.2299	0.630
Social insurance—ESIS	0.2143	−1.5404	0.000
Private plan—Mediclaim	5.1690	1.6427	0.171
Urban resident	0.2855	−1.2536	0.000
Household size (1–4)			
5–6	0.6137	−0.4882	0.169
7–8	0.8579	−0.1533	0.722
9–10	0.9079	−0.0966	0.859
11 or more	0.5836	−0.5386	0.447
Annual household income quintile (lowest)			
2	1.5507	0.4387	0.315
3	1.4488	0.3707	0.409
4	1.8937	0.6385	0.159
5 (top)	4.7391	1.5558	0.003
Constant		1.8405	0.001
Pseudo R^2		0.228	
Number of cases (dependent variable coded as): 1		171	
0		193	

care. As public hospitals are located mainly in urban centers, urban residents have better access and thus showed greater reliance on public services than did their rural counterparts.

Determinants of out-of-pocket expenditures on treatment of ailments, for both ambulatory and inpatient care, are presented in table 9.9. The dependent variable is expressed as the log of out-of-pocket expenditure on treatment. Overall, the direct cost of treatment for ambulatory care was Rs. 286 per episode. For inpatient care, it was Rs. 2,771. Of the 12 variables used in the OLS regression model, 4 depicted health characteristics (chronic ailment, duration of illness, type of provider—private or public—and type of health insurance coverage), 5 personal characteristics (gender, age, education, marital status, and activity status), 2 household characteristics (household size and income quintile), and 1 community variable (area of residence). The mean value of direct out-of-pocket expenditures per episode varied significantly across these characteristics.

The regression results for both ambulatory and inpatient cares are presented in table 9.9. The explanatory power of the model (R^2) was 0.284 for ambulatory care and 0.413 for inpatient care. The following are the main findings.

TABLE 9.9   Determinants of Out-of-Pocket Expenditure on Treatment by Type of Care (Dependent Variable in Log Form)

Predictor	Ambulatory care			Hospitalization		
	Coefficient	Beta	Significance	Coefficient	Beta	Significance
Private provider	0.5502	0.3181	0.000	0.4175	0.3230	0.000
Days of illness	0.0075	0.1735	0.000	0.0111	0.2357	0.000
Whether chronic ailment	0.0830	0.0483	0.108			
Whether hospitalized						
Whether male	0.0982	0.0646	0.025	0.0298	0.0230	0.672
Age	0.0081	0.2212	0.159	0.0098	0.2939	0.266
Age squared	−0.0001	−0.2117	0.095	−0.0001	−0.2696	0.257
Marital status (never married)						
Currently married	−0.0253	−0.0167	0.767	−0.0500	−0.0382	0.657
Widowed/divorced/separated	−0.0528	−0.0207	0.648	0.1315	0.0623	0.421
Education level (0)						
1–4 Std.	−0.0297	−0.0148	0.590	−0.0342	−0.0187	0.708
5–7 Std.	−0.0328	−0.0168	0.574	0.0115	0.0073	0.893
8–9 Std.	0.0722	0.0283	0.322	0.1183	0.0540	0.287
10–12 Std.	0.0539	0.0253	0.417	0.1245	0.0769	0.182
Graduate and above	0.0508	0.0132	0.637	0.1505	0.0449	0.358
Activity status (nonworker)						
Agricultural	−0.0806	−0.0177	0.499	0.1211	0.0275	0.546
Casual labor	−0.0896	−0.0354	0.204	0.1648	0.0808	0.111
Home-based worker	−0.2041	−0.0389	0.119	0.3035	0.0873	0.050
Trade or sales worker	−0.0670	−0.0174	0.509	0.1527	0.0439	0.342
Salaried worker—organized	−0.0179	−0.0066	0.827	0.0641	0.0314	0.588
Salaried worker—unorganized	0.0655	0.0216	0.420	0.0633	0.0289	0.574
Other worker—subsidiary status	0.2297	0.0490	0.050	−0.2883	-0.0694	0.118
Health insurance enrollment (uninsured)						
Community plan—SEWA	0.0145	0.0048	0.855	0.0656	0.0296	0.535
Social insurance—ESIS	−0.3719	−0.2220	0.000	−0.4274	−0.3065	0.000
Private plan—Mediclaim	0.1461	0.0353	0.177	0.3449	0.0784	0.080
Urban resident	−0.2437	−0.1477	0.000	−0.1786	−0.1290	0.007
Household size	−0.0172	−0.0560	0.049	0.0182	0.0673	0.199
Annual household income quintile (lowest)						
2	0.0666	0.0363	0.265	0.0535	0.0337	0.564
3	0.1132	0.0575	0.074	0.1634	0.0981	0.086
4	0.1446	0.0784	0.024	0.1059	0.0697	0.268
5 (top)	0.0515	0.0272	0.466	0.0785	0.0452	0.485
Constant	1.7059		0.000	2.5908		0.000
R^2		0.284			0.413	
Number of illness episodes		1,274			363	

Of the 12 variables used for determining direct out-of-pocket expenditure on ambulatory care, only 7 (type of provider, illness duration, gender, type of health insurance enrollment, household size, income, and area of residence) were found to be significant. Of these, the most important explanatory variables were type of provider, duration of illness, social insurance coverage, and area of residence. Cost of treatment turned out to be higher if treatment were in the private sector and of long duration when the patient was male and resided in a rural area. The cost of care was inversely related to household size and relatively higher among patients in the third and fourth income quintiles. Only social insurance coverage, and not the community plan, provided financial protection. Both the community plan and the private Mediclaim plan cover hospitalization only.

In the case of out-of-pocket expenditures on inpatient care, only 4 of the 11 variables had a significant impact. The cost of treatment for inpatient care was higher if treatment were in a private hospital and of long duration and the patient resided in a rural area. Income effects were not found to be significant. In this case, both social insurance and Mediclaim plans succeeded in providing financial protection whereas the community plan did not meet expectations.

Another way of looking at the financial protection is to explore determinants of annual per capita expenditure on health care at the household level (after obtaining the annual estimates of expenditure on ambulatory care, inpatient care, delivery, and maternal and child health care). Alternatively, one can also estimate the burden of ill health on the household (annual per capita expenditure on health care as a proportion of annual per capita income) and explore how much of this burden is protected through a health insurance mechanism.

Acknowledgments: This chapter further explores household-level data of the NCAER-SEWA study on "Health Insurance for Workers in the Informal Sector." The author is thankful to the Ford Foundation (the sponsor) and SEWA as collaborator in the primary fieldwork in Ahmedabad. The author would also like to thank Ms. Shakun Datta for providing assistance in extracting results of multinomial logit models through STATA software. The author is grateful to the World Health Organization for having provided an opportunity to contribute to the work of the Commission on Macroeconomics and Health and to the World Bank for publishing the material in this chapter as an HNP Discussion Paper.

REFERENCES

Ahmad, E., J. Dreze, J. Hills, and A. Sen, eds. 1991. *Social Security in Developing Countries.* Oxford: Clarendon Press.

Chatterjee, M., and J. Vyas. 1997. *Organizing Insurance for Women Workers: The SEWA Experience.* Ahmedabad: Self-Employed Women's Association (SEWA).

Dave, P. 1991. "Community and Self-Financing in Voluntary Health Programmes in India." *Health Policy and Planning.* 6(1): 20–31.

Gumber, A. 1997. "Burden of Disease and Cost of Ill Health in India: Setting Priorities for Health Interventions During the Ninth Plan." *Margin* 29(2): 133–72.

————. 1998. "Facets of Indian Healthcare Market—Some Issues." *Saket Industrial Digest* 4(12): 11–17.

————. 2000a. "Health Care Burden on Households in the Informal Sector: Implications for Social Security Assistance." *Indian Journal of Labor Economics* 43(2): 277–91.

————. 2000b. "Structure of the Indian Health Care Market: Implications for Health Insurance Sector." *WHO Regional Health Forum* 4(1/2): 26–34.

————. 2001. "Economic Reforms and the Health Sector: Toward Health Equity in India." Paper presented at the National Seminar on Economic Reforms and Employment in the Indian Economy, organized by the Institute of Applied Manpower Research and Planning Commission, New Delhi, March 22–23.

Gumber, A., and V. Kulkarni 2000. *Health Insurance for Workers in the Informal Sector: Detail Results from a Pilot Study.* New Delhi: National Council of Applied Economic Research.

Rahman, K. 2000. "Poverty, Microcredit and Health—What Role Can WHO Play?" *WHO Regional Health Forum* 4 (1/2): 68–80.

Shariff, A., A. Gumber, R. Duggal, and M. Alam. 1999. "Health Care Financing and Insurance Perspective for the Ninth Plan (1997–2002)." *Margin* 31(2): 38–68.

Visaria, P., and A. Gumber. 1994. *Utilization of and Expenditure on Health Care in India, 1986–87.* Ahmedabad: Gujarat Institute of Development Research.

CHAPTER 10

Impact of the Thailand Health Card

Siripen Supakankunti

Abstract: The health insurance card scheme was introduced as the Health Card Project (HCP) in 1983. This program was based on the risk sharing of health expenditures with no cost sharing in a voluntary health insurance prepayment scheme. Frequent adjustments in both the strategies and the objectives of the program have included voluntary risk sharing with cost recovery in addition to service provision. The HCP needs a large enough number of enrollees to ensure a sufficient pool of risks. However, the newly elected government of Thailand has committed to rapidly extending health care coverage to all Thai citizens. All uninsured Thai citizens will have access to required health services for a flat fee of 30 baht (US$0.67), regardless of the type of disease treated. Even though the HCP was suppressed and replaced by this program in October 2001, this study of the determinants of demand for the prepaid health card is still important. The HCP can be assessed as relatively progressive, serving rural areas, poor, and near-poor groups.

This study has found that employment, education, and the presence of illness are significant factors influencing health insurance card purchase. The third factor is related to the program's problem of adverse selection: families with symptoms of sickness are more likely to buy cards and increase their use of health services. The results also show an improvement in accessibility to health care and a high level of satisfaction among cardholders, both key objectives of the program. Problems of program performance include issues of program and financial management, marketing, quality control and cost recovery, ineffective referral systems, and lack of limits on episodes and ceilings for expenses. There is a need for an efficient and consistent health policy, which would involve revised criteria for card use, standard reimbursement agreements with hospitals, government subsidies, and an overall strengthening of the program.

The objective of this chapter is to assess the application of voluntary health insurance, in this case the Health Card Program (HCP) of Thailand, and provide greater understanding of how a voluntary health insurance program performs and how to improve and sustain it more efficiently. Utilizing data collected in Khon Kaen, where the program was implemented in 1983, the following study explores the development, problems, and health service capabilities of a voluntary health insurance scheme, identifies factors influencing project outcomes (accessibility, sustainability, and efficient use of resources), investigates health card purchase and dropout patterns, and evaluates the factors affecting the discrimination between health card purchase and nonpurchase and also affecting dropouts from the continued health card member groups.

To analyze any type of health care financing, it is first necessary to understand its background.

TABLE 10.1   Health Service Utilization Pattern for Reported Ill Persons (Comparing Different Surveys)

Choice of Outlet	1970	1979	1985
No treatment	2.7	4.2	—
Traditional medicine/healers	7.7	6.3	2.4
Self-prescribed drugs	51.4	42.3	28.6
Public health centers	4.4	16.8	14.7
Public hospitals	11.1	10.0	32.5
Private clinics/hospitals	22.7	20.4	21.8

Source: Tangcharoensathien (1995), originally from Health Planning Division, MOPH (1970,1979); Institute for Population and Social Research, Mahidol University (1988).

Health Delivery System

In Thailand, from 1970 to 1985, there was an increasing expectation and use of public outlets staffed by physicians and a decreasing trend in using self-prescribed drugs and traditional medicines, or attendance of healers. This reflects the aim of the Fifth National Health Development Plan (1982–86) to achieve 100 percent district coverage in the country and the three-year compulsory service program at the Ministry of Public Health (MOPH) district hospitals imposed on all medical graduates in 1972. The consequence was an increase in the number of hospitals and doctors at the district level, which undoubtedly began to meet the previously unmet demand for health services in rural areas and led to a significant threefold increase in the use of public hospitals in 1985 compared with 1979 (Tangcharoensathien 1995). Table 10.1 shows the consistent trend in choices of outlets used by ill individuals.

When looking at the employment status and type of health service utilizations in 1986, it is clear that the percentage of health service utilization by self-treatment was highest in all occupational groups. Between the professional and administration groups and those of farmers and miners there were some differences in proportions, that is, self-treatment was more than 50 percent in the farmers' group but lower than 50 percent in the professional group. The professional group has relatively much higher use of private clinics and hospitals than the farmer group, while utilization rates in public facilities were similar.

Trends in Health Expenditure

In 1987, 5.7 percent of the gross national product (GNP) was spent on health, including private household payments and public health expenditures (see table 10.2). Health expenditure has been steadily increasing at a higher rate than the growth of the GNP. In 1984, a 12 percent real-term increase in health expenditure was due to the high capital investment for constructing district hospitals as stated above (Tangcharoensathien 1995). In 1994, 1996, and 1998, 3.53 percent, 3.72 percent, and 3.88 percent of the gross domestic product (GDP) was spent on health respectively (NESDB, 1998).

TABLE 10.2   Trend of Total per Capita Health Expenditure (Public and Private Spending)

1987 Prices

Year	% of GNP on health	Per capita expenditure (Baht)[a]	% Increase health expenditure	% GDP growth (Baht)
1978	3.4	680	—	—
1979	3.6	710	4.4	5.05
1980	3.9	738	3.9	4.57
1981	4.2	798	8.1	5.96
1982	4.6	864	8.3	3.90
1983	4.8	939	8.7	6.76
1984	5.2	1,052	12.0	6.65
1985	5.6	1,132	7.6	3.40
1986	5.6	1,192	5.3	4.30
1987	5.7	1,282	7.6	7.74
Current prices				
1994	3.53	2,186		
1996	3.72	2,858		
1998	3.88	2,924		

Note: The GDP growth rate in 1988 and 1989 was 12.0 percent and 10.8 percent, respectively.

a. 25 Baht:US$1

Source: Modified from Tangcharoensathien (1995), originally from Social Development Project Division, NESDB (1990). NHA Project phase II (2000).

The percent source of health care financing in 1984, 1986, and 1987 at 1987 prices is shown in table 10.3, demonstrating trends in sources of finance during that decade. Public sources of funding play a minor role in financing health services with a decreasing trend from 27.9 percent of total health expenditure in 1984 to 24.2 percent in 1987. The most important source is private out-of-pocket expenditures by households, with an increasing trend from 69.3 percent in 1984 to 73.2 percent in 1987. It must be noted that some of the private household expenditures on health could have been reimbursed from the Ministry of Finance, for government employees and dependents, while others may have been reimbursed from employers. Among the public services, the MOPH is the major provider for the country, providing comprehensive health care mainly in areas outside the Bangkok metropolitan area (Tangcharoensathien 1995). Private household expenditures on health were mainly to pay for curative care either through user fees at government facilities or charges at private clinics and drug stores.

In 1996, of the total 843,200 million baht government budget, 9.1 percent was for agriculture, 10.2 percent for transportation and communication, 20.1 percent for education, 14.3 percent for social services, 12.8 percent for maintenance of national security, and 7.53 percent for public health (see table 10.4). The budget for health remained consistent at the rate of 7.1–7.5 percent of the total public spending during fiscal years 1994–96, compared with 4.1–4.5 percent in the previous decade. All expenses are financed by the government's receipts of revenue and borrowings. In

TABLE 10.3   Percent Source of Health Care Financing in 1984, 1986, and 1987

		1987 Prices	
Sources of funding	1984	1986	1987
Public sources:	27.9	26.0	24.2
MOPH	17.4	15.3	14.1
Other ministries	6.9	6.5	6.0
Public employee medical benefits	3.6	4.2	4.1
Workmen's compensation fund	0.5	0.4	0.4
State enterprise employee medical benefits	0.8	0.9	0.8
Private insurance	0.8	0.7	0.7
Foreign aid	0.8	0.8	0.7
Private households	69.3	71.2	73.2
Total: Percent	**100.0**	**100.0**	**100.0**
Million Baht	**53,032.9**	**62,099.9**	**67,771.3**

Sources: Nittayaramphong and Tangcharoensathien (1994) originally from Health Planning Division, MOPH; National Accounts; Workmen's Compensation Fund, Ministry of Labour and Social Welfare; Controller-General's Department, Ministry of Finance; Financing Health Service and Medical Care in Thailand (1987 report), MOPH.

TABLE 10.4   Budget Expenditures Classified by Program, Fiscal Years 1994–96 (Unit: Million Baht)

	Budget Expenditure (percent)		
Program	1994	1995	1996
Economic development	127,846.4	149,114.3	186,788.3 **(22.15)**
Social development	243,404.2	277,923.7	353,363.7 **(41.91)**
Education	124,457.9	137,641.4	169,560.7 **(20.11)**
Public health	44,335.0 **(7.09)**	52,372.7 **(7.33)**	63,452.2 **(7.53)**
Social services	74,611.3	87,909.6	120,350.8 **(14.27)**
Maintenance of national security and maintenance of internal peace and order	125,063.9	131,886.1	148,304.3 **(17.59)**
General services	70,172.7	111,345.1	106,751.7 **(12.66)**
Debt services	58,512.8	44,730.8	47,992.0 **(5.69)**
Total	**625,000**	**715,000**	**843,200 (100)**

Source: Bureau of the Budget, Office of the Prime Minister.

fiscal year 1996, of the total 843,200 million baht government's estimated receipts, 87.4 percent was from taxes, 7.0 percent from state enterprises, 3.0 percent from sales of assets and services, and 2.6 percent from miscellaneous sources. Only 36.56 percent of government tax revenue came from personal income tax and corporate income tax. All indirect taxes accounted for 71.31 percent: general sales tax 30.54 percent, export-import duties 18.09 percent, and specific sales tax 21.98 percent (calculated from *Thailand in Figures*, 1996).

Health Insurance Development

Health insurance is a means of financial protection against the risk of unexpected and expensive health care. In countries such as Thailand, where the use of government health services is heavily subsidized, governments are implicitly covering the risk of incurring high cost care. This limits the demand for more explicit types of risk-sharing arrangements. Explicit forms of health insurance are widespread in the industrialized or middle-income countries. In some countries, such as Canada and Japan and most European countries, coverage is compulsory and universal and the insurance program is financed from either general government revenue or payroll taxes. In the United States, insurance coverage is voluntary, administered by third parties, not universal, and usually financed by a combination of employer and employee contributions. The expansion of health insurance coverage is usually intended to increase health sector revenues, reduce financial barriers to care, and improve the efficiency of resource allocation and use (Kutzin 1995). How to achieve universal coverage when the proportion of the population in the formal sector is relatively low, for example in a country such as Thailand, is one of the major problems in expanding coverage. Health insurance schemes in Thailand can be classified into three types: welfare and fringe benefit, compulsory, and voluntary health insurance, as discussed below by Piyaratn and Janjaroen (1994) and Tangcharoensathien and Suphachutikul (1993).

There are four health insurance schemes in the welfare and fringe benefit category: Civil Service Medical Benefit Scheme (CSMBS), Free Medical Care for the Low Income Household Scheme (FC/L), Free Medical Care for the Elderly Scheme (FC/E), and the School Health Insurance Scheme (SHI). The CSMBS, initiated in 1980, aims to provide medical care benefits to civil servants and employees, retired pensioners, and their dependents. Dependents include parents, spouses, and up to three children under 20 years of age. Benefits of this scheme include medical consultations, medical treatment, operations and other therapeutic care, drugs, inpatient care, and obstetric delivery expenses. The total population coverage was estimated to be 6.4 million, or 11 percent of the total Thai population in 1993. The FC/L was initiated in 1975 with the twin objectives of creating more equitable access to health services and improving the health status of the poor. The target populations are single persons with income less than 2,000 baht (US$80) per month, 24,000 baht (US$960) per year, and married couples with income less than 33,600 baht (US$1,344) per year per person. The benefits are free medical services from public outlets and hospitals. The population coverage was 11.7 million, or 21 percent of the total population in 1993.

The FC/E was implemented in 1992 with the aim of increasing accessibility to health services and improving the health status of the elderly. The target population is those citizens 60 years old and above who are not covered by other schemes. The benefits include outpatient and inpatient care provided at public facilities. The population coverage was 3.5 million, or 6 percent of the total population in 1993.

Finally SHI, the school health insurance scheme, guarantees medical service to schoolchildren from grade 1 to grade 9 (around 6–14 years old). The population coverage in this scheme was 6.7 million, or 11.5 percent of the total population in 1993. The benefits cover outpatient and inpatient care at public service units. In some areas, dental services are also provided.

Compulsory insurance consists of three insurance schemes: the Workmen Compensation Scheme (WCS), the Social Security Scheme (SSS), and Car Accidental Insurance (CAI). The WCS was introduced in 1974. The objectives of the scheme are to protect workers from illness, injuries, death, and disability caused by work or work-related conditions. The target population is employees in firms with more than 10 workers. Benefits include medical compensation for work-related illness and injuries, temporary and permanent disability benefits, survivor's pension, funeral grants, and rehabilitation expenses. Population coverage in 1992 was 2.8 million, which was 5 percent of the total population.

The SSS was enacted in 1990 and implemented in February 1991. The objectives are to protect workers from nonoccupational illness and injuries and to compensate for maternity, disability, and death. The target population is firms with more than 10 employees. Population coverage was 3.8 million, or 7 percent of the total population in 1993.

The CAI scheme was implemented in 1992, with the main objectives of guaranteeing medical treatment for victims of vehicular accidents. In theory or by law, every vehicle owner, including motorcycle owners, must have this insurance; in practice many are uninsured.

Two health insurance schemes are voluntary: the Voluntary Health Insurance Scheme (VHIS) and Private Health Insurance (PHI). The PHI scheme was introduced in 1978 when the Thai Medical and Health Company Limited was established. The scheme's main objective was to improve security and provide better health care, often by combining life insurance and medical insurance for people in the upper-middle and high-income groups who can afford the premiums. Population coverage was only 0.6 million, or 1 percent of the total population in 1992.

The last scheme is VHIS, commonly known as the Health Insurance Card Scheme, first introduced as the Health Card Project in 1983. The three main objectives of this scheme are to promote community development under the primary health care program, foster the rational use of health services via a referral system, and increase health resources based on a community-financing concept. The Voluntary Health Insurance Scheme has been continuously monitored and evaluated. Frequent adjustments of its strategies and objectives have included voluntary risk sharing with cost recovery in addition to service provision (see table 10.5). The target population is the near-poor and middle-income class in rural areas or those who can afford the premium.

TABLE 10.5 Modification of Health Card Program: Rationale, Objectives, and Activities

	1983	1984–1986	1987–1991	1992–present
Rationale	1. MCH + FP (Community Financing) 1. MCH+FP 2. Referral system	1. PHC 2. Referral system 3. Integrated services 4. MOPH decentralized decisionmaking to provincial level 5. Community Financing 6. To reduce OP visits at provincial hospital	PHC + Voluntary health insurance To provide security to the people PHC	Voluntary health insurance To provide security to the people Coverage all services
1.1 Implementing area	7 provinces 18 villages 1. Khon Kaen 2. Roei 3. Lamphun 4. Nakhon Sawan 5. Phetchaburi 6. Ratchaburi 7. Songkhla	1. At each province selecting 2 villages from one subdistrict 2. Chiang Mai (GTZ) In 1984 implementing in 4 districts, 6 subdistricts, and 33 villages In 1985 whole province	At each province selecting 3 villages from 8 subdistricts in each district	68 provinces
1.2 Coverage	N/A	34% of population 55% of households	36% of households	20% of population 21% of households
1.3 Type and price of card	Medical care and MCH $8 Medical care $4 MCH $4	Family $8 MCH $4	Family $12 Individual $8 MCH $4	Family $20 (member < 5) (MCH included) (Individual is an option)
1.4 Criteria for card use	—	8 episodes (ceiling $80 per episode)	6 episodes (ceiling $80 per episode)	No limit
1.5 Level: health card fund	Village	Village	Village	District Province
1.6 Subsidy	N/A	N/A	$13.50 per card	$20 per card
1.7 Share of health card fund	—	Health service unit 75% Health center 15%, Community hospital 30%, Provincial and regional hospital 30% Health personal 10% Program managing 15%	N/A	Health service unit 80% Incentive & adm. 20% of total monetary amount of card sales revenue (the formula differs slightly from year to year)

Source: Modified from Singkaew (1995, pp. 19–21).

At present, the price of a health insurance card is 1,000 baht (US$40) per year per household of not more than five members. A household contributes half of the price; the other half is subsidized by general tax revenue through the Ministry of Public Health.

The benefits include outpatient care for illness and injuries, inpatient care, and mother and child health services. There is no limit on utilization of the services. The beneficiaries, however, can only go to health care provider units under the MOPH. The first contact is either the health center or community hospital; patients must then follow a referral line for higher levels of care. There is a specific time for card selling at each health card cycle. At present the cycle is one year, and the specific time for card selling depends on the seasonal fluctuations in income. The premium is collected when cash incomes are highest, when, for example, crops are harvested. In 1992 the population coverage by the health card program was 3.6 million, or about 5 percent of the total population.

Summary Information on the Health Card Program

The Health Card Program, introduced in 1983, is based on the risk sharing of health expenditure with no cost sharing in a voluntary health insurance prepayment scheme. Ideally, in a prepayment-insurance scheme, members enroll when healthy, and only those who fall ill make use of services. The success of risk sharing in prepayment-insurance schemes depends upon enrolling a large enough number of people to ensure a sufficient pooling of risks.

Mechanisms for community financing of health resources, one of HCP's three main objectives, include revolving drug funds, nutrition funds, and other funds, which at present are health card funds. The health card program was gradually implemented in rural areas and later, in 1985, started in some urban areas of six pilot provinces. The MOPH health facilities are responsible for providing care to health cardholders. During the HCP implemented nationwide before 1992, the MOPH decentralized decisionmaking to the provincial level, allowing health agencies to define their own prices for health cards and policies of disease coverage, number of episodes, number of members, the level of compensation to providers, and the percentage of HCF kept in the community. The number of members covered by a card varies by provinces, but the premium is generally the same (Tangcharoensathien 1995). In 1995, there were many adjustments in the program. Some were that no HCF is kept in the community, the maximum number of members per card is five, no limit is set on the number of episodes, and no ceiling is set on health care expense. The price of a card is fixed at 500 baht (US$20 in 1995). MOPH set a general formula for allocating HCF, that is, to compensate the providers for administrative costs and for incentives to sell cards, but kept decentralized decisionmaking at the provincial levels, allowing those levels to design details of HCF allocation. In 1985–86, there was strong support from MOPH for the Health Card Program. In 1986, the program was described to the parliament as a key strategy toward a voluntary health insurance. Unfortunately,

HCP was a low priority for MOPH support from 1989 until 1995. This reflects the overall HCP situation during 1988–1992. In 1990, the area coverage rate in terms of population by HCP was 4.49 percent in 1988 and decreased to 2.6 percent in 1992. HCP covered 20.3 percent of villages in 1988 and increased to 33.6 percent in 1992; 48.2 percent of subdistricts in 1988 decreased to 30.2 percent in 1992; covered 79.7 percent of districts in 1988 and decreased to 58.8 percent in 1992 (Health Insurance Office report 1992; Kiranandana and Apairatr 1990).

Assessments and Studies of HCP

Demand for health cards has changed over time due to various factors in both the demand and supply sides, particularly government health policies. There are likewise many studies on the performance of the program.

The Health Card Program in Chiang Mai is the pilot phase of a national health insurance system in Thailand. In 1985, 1986, and 1988, the pilot project for the Health Card Program and Social Research Institute (SRI) of Chiang Mai University conducted three household surveys. The surveys investigated household health care expenditure and utilization patterns, health card knowledge, attitudes of the target groups regarding the health card system, and fund management. In 1988, Adeyi studied the Health Card Program in Chiang Mai and found three main factors affecting health card purchase: the expectations of free treatment, reduced waiting time at referral centers, and subsidized drugs. Since the present program has many changes, some of these factors may no longer affect the health card purchase.

The main reason for buying a health card has been examined in various studies. Kiranandana (1990) evaluated the HCP situation using a national census of all HCFs and health facilities and found that the main reason was not to ensure future coverage for the possible illness of a household member, but either awareness that a family member was currently becoming sick or influence from others. In 1994, Veeravongs analyzed the HCP in the Phuket Province and found that the influencing factors of health card purchase were coverage by alternative health insurance, accessibility to health care, card purchaser's place of origin and sex, age of the household head, level of education of the household head and religious group affiliation, marital status of the household head, number of household members, number of sick household members, and problems experienced with health expenditure. In summary, the reasons to buy a card are economic conditions, benefits of the program, family size, presence of illness in the family, expectation of received health care, and the way the program is publicized (Hongvivatana and others 1986; Santampol 1990; Supakankunti, Janjaroen, and Sritamma 1996). When HCP has been implemented in its current revised form (1995 to date), a research question arises: What are the current reasons for a household to buy the health card? These problems of moral hazard and adverse selection are also found in other countries with similar programs. For example, in Burundi, if insurance is sold for short periods to accommodate families' fluctuations in income, then people may buy the "health card" entitling them to services only when they are already sick or can anticipate a medical need (McPake, Hanson and Mills 1992).

The reasons not to buy a card have also been studied and identified as follows: trend of the number of card users decreases because people do not have enough money to pay for the card, because of the health workers or the inefficiency of the referral system, because they do not receive enough information about the card, because they have alternative health insurance, never used a previous card, no one sells the card, or it is difficult to use card (Manopimoke 1993).

The attitude of households toward the program is a main factor for program sustainability. Hongvivatana and Manopimoke (1991) found that more than 50 percent of the people knew about the benefits of the program. When there were changes in the price of the card, including the benefits and criteria for card use in 1993, more than 50 percent of the people knew about the changes. Nonetheless, between card users and nonusers there was a significant difference, with the card user group having better knowledge than the nonuser group.

Behavior of card users had been examined in various studies, but there is no clear evidence of the changes in behavior before and after the implementation of the program. In addition, the episodes of card use and the referral systems have been studied in various ways. Even though the health center and community hospital can screen patients before referring them to a higher level, Kiranandana and Apairatr (1990) found that more than 50 percent of the patients at community and regional hospitals did not follow the referral system. The health center bypass rate (without a referral letter) was 52 percent for outpatients (OPs) and 40 percent for inpatients (IPs), respectively. Health centers could screen 62 percent of the OP consultations (38 percent were referred), while community hospitals could screen up to 97 percent of the OP visits, with only 3 percent referred. These findings are consistent with those in other studies, which have found that people still do not follow the referral system.

The sustainability of the program also depends on program financial viability, which is in turn dependent upon relatively stable and adequate demand to ensure a sufficient pooling of risks. Therefore the cost of providing health care at all levels, usage rates, and utilization patterns of cardholders, apart from purchase patterns, have been studied. Different unit costs in different regions and years from several studies are shown in table 10.6.

Cost recovery also has been studied in various regions and years. The cost recovery for community and provincial hospitals is still quite low. Permpoonwatanasuk (1985) looked at cost recovery in the Ratchaburi Province and found it to be 32.62–47.76 percent; while in the Health Card Program in Chiang Mai (1989) it was 31 and 39 percent in 1987 and 1988, respectively (only material cost). Kiranandana and Apairatr (1990) found that cost recovery for drugs was 40 percent for community hospitals and 46 percent for provincial hospitals. Manopimoke (1993) found that for outpatients at community and provincial hospitals cost recovery was 60 percent and 59 percent, respectively, for an average of 70 percent. The inpatient average was 54 percent, and cost recovery at health centers was 108 percent.

TABLE 10.6   Unit Cost at Health Service Unit Used by Health Card Member (Unit: Baht)

Case study	Index	Health Service Units			
		Health center	Com. hosp.	Prov. hosp.	Reg. hosp.
Ratchaburi	Cost/outpatient visit	23.61	77.35	86.11	—
(1985)	Cost/inpatient day	—	283.85	466.25	—
Ubon-	Cost/outpatient	10.11[a]	69.31[d]	—	137.34
Ratchathani		7.17[b]	60.01[e]	—	—
(1984)		15.09[c]	63.10[f]	—	—
	Cost/inpatient	—	733.99[d]	—	1,431.34
		—	419.04[e]	—	—
		—	556.09[f]	—	—
Chiang Mai*	Cost/visit	23.85	66.12	52.62	—
(1987)	Cost/admission	—	364.15	724.99	—
	Cost/green card/year				
	outpatient	74.87	112.40	4.21	—
	inpatient	—	29.13	28.96	—
Chiang Mai**	Cost/visit	26.11	67.27	50.39	—
(1987)	Cost/green card/year				
	outpatient	65.28	107.63	9.07	—
	inpatient	—	27.30	77.84	—
(1988)	Cost/visit	30.44	64.60	76.01	—
	Cost/green card/year				
	outpatient	32.27	38.76	28.88	—
	inpatient	—	39.28	91.21	—
Chiang Mai***	Cost/outpatient	100	182	212	—
(1996)	Cost/outpatient visit	34	96	118	—
	Cost/inpatient	—	1,100	1,102	—
	Cost/inpatient day	—	303	522	—
9 provinces	Cost/person/year	9.98	34.27	17.84	17.74
(samples)	Cost/card/year	36.71	114.84	79.09	79.09

Note: Districts in Ubon Ratchathani: a. Sa Tuek, b. Non Rung, c. Som Sa Ard, d. Tra Karn Puech Phol, e. Khueng Nai, f. Dech Udom.

Sources: Ratchaburi: Chaisak Permpoonwatanasuk (1985); Ubon Ratchathani: Penjant Pradabmuk (1984); Chiang Mai*, Thai-German Technical Cooperation for Health (1987); Chiang Mai**, Health Card Program in Chiang Mai (1989); Chiang Mai***, Pravuth Vechrak (1996); sample of 9 provinces: Vachiraphan Chantamars (1989).

The card usage rate from the Thai-German Technical Cooperation for Health (1987) found that the averages of outpatient visits per case at health centers, community hospitals, and provincial hospitals were 0.5, 0.38, and 0.12, respectively. Kiranandana and Apairatr (1990) found on average, in a health card fund, 207 outpatient visits were made, 44 percent at a health center, 33 percent at a community hospital, and 23 percent at a provincial hospital (nine inpatients were admitted to the hospitals). Thus the health card usage rate was 6.63 services per card per year.

The success of the program depends on several factors implicit in health service utilization and health card purchasing patterns, as well as government policy: personal health management, the effectiveness of HCP, and community participation. A review of this scheme identified four critical factors for success: (1) strong government support, (2) managerial capability and supervision by local health staff, (3) strong community involvement and capacity, and (4) administrative simplicity of the scheme (Wibulpolprasert 1991 cited in Kutzin 1995). Before 1995, the main difference between HCP and other health insurance programs was that the financial management of the HCP was in the hands of responsible committees at village level, under the supervision of health workers. The committee could manage revenue collected as a revolving fund for income-generating activities initiated by villagers to promote PHC (Veeravongs 1994). According to the records, some villages had success in managing the fund, while some encountered many problems. Therefore this was removed under the most recent form of the HCP. The committee is now at the district and provincial levels and cannot use the fund to generate income. In addition to this change, the price and type of card and the criteria for card use have changed. Therefore this study is different from previous studies, which analyzed the former program.

METHODS

Study Area

Khon Kaen Province has had, and has developed, experience with voluntary health insurance since 1983. In 1995, Thailand had 76 provinces in total. Khon Kaen is a large province located in the northeastern part of the country. In 1995, it had a population of 1,652,030, population rank per total was 4/76, and population per square kilometer was 152. The population age structure in the year 2000 has been estimated for age groups 0–9, 10–19, 20–39, 40–59, and 60+ as 19.0, 19.1, 37.0, 18.0, and 6.9, respectively. Its area accounts for 10,886 square kilometers and area rank per total was 15/76. For the economic status, Khon Kaen's gross provincial product (GPP) in 1993 was 38,688 million baht. GPP rank per total was 12/73, and GPP per capita was 23,519 baht. The industry that has the highest share in the GPP is the wholesale and retail trade sector, with growth in the transport, communication, and service sectors, and a decrease in the agriculture sector. Khon Kaen was designated a major city in the northeastern part of Thailand along the country development plan. In the province there are a regional university and several public health facilities: 1 regional hospital, 7 specialist centers or health services, 19 community hospitals, 212 health centers, and 1 municipality health center. There are also many private clinics and hospitals.

The card project involved in this study was implemented in six districts in Khon Kaen Province. The target population was identified by the research team and the provincial health office. The provincial and district health officers and the research team went to the six districts to explain the program to the communities and to investigate the readiness of the communities. A sample of 1,000 households from the target population were selected by health officers. In this study, investigations were conducted first to examine differing characteristics of card purchasers and nonusers as well as of card dropouts and continuing card users. There are four groups of house-holds in the sample: (1) individuals who had not purchased a health card during the period 1993–1995, or *card nonpurchase;* (2) individuals who had purchased a health card for the first time in 1995, or *new card purchase;* (3) individuals who had repur-chased a health card, or *continued card purchase;* and (4) individuals who had not repurchased a health card, or *health card dropouts.* Further examination of the attitudes toward the health card program of card and non–card users at health centers and community hospitals will be carried out, using information from the questionnaires.

Data Sources

This chapter is based in part on the data collected from the research project on voluntary health insurance in Khon Kaen Province. The project implemented in Khon Kaen was a pilot project, the main objective of which was to provide health insurance for the uninsured in the province to achieve universal cover-age. The study period was 1994–95. The unit of study was households in selected rural areas. Health officers at both provincial and district levels were trained to conduct field interviews in six districts (study areas). There were four types of questionnaires used in the study:

- Interview questionnaire of subdistrict and village leaders and volunteer health workers

- Interview questionnaire of households in the sample areas

- Interview questionnaire about the attitude toward the program of card and non–card users

- Cost data obtained from the health center and community hospital.

In addition to these primary data, there is secondary data, namely the statistics of card-usage rate at all levels, utilization rates, retrospective reimbursement from providers, and the number of insured and uninsured in the province before and after the implementation of the program, by type of insurance schemes. Data from the reports from each district in which the card project was imple-mented are also used in the study.

The primary data of households and health facilities consists of:

- Socioeconomic information, that is, number of household members, marital status, gender, age, number of dependents, number of unemployed members, use of alternative health insurance, education, occupation, income, type of expenditure and income, problem of health care payment, presence of illness (in past three months), number of members having chronic illness

- Health care seeking behavior, that is, choice of providers, type of communica-tion, health card knowledge, decision to buy health card

- Health care services utilization, that is, health card utilization rate, hospital utilization rate

- Source of health care financing, that is, out-of-pocket, relative, health insurance

- Attitude of the target groups regarding the health card system

- Utilization rate and reimbursement of health care expenditure from providers.

Analytic Methods

This study employed both qualitative and quantitative methods. The data were entered from the interview questionnaires into coding form, and verification of the database was carried out using spreadsheet software. Data processing involved use of the statistical package for Social Science (SPSS/PC+, Marija J. Norusis/SPSS Inc., 1993).

The analysis of the data involved the investigation of the factors influencing health card purchases and dropout patterns including continuity of card use as well as attitude of card users. The nonparametric test, that is, Chi-square statistic and parametric t-test statistic, were used initially to identify the various variables in both socioeconomic and psychological factors. These significant factors provide more understanding of demographic and socioeconomic patterns between card purchase and nonpurchase groups, and of subsequent repurchase and non-repurchase groups. The logistic regression model was then used to identify significant predictors of health card purchase and nonpurchase patterns as well as the continuation of card purchase. Card utilization patterns and attitudes toward the health card will also be analyzed for a better understanding of the future prospect of voluntary health insurance in Thailand.

Results

The total number of response households was 1,005. The number of households that reported having not purchased a health card at any time over the 1993 to 1995 period was N = 495 (49.3 percent) as *non–card purchase* and N = 510 (50.7 percent) as *card purchase*. Of the 510 cards purchased, N = 297 (58.2 percent) as *new card purchase*, N = 132 (25.9 percent) as *continued card purchase,* and N = 81 (15.9 percent) as *health card dropout* (no longer cardholders).

Description of the Data

The demographic, socioeconomic, and cultural characteristics of card purchase and nonpurchase, and of subsequent repurchase groups are shown in tables 10.7–10.10. Results shown in the tables may be interpreted in different ways, since the program has undergone many changes, for example, in price and type of card, card usage criteria, and financial management, as stated above. Some characteristics between the health card nonpurchase and new card purchase groups are different (see table 10.7). The results show that compared with the nonpurchase group, those in the health card new purchase group were older,

TABLE 10.7   Demographic and Socioeconomic Characteristics of Health Card New Purchase and Health Card Nonpurchase

Demographic Socioeconomic Characteristics	Health Card Nonpurchase (495)	Health Card New Purchase (297)
Marital status		
Single/widowed/divorced	2.4	2.7
Married	97.6	97.3
Educational level **		
Lower 6 grade	87.1	93.9
Higher	12.9	6.1
Number of household members		
Under 5	66.9	70.2
6 and above	33.1	29.8
(average)	(5.03)	(5.01)
Average number of employed members	2.32	2.83
Average household income/baht/year	60,253.17	50,580.00
Presence of illness***		
Yes	47.5	57.2
No	52.5	42.8
Number of sick members with chronic illness		
None	78.4	78.5
1–2	20.6	21.5
More than 2	1.0	0.0
Family economic problems during sickness of family members		
Have problems	13.6	17.5
Never have problems	86.4	82.5

Note: *$p<.05$, **$p<.01$, and ***$p<.001$

had a higher average number of employed members in the family, had a higher percentage of presence of illness, had a higher percentage of family economic problems during sickness of family members, and had a lower level of education and household income per year. Only two of these factors are significant, namely educational level and presence of illness.

In addition, among the health card dropout group and continued health card purchase group, the results show that compared with the health card dropout group, the continued card purchase group tended to get married at a higher rate, have a lower educational level, have a higher average number of employed members in the family, have a smaller number of household members, have a higher household income per year, have more members with chronic illness, have a higher percentage of presence of illness, have a higher percentage of having family economic problems during sickness of family members, and have a higher percentage of card use (see table 10.8). But only one factor is significant—presence of illness. Interestingly, these findings are consistent with the above comparison between health card nonpurchase and health card new purchase

TABLE 10.8   Demographic and Socioeconomic Characteristics of Health Card Dropout and Continued Card Purchase

Demographic socioeconomic characteristics	Health card dropout (81)	Continued card purchase (132)
Marital status		
Single/widowed/divorced	4.9	3.1
Married	95.1	96.9
Educational level		
Lower 6 grade	87.5	93.1
Higher	12.5	6.9
Number of household members		
Under 5	63.0	71.8
6 and above	37.0	28.2
(average)	(5.15)	(4.86)
Average number of employed members	2.52	2.88
Average household income/baht/year	44,964.35	52,207.26
Presence of illness**		
Yes	48.1	66.7
No	51.9	33.3
Number of sick members with chronic illness		
None	82.7	77.3
1–2	16.0	19.7
More than 2	1.2	3.0
Family economic problems during sickness of family members		
Have problems	13.5	15.4
Never have problems	86.5	84.6

Note: *p<.05, **p<.01, and ***p<.001

groups except for the data on income per year, marital status, and number of sick members with chronic illness.

Between the health card nonpurchase group and the health card dropout group, the results show that compared with the health card nonpurchase group, the health card dropout group had a lower income per year and a lower number of sick members with chronic illness (see table 10.9). As expected, there were no significant differences between these groups; both groups had similar characteristics, and they did not purchase the card during the current year.

It is important to note that the association between chronic illness and health card purchase or insurers has been previously observed. For example, Hongvivatana and others (1986) found that there was significantly more chronic illness in a health card user family, as did Veeravongs (1994). But in this study even though there were differences—a higher percentage of sick members with chronic illness in the new health card purchase group than in the nonpurchase group, likewise a higher percentage in the continued card purchase group than in the health card dropout group, and also higher in the health card nonpur-

TABLE 10.9   Demographic and Socioeconomic Characteristics of Health Card Nonpurchase and Dropout Groups

Demographic socioeconomic characteristics	Health card non-purchase (495)	Health card dropout (81)
Marital status		
Single/widowed/divorced	2.4	4.9
Married	97.6	95.1
Educational level		
Lower 6 grade	87.1	87.5
Higher	12.9	12.5
Number of household members		
Under 5	66.9	63.0
6 and above	33.1	37.0
(average)	(5.03)	(5.15)
Average number of employed members	2.32	2.52
Average household income/baht/year	60,253.17	44,964.35
Presence of illness		
Yes	47.5	48.1
No	52.5	51.9
Number of sick members with chronic illness		
None	78.4	82.7
1–2	20.6	16.0
More than 2	1.0	1.2
Family economic problems during sickness of family members		
Have problems	13.6	13.5
Never have problems	86.4	86.5

Note: $*p<.05$, $**p<.01$, and $***p<.001$

chase group when compared with the health card dropout group—there were no significant differences between any of these groups. After testing for the mean of numbers of chronic illness in the family between the health card nonpurchase group and the combined other three groups, no significant difference was found.

For further investigation of the factors influencing the purchase pattern, the response households were divided into two groups: the nonpurchase (never purchase) group and the purchase either current or continued purchase group. In table 10.10, the results show that when the nonpurchase group was compared with the purchase (currently purchase, continued, and dropout) group, the purchase group was older, had a higher average number of employed members in the family, had a higher percentage of presence of illness, had a higher percentage of family economic problems during sickness of family members, and had a lower average income per year and educational level. In terms of access to health facilities, the results show that the purchase group had more convenient access to a community hospital when needed than the nonpurchase group, and no different access for other places, such as health centers, private clinics, or hospitals.

TABLE 10.10   Demographic and Socioeconomic Characteristics of Health Card Nonpurchase and Health Card Purchase (Dropout/Continued/New Purchase Groups)

Demographic socioeconomic characteristics	Health card nonpurchase (495)	Health card purchase (510)
Marital status		
Single/widowed/divorced	2.4	3.2
Married	97.6	96.8
Educational level**		
Lower 6 grade	87.1	92.7
Higher	12.9	7.3
Number of household members		
Under 5	66.9	69.4
6 and above	33.1	30.6
(average)	(5.03)	(4.99)
Average number of employed member**	2.32	2.80
Average household income/baht/year**	60,253.17	50,099.12
Presence of illness**		
Yes	47.5	58.2
No	52.5	41.8
Number of sick members with chronic illness		
None	78.4	78.8
1–2	20.6	20.2
More than 2	1.0	1.0
(average)	(0.23)	(0.22)
Family economic problems during sickness of family members		
Have problems	13.6	16.3
Never have problems	86.4	83.7

Note: *$p<.05$, **$p<.01$, and ***$p<.001$

Only four of these factors are significant, namely educational level, income per year, number of employed members in the family, and presence of illness.

Interestingly, the significant factors between the health card nonpurchase group and the health card new purchase group are educational level and presence of illness. The latter factor also was significant between the health card dropout and continued card purchase group and between the purchase and nonpurchase groups. As expected, it was not significant between the health card nonpurchase and the health card dropout group. This strongly confirms the problem of adverse selection among health card purchase and nonpurchase groups. The family with presence of illness tended to purchase and repurchase the health card. This crucial finding indicates a factor that will jeopardize the sustainability of the HCP in the future if the program continues to be implemented without improvement.

Some of the psychological factors affecting card use were found to be particularly related to the continued and dropout groups. The continued card purchase group reported greater knowledge regarding the referral system, greater ability to seek treatment, greater convenience in buying a card, greater use of the health card, and greater satisfaction in using a card. They were more likely to have been persuaded by a health officer rather than a HCF committee or village leader to buy a health card. By receiving a clear explanation about the card in advance from a health officer, they were able to make a decision to buy a card immediately. They had better access to health centers, while those in the card dropout group had better access to a community hospital. Finally, they wanted to buy a card, although no one persuaded them when compared with the dropout group, which has a higher percentage of having been persuaded to buy a card at home. But only a few factors are significant: convenient access to health care, persuasion by a health officer to buy a card, reception of clear advance information about the health card from a health officer, health card usage in the last year, satisfaction with the health card, and persuasion by a neighbor to buy a card. These factors clearly demonstrate how to make cardholders continue to buy a card. The effort needs active health officers who will explain about the health card, but it also depends on how convenient health care access is for people, and what card use experience they have had.

Logistic Regression Model

In the first part of the analysis, the factors influencing card purchase and nonpurchase were identified by using t-test and Chi-square analyses. The analysis was performed separately for the following four pairs:

- The nonpurchase and purchase group

- The health card dropout and continued card purchase group

- The nonpurchase and new card purchase group

- The nonpurchase and health card dropout group.

Only five significant demographic and socioeconomic factors were identified, namely, educational background, number of employed members in the family, household income per year, presence of illness, and convenient access to health care—that is, health center, community hospital, private health facilities, provincial hospital. These factors were included in the logistic regression models to estimate their relationships to the following health card purchase patterns: (1) the nonpurchase versus purchase (dropout/continued/new purchase) group, (2) the nonpurchase and health card dropout group versus continued and new card purchase group, (3) the nonpurchase versus new card purchase group, (4) the health card dropout versus continued card purchase group, and (5) the new card purchase and continued card purchase versus health card dropout group. In models 4 and 5, nine more factors were added to estimate the pattern of card purchase. The additional factors added were who persuaded the cardholder to buy a card (health officer, village health volunteer, village leader); who gave a clear explanation of the health card; health card usage; satisfaction with the health card; and persuasion by a neighbor to buy a health card.

The following factors were used to estimate the various models of the logistic regressions to identify the best set of predictors for each model:

Marital status

- Single/widowed/divorced
- Married

Age in years

- Under 40
- 41 and above

Educational level

- No school/primary
- Secondary
- Higher

Proportion of employed persons to total family members

Household income per year

- Less than 33,600 baht
- More than 33,600 baht

Presence of illness

Number of sick members with chronic illness in the family

Family economic problems during sickness of family members

The most convenient place to access health care

- Health center
- Community hospital
- Private hospital/private clinic/drugstore
- Other

Who influenced card purchase

- Village health volunteer
- Health center personnel
- Village head
- Other

Who explained clearly and in advance about health card program

- Village health volunteer
- Health center personnel
- Village head
- Other

How the person persuaded cardholder to buy a card

- Arranged meeting at village
- Came to your home

- None
- Other

Who made the decision to buy a health card
  - Household head
  - Spouse or household members
  - Card bought from whom
  - Village health volunteer
  - Health center personnel
  - Village head
  - Other

Health card usage
  - Satisfaction with the card
  - Persuaded neighbors to buy a card

The Coefficients of the Logistic Regression Model

In logistic regression the probability of an event occurring, such as card purchase, can be directly estimated from the model. For the case of multiple independent variables, the logistic regression model can be written as

(10.1)   Prob (card purchase) $= 1/1 + e^{-Z}$,

where Z is the linear combination

$Z = B_0 + B_1 X_1 + B_2 X_2 + \dots\dots\dots\dots + B_P X_P$.

The probability of the event not occurring is estimated as

Prob (not purchase) $= 1 -$ Prob (purchase).

Xi are the independent variables in the model, such as the demographic-socioeconomic factors or psychological factors among health card purchasers and nonpurchasers. The interpretation of the logistic regression coefficient is not straightforward as in the regression model. The logistic model can be rewritten in terms of the odds of an event occurring. The odds of an event occurring are defined as the ratio of the probability that it will occur to the probability that it will not. The value of the coefficient for each variable indicates the changes in the log odds when the value of a particular variable changes by one unit and the values of the other independent variables remain the same (SPSS/PC+, Marija J. Norusis/SPSS Inc. 1993).

DISCUSSION

Results from the various models of the health card groups described above are interesting and should prove valuable from several aspects. Tables 10.11–10.14 show that the statistically significant factors distinguishing purchase groups (dropout, continued, and newly purchase groups) from nonpurchase groups are educational level, proportion of employed persons to total family members,

TABLE 10.11   Variables that Predict People Who Ever Purchased a Health Card Versus Nonpurchase Group

Variable	Coefficient	Standard error	Significance	Exp. (β) odds ratio
Marital status				
Single	0.7467	1.4994	0.6185	2.1100
Married	0.4360	1.4416	0.7623	1.5465
Widowed	0.3409	1.4984	0.8200	1.4062
Separated	−0.4263	2.0675	0.8367	0.6530
Age	−0.0003	0.0079	0.9727	0.6530
Gender	0.0888	0.1662	0.5934	1.0928
Educational level				
Primary	2.0272	0.8406	0.0159	7.7924
Secondary	1.5163	0.8711	0.0817	4.5552
Proportion of employed in household	−0.7015	0.1565	0.0000	0.4959
Household income				
Quintile 1	0.6477	0.2435	0.0078	1.9111
Quintile 2	0.3913	0.2355	0.0966	1.4789
Quintile 3	0.6207	0.2350	0.0082	1.8602
Quintile 4	0.5828	0.2305	0.0115	1.7910
Presence of illness in the past 3 months	0.4545	0.1515	0.0027	1.5754
Number of sick with chronic illness				
None	0.6365	0.6829	0.3513	1.8898
1–2	0.6049	0.6984	0.3864	1.8311
Economic problems during sickness	0.0329	0.2112	0.8763	1.0334
Most convenient access to health care				
Health center	−0.6580	0.2602	0.0115	0.5179
Community hospital	−0.7958	0.3046	0.0090	0.4512
Provincial hospital	0.0801	1.1992	0.9467	1.0834
Drugstore	0.2289	0.5545	0.6797	1.2572
Private hospital	−1.2076	1.4773	0.4137	0.2989
Private clinic	−2.0717	0.6338	0.0011	0.1260
University hospital	−5.3682	5.8082	0.3554	0.0047
Constant	−2.6297	1.8332	0.1514	

household income, presence of illness, and a convenient community hospital. Interestingly, the significant differences related to purchase patterns in the current year between currently nonpurchase (never purchase and dropout groups) and currently purchase (continued and new card purchase) are the first four as well, but the fifth, the most convenient place to access health care, is no longer significant in the model. This is consistent with the model of card purchase between the nonpurchase and new purchase groups. The finding clearly and strongly demonstrates that health card purchase in Khon Kaen in the current year is influenced by the following four factors: proportion of employed to total in family, education, household income, and presence of illness. The last factor

TABLE 10.12 Variables that Predict Health Card Nonpurchase and Dropout Groups Versus Continued and New Card Purchase Groups

Variable	Coefficient	Standard error	Significance	Exp. (β) odds ratio
Marital status				
Single	0.3945	1.4957	0.7920	1.4836
Married	0.3018	1.4401	0.8340	1.3523
Widowed	0.6496	1.4972	0.6644	1.9148
Separated	−0.3808	2.0320	0.8514	0.6833
Age	−0.0102	0.0080	0.2029	0.9898
Gender	0.1677	0.1681	0.3186	1.1826
Educational level				
Primary	1.7220	0.8331	0.0387	5.5957
Secondary	0.8842	0.8698	0.3093	2.4210
Proportion of employed in household	−0.6352	0.1563	0.0000	0.5298
Household income				
Quintile 1	0.3476	0.2469	0.1591	1.4157
Quintile 2	0.3002	0.2397	0.2105	1.3501
Quintile 3	0.5018	0.2370	0.0342	1.6517
Quintile 4	0.7239	0.2323	0.0018	2.0625
Presence of illness in the past				
3 months	0.4972	0.1524	0.0011	1.6442
Number of sick with chronic illness				
None	0.6449	0.6063	0.3473	1.9059
1–2	0.8206	0.7020	0.2424	2.2718
Economic problems during sickness	−0.0054	0.2108	0.9797	0.9946
Most convenient access to health care				
Health center	−0.6941	0.2473	0.1640	0.7088
Community hospital	−0.3441	0.2983	0.0200	0.4995
Provincial hospital	−6.5534	11.0855	0.5544	0.0014
Drugstore	0.5353	0.5292	0.3117	1.7080
Private hospital	−0.7154	1.4422	0.6199	0.4890
Private clinic	−1.4901	0.6292	0.0179	0.2254
University hospital	−5.8800	9.4998	0.5359	0.0028
Constant	−2.4282	1.8287	0.1842	

demonstrates the problem of adverse selection in the program, particularly significant since the health card program was introduced in the country in 1983, and Khon Kaen was one of seven provinces in the implementing areas in that year, has thus had experience with voluntary health insurance, and has undergone development of its program throughout the years.

The various previous studies of card purchase patterns showed the important factors for card purchase to be gender, age, chronic illness, alternative health insurance, family size, income, and health service satisfaction. Veeravongs (1994) found that females tended to purchase health cards more than males because this related to greater maternal and child health care card use, and that there was also an association

TABLE 10.13   Variables that Predict Health Card Nonpurchase Versus New Card Purchase Group

Variable	Coefficient	Standard error	Significance	Exp. (β) odds ratio
Marital status				
Single	0.0611	1.5223	0.9680	1.0630
Married	−0.1779	1.4451	0.9020	0.8370
Widowed	0.2639	1.5052	0.8608	1.3019
Separated	−7.1747	36.6851	0.8449	0.0008
Age	−0.0065	0.0093	0.4838	0.9935
Gender	0.3009	0.2000	0.1324	1.3511
Educational level				
Primary	2.2894	1.1173	0.0405	9.8693
Secondary	1.5669	1.1540	0.1745	4.7918
Proportion of employed in household	−0.5981	0.1781	0.0008	0.5494
Household income				
Quintile 1	0.4567	0.2846	0.1085	1.5789
Quintile 2	0.2161	0.2749	0.4318	1.2412
Quintile 3	0.6155	0.2658	0.0206	1.8505
Quintile 4	0.4982	0.2655	0.0607	1.6457
Presence of illness in the past				
3 months	0.4498	0.1744	0.0099	1.5680
Number of sick with chronic illness				
None	6.8014	16.1808	0.6742	899.0828
1–2	6.8769	16.1819	0.6709	969.5739
Economic problems during sickness	0.0405	0.2403	0.8660	1.0414
Most convenient access to health care				
Health center	−0.4297	0.3097	0.1653	0.6507
Community hospital	−0.4881	0.3571	0.1717	0.6138
Provincial hospital	−7.2429	36.6599	0.8434	0.0007
Drugstore	0.6634	0.5983	0.2675	1.9415
Private hospital	−7.2481	36.6596	0.8433	0.0007
Private clinic	−1.5246	0.7145	0.0329	0.2177
University hospital	−6.7581	15.5401	0.6636	0.0012
Constant	−9.0499	16.2870	0.5784	

between gender and chronic illness. Another important factor is family size, which some researchers have indicated (Veeravongs 1994; Hongvivatana and Manopimoke 1991; Suwanteerangkul 1992). This was not confirmed in this study since many aspects of the program have been changed. The gender and family-size factors were not statistically significant, perhaps because the average Thai family size is five persons and the sample shows, on average, household size is also five. More important, the health card is now a household card, which allows five members per card. The family-size factor was also not significant between groups, as tested above. Therefore the proportion of employed persons to total family members factor was selected in estimating the model to reflect the dependency among the family members. Interestingly, it was one of the significant factors found in this study.

TABLE 10.14   Variables that Predict New and Continued Health Card Purchase Versus Health Card Dropout Group

Variable	Coefficient	Standard error	Significance	Exp. (β) odds ratio
Marital status				
Single	−5.8711	60.4411	0.9226	0.0028
Married	−4.9461	60.4371	0.9348	0.0071
Widowed	1.4894	62.3793	0.9810	4.4344
Separated	0.7680	85.4692	0.9928	2.1555
Age	−0.0533	0.0182	0.0034	0.9481
Gender	−0.2368	0.3581	0.5084	0.7892
Educational level				
Primary	−6.5208	60.4342	0.9141	0.0015
Secondary	−7.9935	60.4356	0.8948	0.0003
Proportion of employed in household	−0.4364	0.3287	0.1843	0.6464
Household income				
Quintile 1	−0.8185	0.4989	0.1008	0.4411
Quintile 2	−0.0655	0.5323	0.9020	0.9366
Quintile 3	−0.1471	0.4944	0.7660	0.8632
Quintile 4	0.5668	0.5491	0.3020	1.7626
Presence of illness in the past				
3 months	0.1946	0.3395	0.5665	1.2149
Number of sick with chronic illness				
None	1.2969	1.3407	0.3334	3.6579
1–2	2.0872	1.3838	0.1315	8.0627
Economic problems during sickness	−0.3714	0.4572	0.4166	0.6898
Most convenient access to health care				
Health center	0.1308	0.4563	0.7744	1.1397
Community hospital	−0.4435	0.5730	0.4389	0.6418
Provincial hospital	−9.3719	42.7032	0.8263	0.0001
Drugstore	0.8040	1.1644	0.4899	2.2345
Private hospital	6.5944	29.1878	0.8213	730.9802
Recommendation to neighbors	−0.3269	0.4092	0.4243	0.7211
Purchase health card from				
HCF committee member or village				
health volunteer	−1.5333	0.6830	0.0248	0.2158
Heath center personnel	−0.4324	0.6372	0.4974	0.6490
Village head	−1.7454	0.8440	0.0386	0.1746
Health card usage	0.1527	0.3580	0.6696	1.1650
Who made decision to buy health card				
Household head	0.0110	0.4140	0.9787	1.0111
Spouse	−0.2649	0.4630	0.5673	0.7673
Constant	15.5619	85.4793	0.8555	

The households that had a higher proportion of employed persons tended to purchase more cards than the households with a lower proportion. This might be because the former can afford the price of the card, which must be prepaid, although the income factor was not of overall significance in this study. The proportion of employed to total in family factor might represent the income class, a higher proportion reflects the lower income class, which tended to buy health cards. This would also relate to alternative insurance schemes such as the Elderly Scheme (FC/E) and the School Health Insurance Scheme (SHI) since unemployed persons in the family might be eligible for these schemes. Moreover, most of the employed persons in rural areas are not covered by any of the health insurance schemes.

As stated above, income was not shown to be a strong determinant of card purchase. This was confirmed by Veeravongs (1994). However, other studies have found that economic status was a significant indicator of the ability to purchase a health card (Hongvivatana and Manopimoke 1991). There was not much difference in income among households in this study, the subjects of which were rural residents, even though there were observable trends by income among the groups. For example, the dropout group tended to have incomes lower than the continued card purchase group.

The other significant factor is education. Those with lower levels of education tended to purchase cards, since lower education means lower income and thus usually not covered by any of the health insurance schemes. The only health insurance for which these persons are eligible is the health card program. The number of members with chronic illness in the family, marital status, age, and problems with health expenditures were not significant in determining card purchase in this study.

The satisfaction with health services factor was indicated in previous studies as a determinant factor for card purchase, but in this study the factor was not significant. The results found little difference among households and found most to be satisfied with the services. This is discussed in detail below.

It was difficult to make a comparison between studies since the studies were of different areas and conducted at different times. Of most importance, however, are the differences in health card rationale, type and price of card, criteria for card use, health card fund management, government subsidies, and share of the health card fund.

Continuity of Card Purchase

The sustainability of the program depends on various factors, a very important one being is satisfaction of the card users to continue to buy. The findings indicate that the continuity of card purchase in the study was associated with these factors: marital status, lower levels of education, number of employed in the family, income, presence of illness, problems with health expenditure, most convenient place to access health care, health card usage, the persuasion of a household to buy the card at home, health center personnel, and persuasion by a neighbor to buy a card. Of these, the significant factors were persuasion by a neighbor to buy a card, age, education, income, health center personnel explained clearly about card, and persuasion of a household to buy the card at home.

To analyze the satisfaction of card users with health care services requires more data; therefore, this study utilized the data from another set of questionnaires distributed when the program had been implemented for one year. The sample is health care seekers at health center and community hospitals: possession or nonpossession of a health card. They were interviewed about their attitudes toward the health card program when seeking care at health centers and community hospitals and about their health-seeking behaviors in the past three months. Below is the summary of demographic and socioeconomic characteristics between individuals who held cards and those who did not hold cards.

Results in table 10.15 show that the statistically significant factors related to health card users and non–card users are education, number of household members, presence of illness, problems with health expenditure, and the most convenient place to access health care and seek care when sick. Card users tended to have a lower education, a lower average income per year, a lower health expenditure per year—but in terms of the proportion of total expenditure to total income it is higher. Moreover, card users had not had many problems with health expenditure and had more members in the family, had more presence of

TABLE 10.15   Demographic and Socioeconomic Characteristics of Health Care Seekers* by Whether or Not They Possess Health Card

Demographic socioeconomic characteristics	Health card (non-possession) (464)	Health card (possession) (500)
Marital status		
Single/widowed/divorced	15.1	12.8
Married	84.9	87.2
Educational level***		
Lower 6 grade	79.6	87.8
Higher	20.4	12.2
Number of household members**		
Under 5	72.9	70.2
6 and above	27.1	29.8
(average)	(4.78)	(5.07)
Gender		
Male	35.3	38.6
Female	64.7	61.4
Average household income/baht/year	63,453.84	58,572.21
Average household expenditure/baht/year	41,099.33	39,401.24
Average household health expenditure/baht/year	4,294.71	3,945.20
Average proportion of total expenditure to total income	0.7372	0.9477
Average proportion of health expenditure to total expenditure	0.1157	0.1123

(continued)

TABLE 10.15   Continued

Demographic socioeconomic characteristics	Health card (non-possession) (464)	Health card (possession) (500)
Presence of illness**		
Yes	42.1	52.0
No	57.9	48.0
(average)	(0.4213)	(0.5200)
Having chronic illness		
Yes	19.5	25.2
No	80.5	74.8
Family economic problems during sickness of family members**		
Have problems	38.4	30.2
Never have problems	61.6	69.8
Most convenient place to access health care		
Health center	75.1	81.0
Community hospital	16.5	15.2
Private clinic/hospital***	8.0	2.8
Other	0.4	1.0
Type of chronic illness	(86)	(127)
Diabetes	38.0	62.0
High blood pressure	58.8	41.2
Asthma/respiratory	39.4	60.6
Other	38.9	61.1
Seek care**		
Yes	69.9	78.6
No	30.1	21.4

Note: *Patients who visited health center or community hospital.

Note: * $p<.05$, ** $p<.01$, and *** $p<.001$

illness, had more chronic illness, sought more care when sick, and had a health center as the most convenience place of access. This shows that the health card eased their health expenditure burden, despite the fact that there was more illness among card users. The proportion of health expenditure to total expenditure on average was not different when compared with that of non–card users. Nonetheless there remained a problem of adverse selection among card users.

To improve the program, officials must know how often and what factors influence health card utilization. Table 10.16 shows that 69.4 percent of cardholders have used the cards 1–5 times, while only 4.2 percent never used it. In addition, 74.5 percent of card users tended to visit health centers while 23.8 percent with a common illness such as fever, cough, flu, and ulcer visited community hospitals. Interestingly, 94.8 percent were satisfied with health services, leaving only 5.2 percent not satisfied. Of those not satisfied, 63 percent had dissatisfaction with the referral system and 28 percent with the quality of care. Of the sample, 90 percent will purchase a health card again next year. Since this is related to the problem of illness, they definitely will utilize health cards.

The results in table 10.17 show that non–card users tended to receive no treatment when sick, have more self-prescription, and sought care at private clinics or hospitals, but sought care at health centers and public hospitals less than the card users. This health care seeking pattern among card users and non–card users strongly supports the importance of accessibility to health care among the card user group. However, it still leaves risk-sharing and card-utilization pattern problems to consider in making the program more sustainable and efficient. Therefore the health card utilization patterns will be studied in detail to provide more information on card usage.

TABLE 10.16   Frequency of Card Use among Card User Group

		N=451
Card utilization rate	Frequency	Percent
Never used	19	4.2
1–5	313	69.4
6–10	91	20.2
More than 10	28	6.2

TABLE 10.17   Health Care-Seeking Pattern in the Past 3 Months among Card Users and Noncard Users

	Percent of Health Care Seekers at Different Facilities		Number of Visits (average)		Drug Expenditure (Baht) (average)	
	Card users (500)	Non–card users (464)	Card users (500)	Non–card users (464)	Card users (500)	Non–card users (464)
Sick but no treatment	16.4	18.6	—	—	—	—
Self-prescription	12.0	19.5	2.16	2.37	89.00	72.80
Sick and received treatment at private clinics and hospitals	5.8	8.2	2.47	2.11	252.86	241.94
Sick and received treatment at health center	50.0	41.5	2.49	2.35	61.02	47.06
Sick and received treatment at public hospitals	18.6	14.4	2.32	2.46	645.42	257.02

The main purposes of estimating health card utilization patterns were twofold: investigate the factors affecting the frequency of card use through a multiple regression model, and investigate the factors affecting the use or nonuse of health cards through a logistic regression model.

The variables listed below were selected in estimating health card utilization patterns:

- Marital status
- Gender
- Educational level

- Number of household members
- Proportion of total household expenditure to total income
- Proportion of total household health expenditure to total expenditure
- Presence of illness
- Having chronic illness
- Family economic problems during sickness of family members
- Most convenient place to access health care.

Results

Multiple Regression Model

The model in table 10.18 shows that the significant factors related to card usage rate are having chronic illness and convenient access to a health center. This is not surprising since the chronically ill will seek care regularly and usually at a health center located in the village near their homes, where they will use cards. This is related to the problem of adverse selection in the program.

TABLE 10.18   Multiple Regression Model

Variable	B	SE	Beta	T	Sig T
Chronic	1.622212	0.563359	0.156944	2.880	0.0043
Health center	1.915122	0.593073	0.175999	3.229	0.0014
Constant	2.613482	0.555544		4.704	0.0000

Logistic Regression Model

The results from table 10.19 show that the significant factor related to card use is the presence of illness; the others are not statistically significant. This confirms once again the problem of adverse selection in the program since the one who has the presence of illness tended to buy a card and affected the card usage.

In addition, other models were estimated to investigate the impact of having or not having a card to the health care seeking behavior among the households. Interestingly, the results show that possession or nonpossession of a health card was not a significant factor at the beginning of the program. But when the program had been implemented for one year, among health care seekers, possession of a health card was a significant reason to visit the health centers or community hospitals. This evidence strongly supports the importance for cardholders of accessibility to health care. Problems concern the risk sharing among the target population and card overutilization. The problem of card overutilization, confirmed in this study, has implications for the sustainability and efficiency of the program. The results show that among card users 41.6 percent tended to visit health facilities more than before having a card, 48.4 percent the same as before, only 7.2 percent less than before, and 2.8 percent do not remember.

TABLE 10.19   Logistic Regression Model: Variables that Predict Health Card Usage among Card Users

Variable	Coefficient	Standard error	Significance	Exp. (B) odds ratio
Marital status	0.0245	1.0413	0.9812	1.0248
Gender	0.3981	0.6898	0.5639	1.4889
Age	−0.0275	0.0325	0.3973	0.9728
Educational level	1.2836	0.9249	0.1652	3.6097
Number of family members	0.0262	0.1986	0.8950	1.0266
Proportion of total household expenditure to total income	0.0270	0.1618	0.8673	1.0274
Proportion of total household health expenditure to total expenditure	0.2636	2.7682	0.9241	1.3016
Presence of illness	1.8629	0.8417	0.0269	6.4422
Having chronic illness	−0.4791	0.8084	0.5534	0.6193
Family economic problems during sickness of family members	0.8375	0.8334	0.3160	2.3064
Most convenient place to access health care				
Health center	1.9755	1.4112	0.1616	7.2100
Community hospital	1.2323	1.4958	0.4100	3.4292
Constant	0.4165	1.8298	0.8200	

Attitudes toward the Health Care Program among Cardholders and Noncardholders

Among the health care seekers, cardholders and noncardholders at health centers and community hospitals were interviewed about their attitudes toward the health card program. The main results are shown in tables 10.20–10.21.

Cardholders had greater prior knowledge about the health card program before health officers explained it to them than did noncardholders, and they had more satisfaction with the explanations from health officers. This confirms the idea that knowledge of the health card was a strong determinant of card purchase. Even more important, the attitude about the usefulness of the health card to them or their family was different in the two groups. The cardholder group had greater satisfaction with the health card than the noncardholder group, and the cardholders tended to be satisfied with the price of the card more than were the noncardholders. This strongly explains the role of attitude. Cardholders said they would buy a new card next year, while noncardholders were not likely to buy. It is important to note that the decision to purchase a health card was not dependent solely on the price of the card but was also influenced by other factors, such as the quality of drugs received, the quality of medical services provided,

TABLE 10.20 Attitudes toward Health Card Program of Cardholders and Noncardholders

| Context | Cardholders | | | | | Noncardholders | | | | |
| | Level of scale | | | | | Level of scale | | | | |
	1	2	3	4	5	1	2	3	4	5
Prior knowledge about HCP	11.2	44.2	31.2	12.4	1.0	4.3	24.0	41.5	21.7	8.5
Card seller clearly explained HCP limits and benefits	13.2	64.1	17.6	4.7	0.4	5.2	37.8	34.7	16.9	5.4
Satisfaction with explanation	12.0	55.8	29.6	2.2	0.4	4.3	31.5	40.8	19.6	3.8
Benefits of health card to family	33.5	53.0	12.8	0.2	0.4	11.9	26.9	28.5	24.0	8.7
Price of card (500 baht) is appropriate	23.6	44.7	29.1	2.2	0.4	14.8	38.3	35.9	9.2	1.8
Coverage for 1 year appropriate	18.9	42.6	30.2	6.9	1.4	11.7	38.1	35.9	12.2	2.0
Worried will receive substandard medical services when using card	4.3	15.4	27.8	37.1	15.4	5.0	19.9	39.7	27.5	7.9
Worried about the possible longer waiting time for care when using card	3.1	11.0	40.7	32.8	12.4	2.7	17.8	42.9	28.0	8.6
Worried about expected low quality of drugs received with card	3.7	15.5	27.7	38.5	14.7	4.3	18.7	37.5	29.1	10.4
Will buy card next year	41.2	33.5	22.2	2.0	1.0	15.3	25.3	37.5	14.7	7.2

Note: Level 1 most likely (very satisfactory), and level 5 most unlikely (very unsatisfactory).

TABLE 10.21   Attitudes toward Health Card Program of Cardholders and Noncardholders (Mean Score)

Context	Cardholders Mean score	Noncardholders Mean score
Prior knowledge about HCP	2.479	3.063
Card seller clearly explained HCP limits and benefits	2.150	2.795
Satisfaction with explanation	2.233	2.872
Benefits of health card to family	1.809	3.092
Price of card (500 baht) is appropriate	2.112	2.448
Coverage for 1 year appropriate	2.294	2.546
Worried will receive substandard medical services when using card	3.440	3.135
Worried about the possible longer waiting time for care when using card	3.138	3.219
Worried about expected low quality of drugs received with card	3.450	3.226
Will buy card next year	1.882	3.269

and whether the subjects had alternative health insurance. This study found that the problem of expectations about substandard medical services, low quality of drugs, and longer waiting time for care with cards were similar in the two groups, except that the noncardholders tended to worry more than the cardholders.

Even though some studies have indicated that health service satisfaction is the most important factor influencing the use of health services and dissatisfaction among health card users was one significant factor influencing the dropout group (Adeyi 1988; Silapasuwan 1989; Suwanteerangkul 1992). This was not confirmed with the study by Veeravongs (1994), which found that both continuing card users and dropouts were satisfied with their current health service and there were no differences between them in terms of card knowledge obtained from village health volunteers and health card committee members. This study had similar findings as stated above. Actually, knowledge regarding the benefits of the program, and better knowledge about the principle of health insurance and the health system among the households are more important to the program in terms of the efficient use of resources, encouragement of households to participate in the program, and the sustainability of the program.

In organizing a voluntary health insurance program there are important implications concerning the allocation of resources used and the technical efficiency with which they are used. These relate to the type of medical services provided in the program, its referral system, the use of medical technologies, and mechanisms to allocate the resources. Some studies have shown similar problems in organizing health insurance, particularly for rural populations. Economic pressure is key to bringing about health care financing reform in various countries, and one way of doing so is through the health insurance schemes, either compulsory or voluntary. It is important to realize that the existence of any scheme will be unstable if the scheme attracts a special subset of the population with unusually high health care costs or with greater sickness.

Health Card Fund

The current formula to allocate HCF to compensate providers and for administrative costs is set at 80 percent and 20 percent of the monetary amount of health card sales revenue (this differs slightly from year to year). The revenue is generated by health card sales (US$20 per card) and subsidized US$20 per card from the government budget. After one year of implementation of the health card program in Khon Kaen, operating cost data at health centers and community hospitals in six districts were collected; including the utilization rate with these data will provide better understanding about the health card fund and its viability.

At community hospitals, the unit cost per case for inpatients is 1,356 baht, and the unit cost per visit for outpatients is 168 baht. At health centers, the unit cost per case is 71 baht, and the unit cost per visit is 37 baht. When card usage rates in this study are compared with those in the previous study (Kiranandana and Apairatr, 1990), the *rates per case* for outpatient visits at health centers and community hospitals are higher by as much as 50 percent and 94 percent, respectively (see table 10.22). The *rates per card* for outpatients at health centers and community hospitals are also higher by 15 percent and 48 percent, respectively. Likewise, the card usage rate for inpatients is higher both per case and per card, but not by such a high percentage. Nonetheless, considering the difficulties of comparing the present study directly with other studies (they were conducted in different areas, times, and most importantly, under different rationales, types, card prices, and criteria for card usage), the average card usage rate per card for all services at health centers and community hospitals was not greatly different.

TABLE 10.22   Health Card Utilization Rate

Utilization rate	Health center		Community hospital	
	Card	Case	Card	Case
Outpatient	3.2	0.72	3.11	0.70
Inpatient	—	—	0.17	0.04
Inpatient days	—	—	0.66	0.15

However, the results did show that under the new criteria for card use, with no limit on episodes and with the first contact at either a health center or community hospital depending on convenient location, the rate of usage is increasing greatly, especially at community hospitals. This result in the major workload and cost of care is borne by community hospitals. The cost of care compared with unit cost in Chiang Mai in the same year revealed a similar pattern. The data show that providers, health centers, and community hospitals need to reimburse their expenses (based on price schedules rather than cost) in amounts greater than the health card fund committee can allocate from the fund, which is financed from the total monetary amount of card sales revenue alone. The collected data show that health centers and community hospitals can receive only 58 percent of their reimbursement (the government subsidy was not included in this statistic because there was a delayed subsidy from the government in 1996). The existing program formula is set at 80 percent of the total monetary amount of card sales revenue. If no subsidy from the government was allocated to the providers, the expense would be borne by providers. There is a problem of equity since only the health cardholders are better off if community hospitals must subsidize cardholders by the former's own revenues.

It is essential that the formula of reimbursement from HCF to compensate providers should be developed. HCF should establish reimbursement agreements with public hospitals based on a combination of expected outputs and costs, and all agreements might contain either a cost or a volume ceiling. This policy must be developed for the country as a whole to assist the HCF committee in each province in applying a standard criteria for allocation of funds.

Program Sustainability

In Khon Kaen Province there were a series of meetings during the year of this study between the research team, provincial health officers, and district health officers, including the health care providers in the province. In the meetings, there were discussions of how to organize the program, how to improve the program, problems in the field, government policy, budget, and how to sustain the program. The discussions give valuable suggestions for improving the existing program in areas such as program management, marketing management, financial management, and quality of services.

Program management:

- Build up an effective organization at all provincial and district levels. Problems may arise in the large district areas.

- Make the health card project more prominent among the various ongoing projects being implemented in the province.

- Improve the objectives and plan more efficiently.

- Create positive attitudes toward the health card program among managers and officers at all levels of the health system. Encourage effective coordination among health officers at all levels of the system to promote greater knowledge and better understanding of the health card program. This will help address the problem of providers being reluctant to participate in the program because of insufficient reimbursements. The public facilities under MOPH must participate, even though some of them are unwilling. This indicates the problem of coordination among health officers at all levels.

- Make the health insurance information system more effective.

Marketing:

- Work toward a goal of 100 percent coverage in an appropriate way.
- Improve marketing strategies, for example, using the social marketing concept.
- Develop a serious and continuous advertising campaign for the health card program.
- Create incentives to sell the health card.

Financial management:

- Establish monitoring committees at all levels.
- Improve the regulation of monitoring committees.
- Set penalty rules.
- Abandon the installment payment for health cards.

Quality of services:

- Strengthen the health care service units to achieve a high quality of care.
- Create good attitudes toward provider; provide services of equity and merit.

These problems are similar to those in other countries where voluntary health insurance for rural people is implemented. Dave (1991) studied the community and self-financing in voluntary health programs in India and found that mixed success with financing efforts. The financing methods, including user charges, community-based prepayment schemes, fundraising, commercial schemes, and in-kind contributions can be further strengthened with better planning, management, monitoring, and evaluation. Chabot, Boal, and da Silva (1991) studied national community health insurance at the village level and found that the experience of a voluntary levy scheme in Guinea-Bissau may be feasible and manageable in rural parts of Africa, if the village population is allowed to decide on the amount of money and method of collection and if the government supports the scheme by guaranteeing sufficient drugs, low prices, and effective control measures. A review of case studies carried out by the Bamako Initiative in five countries noted that the extension of insurance coverage to rural populations is a strategy that can improve equity (McPake, Hanson, and Mills 1992).

The main problem areas concerned in the program are as follows:

- Program management: marketing, financial, quality of care
- The adverse selection or self-selection problem, that is, how to increase the number of people enrolled to ensure a sufficient pooling of risks
- Operational policies: choices about the type of services included in the program, number of episodes per card, reimbursement from providers, and effective referral systems
- Communications: providing people with greater knowledge and better understanding of HCP, that is, sustainability (strong promotion of the program).

Problems of program management are related to the effectiveness of health officers, government health policies, and many adjustments in the program as stated above. The problem of risk sharing with no cost sharing needs a sufficient number of people or communities participating in the program. Households have been encouraged to participate in the program in various ways.

The percentage of HCF kept in community (village): In 1984–1986, there were village committees responsible for selling the health cards and collecting premiums. These funds were kept at the village because a HCF with a minimum enrollment base of 35 percent of the households in each village was required to ensure risk sharing. These committees also manage revenue collected as a revolving fund for income-generating activities initiated by villagers to promote PHC. A fixed rate of 75 percent of HCF is reimbursed to compensate the providers in the referral line at the end of the year. In FY 1987, premiums collected were 182.9 million baht and the approximate medical expenses were 267.5 million baht (Tantiserani and Prompakdi, 1988, cited in Tangcharoensathien 1995); the health card fund decreased to 81.3 million baht in 1992. This also related to the MOPH's inconsistent support for the program, as stated above, which reflects an inadequate sales promotion. At present the HCFs are kept at district and provincial levels, with no income generating from the funds.

The renewability of unused cards: This was abolished after 1985.

No limit of criteria for card use from 1992 to present: There has been no limitation imposed on the number of episodes and no ceiling on expenses per episode.

The problem of adverse selection or self-selection or selection bias is a common problem in voluntary health insurance schemes. In this study, this problem is quite apparent. The research results show that the presence of illness was one of the significant factors related to card purchase and card utilization patterns. This suggests that the selection bias from this source may influence card purchase.

Another problem is the bypassing of health centers due to peoples' perception of the low quality of services provided there. In any case, free services were provided to cardholders at all levels in the referral line, and thus cardholders chose free services at hospitals rather than at health centers. Some studies (Hongvivatana and others 1986) have suggested that cost sharing, either as a deductible or a fixed percent of the bill (coinsurance), should be imposed at community hospitals and higher levels but not at the health center. This would encourage greater use at the subdistrict level and more rational use of higher unit cost care at higher levels and would also generate more revenue to the providers. Yet it might deter the demand for cards. The renewability of unused cards, which was abolished after 1985, was a successful incentive for avoiding unnecessary use of health cards. In the present program, the first contact in which the cardholders can choose is either a health center or a community hospital, which might be one factor influencing health cardholders to bypass the health centers, as stated above.

The problem of case-based reimbursement of providers, which is a retrospective reimbursement in the program, requires substantial administrative capacity and a highly developed information infrastructure. HCF should be aware of the sophisticated nature of such a system when establishing reimbursement agreements with public hospitals based on a combination of expected outputs and costs.

Finally, a continuing problem of the HCP is dissemination of knowledge about HCP and a better understanding of health insurance in principle among the Thai people. This requires consistent sales promotions and strong annual campaigning about the HCP, a problem separate from that of the frequent adjustments in the program.

CONCLUSIONS AND RECOMMENDATIONS

Although the health card program has been in operation for more than 15 years and has undergone many adjustments, whether or not the project is a success is still unclear. Thailand's economic structure is changing toward more industrialization with multiple effects on society. The transition poses difficult questions for planners and affects many key issues in the health sector. The country faces many problems, such as how to increase, or at least sustain, economic growth, income distribution, political instability, and incompetence. The overall performance of the economy remains a major concern. Likewise, in the health sector, financing is still the main problem. The objective of this chapter was to assess the future potential for application of voluntary health insurance, the Health Card Program scheme, in Thailand by utilizing data collected in Khon Kaen, where the recent program was implemented. This study has indicated the problems, development, and health service capability in the application of the Health Card Program, identified factors influencing project outcomes, investigated the card purchase and dropout pattern, and evaluated the factors affecting the discrimination between health card purchase, nonpurchase, and dropouts from continued health card member groups. The results of the study will provide more understanding of how the program performs and how to sustain it more efficiently, as well as suggesting alternative ways to improve it. Both qualitative and quantitative statistical techniques have been applied to provide complementary approaches to investigating the factors affecting the performance of the program. The research results show that the statistically significant factors related to new card purchase and nonpurchase groups are education level and presence of illness. Between the health card dropout and continued card purchase groups, the significant factor is again the presence of illness. Moreover, there were four significant factors related to non–card users and card users: educational level, income per year, number of employed members in the family, and presence of illness.

A study of health card purchase patterns and health card utilization patterns (health utilization behavior) demonstrates clearly and strongly that health card purchase in Khon Kaen has been influenced by the following factors: proportion of employed persons to total family members, education, and presence of illness. The last factor confirms the problem of adverse selection in the program, particularly significant in the health card program implemented in Khon Kaen, since the program was introduced in the country and that province in 1983, giving Khon Kaen extensive experience with voluntary health insurance and its development throughout the years.

The sustainability of the program depends on various factors, one of which is a level of satisfaction among card users that leads them to continue to buy in the following years. The findings indicate that the continuity of card purchase in the study was associated with the following factors: age, education, and income, and obtained knowledge on HCP from health center personnel. Moreover, the cardholders who had been persuaded to buy a card at home and had been persuaded by a neighbor to buy a card were more likely to be continued users.

This study also investigated the health care seeking pattern among card users and non–card users. The results indicate clearly the importance of accessibility to health care among the card user group. However, the program still has the risk-sharing and card utilization pattern problems to consider in order to become more sustainable and efficient. The results also show that the significant factors related to card usage rates are having chronic illness and convenient access to a health center. This is not surprising since the chronically ill will seek care regularly.

Recommendations

The uninsured have to pay out of pocket for medical services either in public or private facilities. A proper voluntary health insurance scheme is a choice for people, especially for the poor, who are not covered by any schemes and are thus not protected from financial difficulties due to the high cost of care. The health card program can be a choice for these people, who are in rural areas or some urban areas. To expand this program for urban residents, it would need many adjustments because there are no community hospitals provided in such areas, only municipal health centers, provincial hospitals, and regional hospitals. The cost of care and types of care are different.

If the existing health card program continues to be implemented without any of the adjustments suggested above, it might destabilize the whole health system. This study suggests another possibility to adjust the program as a compulsory program. It could be implemented in rural areas as a community-based compulsory insurance scheme. The services in the program would cover catastrophic cases only, the household would pay out-of-pocket for outpatient care because the various studies, including the present one, show that the cost of such care is not very high. Low-income households will be eligible for the FC/L scheme, which provides free medical care for the low-income households. Aside from that there must be an essential package of health services provided free at the public facilities to guarantee basic care for the people. Given the low probability of hospitalization and the compulsory enrollment, premiums will be low and affordable. For the urban areas it must be linked to health service facilities now provided and will require more information and further studies to establish. This might be an alternative way to assist the uninsured for high cost care.

To summarize, the findings reported in this study show that improvements to the existing health card program require:

- Efficient and consistent health policy

- Revision of the criteria for card use such as number of episodes, type of services, ceiling on expenses, and effective referral system (problem of bypassing the health centers)

- Development of reimbursement agreements with public hospitals based on a combination of expected outputs and costs to assist the HCF committee in allocating funds to compensate the providers

- A subsidy from the government budget

- The strengthening of public health service units

- The securing of the health card program as the base for universal health insurance.

Finally, the findings in this study can provide more information on HCP performance and its prospects for the future beyond a pilot project of voluntary health insurance: a prepayment with no cost-sharing scheme. The project aims to achieve the universal coverage that the government has taken as its goal. It is hoped that the results and recommendations emerging from the careful investigations in this chapter may assist policymakers to improve and to expand the existing health card program as the base for universal insurance.

Acknowledgments: The author is grateful to the World Health Organization (WHO) for having provided an opportunity to contribute to the work of the Commission on Macroeconomics and Health and to the World Bank for having published the material in this chapter as an HNP Discussion Paper. Part of this research was supported by the Health Insurance Office, Ministry of Public Health (MOPH), Thailand. The study was conducted under the auspices of the College of Public Health and the Centre for Health Economics, Faculty of Economics, Chulalongkorn University. The author thanks the staff of the Department of Population and International Health, Harvard School of Public Health, for their valuable comments and support. The findings, interpretations, and conclusions expressed in the chapter are entirely those of the author and do not necessarily represent the views of the World Bank, its Executive Directors, or the countries they represent.

REFERENCES

Adeyi, O. 1988. "Requirement for the Health Card? Sustaining the Demand for Rural Health Insurance in Thailand: A Case Study from Chiang Mai Province." Master's thesis, Liverpool School of Tropical Medicine.

Buisai, S. 1995. "Urbanization and the Health Systems." Health System in Transition, Contemporary Health Issue. No. 1. Health Systems Research Institute, Thailand.

Chabot, J., M. Boal, and A. da Silva. 1991. "National Community Health Insurance at Village Level: the Case from Guinea-Bissau." *Health Policy and Planning* 6(1): 46–54.

Dave, P. 1991. "Community and Self-Financing Voluntary Health Programmes in India." *Health Policy and Planning* 6(1): 20-31.

Hongvivatana, T., and S. Manopimoke. 1991. *A Baseline Survey of Preference for Rural Health Insurance*. Bangkok: Center for Health Policy Studies, Mahidol University.

Hongvivatana, T., P. Tantiserrani, P. Predaswat, S. Prompakdee, P. Leerapan, and others. 1986. *Health Services Utilization under the Health Card Program*. Mahidol University, Monograph of Center for Health Policy Studies No. 4. Bangkok.

Janjaroen, W. S., and S. Supakankunti. 1994. *Voluntary Health Insurance (Health Card): A Mechanism to Ease up Household Health Care Expenditure Burden*. Paper prepared for the VII International Congress, World Federation of Public Health Associations in Bali, Indonesia, December 4–8.

———. 1996. *Economic Evaluation of Voluntary Health Insurance: A Case Study from Chiang Mai Province*. Bangkok: Chulalongkorn University.

Kakwani, N., and M. Krongkaew. 1996. "Big Reduction in 'Poverty'." *Economic Review Year-End '96, Bangkok Post*. Bangkok.

Keeratipipatpong, W. 1996. "Expansion by Healthy Rate." *Economic Review Year-End '96, Bangkok Post*. Bangkok.

Kiranandana, T. 1993. "Voluntary Health Insurance in Thailand." Proceedings of a National Workshop on Health Financing in Thailand. Bangkok.

Kiranandana, T., and S. Apairatr. 1990. *Evaluation of Health Card Project: A National Census*. Bangkok: Military Welfare Organization.

Kutzin, J. 1995. *Experience with Organizational and Financing Reform of the Health Sector*. WHO, SHS Paper No. 8. Geneva.

Maddala, G. S. 1991. *Limited-Dependent and Qualitative Variables in Econometrics*. New York: Cambridge University Press.

Manopimoke, S. 1993. *Financial and Social Sustainability of the New Health Card Approach*. Bangkok: Thai-German Cooperation for Health.

McPake, B., K. Hanson, and A. Mills. 1992. "Experience to Date of Implementing the Bamako Initiative: A Review and Five Country Case Studies." London School of Hygiene and Tropical Medicine, Department of Public Health and Policy, Health Policy Unit.

MOPH (Ministry of Public Health). 1989. *Health Card Programme–HCP Chiangmai Pilot Project 1985–1988: Summary of Main Results and Conclusions*. The Health Card Programme Center and the Thai-German Cooperation for Health (GTZ), Bangkok.

———. 1992–96. *Health Development Plan under the Seventh*. National Economic and Social Development Plan, Health Development Planning Committee, Bangkok.

Musgrove, Philip. 1996. "Public and Private Roles in Health: Theory and Financing Patterns." World Bank, Discussion Paper No. 339. Washington, D.C.

NESDB (National Economic and Social Development Board), UNDP (United Nations Development Programme), and TDRI. 1991. *National Urban Development Policy Framework Final Report,* vol. 1. Bangkok.

Nittayaramphong S., and V. Tangcharoensathien. 1994. "Thailand: Private Health Care Out Of Control?" *Health Policy and Planning* 9(1): 31–40.

Norusis, Marija J. 1993. SPSS/PC+ Advanced Statistics version 5.0.

Office of the Prime Minister, National Statistical Office. 1986–90. *Statistical Yearbook Thailand*. Bangkok: Ladprao Teachers' Association Press.

———. 1992a. *Preliminary Report of the 1992 Household Socio-Economic Survey*. Bangkok.

———. 1992b. *Survey of Private Hospital and Clinic*. Bangkok.

Pempoonwatanasuk, C. 1985. *The Health Card Programme in Ratchaburi Province: A Case Study*. Master's thesis, Thammasat University.

Piyaratn, P., and W. S. Janjaroen. 1994. *Health Insurance in Thailand*. Paper presented at the National Seminar on Health Sector Development in Hanoi, Vietnam, October 4–7.

Pradabmuk, P. 1984. "The Health Card Program in Ubol Ratchatani: A Case Study." In T. Hongvivatana and others, eds. *Health Services Utilization under the Health Card Program*. Center for Health Policy Studies, Mahidol University.

Puntachart, P., and others. 1988. *An Evaluation of Chiangmai Health Card Project*. Research Report No. 34. Research and Development Center, Payub University, Chiangmai, Thailand.

Santampol, J. 1990. "Comparative Analysis of Expenses Related to Care Providing, at Several Levels of Health Card Program: A Case Study of Chiang Mai Province." Master's thesis, Chulalongkorn University.

Silapasuwan, V. 1989. "Factors Affecting Health Card Program Utilization among People in Rural Thailand." *Journal of Primary Health Care and Development* 2 (December): 84–95.

Singkaew, T. 1995. "Comparison between Voluntary and Compulsory Health Insurance in Thailand." *Health Insurance Office Report 1992*. Ministry of Public Health, Thailand.

Supakankunti, S. 1994. *Structural Change: Impact on Urbanization Process in Thailand*. Faculty of Economics. Bangkok: Chulalongkorn University.

Supakankunti, S., W. S. Janjaroen, and S. Sritamma. 1996. *Economic Analysis of Voluntary Health Insurance Schemes in Khon-Kaen Province*. Bangkok: Chulalongkorn University.

Suwanteerangkul, J. 1992. "Factors Influencing Drop Out in Health Cardholders: A Case Study of Mae Rim District, Chiang Mai Province, 1989–1991." Master's thesis, Chulalongkorn University.

Tangcharoensathien, V. 1995. "Health Care Financing in Thailand." *Health System in Transition, Contemporary Health Issue*, No. 1. Health Systems Research Institute, Thailand.

Tangcharoensathien, V., and A. Suphachutikul. 1993. "Health Insurance in Thailand: Present and Future." In MOPH, Office of Undersecretary, *Report of Health Insurance Office: 1992 Performance*. Bangkok.

Terdudomtham, T. 1996. "Analysts Taken by Surprise." *Economic Review Year-End '96, Bangkok Post*. Bangkok.

Thailand Economic Information Kit. 1994. Thailand Development Research Institute. Bangkok.

Thailand in Figures. 1996. Alpha Research Co., Ltd. Sukhum and Sons Co., Ltd. Bangkok.

Thailand Public Health. 1995. Alpha Research Co., Ltd. and Manager Information Services Co., Ltd. Sukhum and Sons Co., Ltd. Bangkok.

UNDP (United Nations Development Programme). 1995. *Human Development Report.* New York: Oxford University Press.

Veeravongs, S. 1994. "Factors Influencing Health Card Purchase and Continuity: A Case of Voluntary Health Insurance in Phuket Province, Thailand." Takemi Research Paper No. 89. Takemi Program in International Health. Harvard School of Public Health. Harvard University.

Wibulpolprasert, S. 1991. "Community Financing: Thailand's Experience." *Health Policy and Planning* 6(4): 354–60.

World Bank. *World Development Report 1993: Investing in Health.* New York: Oxford University Press.

CHAPTER 11

Deficit Financing of Health Care for the Poor

Alexander S. Preker, John C. Langenbrunner, and Emi Suzuki

Abstract: What is the optimal amount of health care spending needed to achieve a given outcome, and how much is a country able and willing to afford? Health sector experts and policymakers have asked these questions for decades. In recent years, the Millennium Development Goals (MDGs) have become a quantitative set of targets for poverty reduction and improvements in health, education, gender equality, the environment, and other aspects of human development. To help focus national and international priority-setting, the goals and targets selected were intended to be limited in number, be stable over time, and be easily communicated to a broad audience. This chapter attempts to estimate the expenditure needed to achieve the health-related targets set by the MDGs—reducing the number of children who die before their fifth birthday and women who die from complications of childbirth, and reversing the spread of HIV/AIDS, malaria, tuberculosis, and other major diseases—using a production frontier technique. The chapter compares this expenditure estimate with current expenditure trends in low- and middle-income countries.

D uring recent years, the Millennium Development Goals (MDGs) have become a quantitative set of targets for poverty reduction and improvements in health, education, gender equality, the environment, and other aspects of human development (see box 11.1).[1] This chapter attempts to estimate the expenditure needed to achieve the MDGs health-related targets—reducing the number of children who die before their fifth birthday and women who die from complications of childbirth, and reversing the spread of HIV/AIDS, malaria, tuberculosis (TB), and other major diseases—using production frontiers as an analytical technique. The chapter compares this expenditure estimate with current expenditure trends in low- and middle-income countries to arrive at an estimate of the global health care expenditure gap.

PROGRESS TOWARD ACHIEVING THE MDGS

Progress since 1990 in achieving the MDGs has been uneven across countries and regions and uneven among the goals themselves (Devarajan, Miller, and Swanson 2002) and (Preker, Langenbrunner, and others 2001). The United Nations set 1990 as the baseline year for monitoring the targets and 2015 as the target date for achieving the goals.

In 1990, 29 percent of the global population—1.3 billion people—lived in extreme poverty (first component of Goal 1). This had dropped to 22.7 percent of

---

BOX 11.1   MILLENNIUM DEVELOPMENT GOALS (1990–2015)

1. **Eradicate extreme poverty and hunger**
   - halve the proportion of people living on less than US$1 a day
   - halve the proportion of people who suffer from hunger

2. **Achieve universal primary education**
   - ensure that boys and girls alike complete primary schooling

3. **Promote gender equality and empower women**
   - eliminate gender disparity at all levels of education

4. **Reduce child mortality**
   - reduce by two-thirds the under-five mortality rate

5. **Improve maternal health**
   - reduce by three-quarters the maternal mortality ratio

6. **Combat HIV/AIDS, malaria, and other diseases**
   - halt and reverse the spread of HIV/AIDS
   - halt and reverse the spread of malaria and tuberculosis

7. **Ensure environmental sustainability**
   - integrate sustainable development into country policies and reverse loss of environmental resources
   - halve the proportion of people without access to potable water
   - significantly improve the lives of at least 100 million slum dwellers

8. **Develop a global partnership for development**
   - increase official development assistance, especially for countries applying their resources to poverty reduction
   - expand market access
   - encourage debt sustainability

---

the population—1.15 billion people—by 1999. During the same time period, the undernourished dropped from 22 percent of the global population to 18 percent—780 million people (second component of Goal 1). The global targets for both poverty reduction and hunger are broadly on target (see figure 11.1a).

The income poverty indicator is important, since it correlates highly with the overall social indicators such as health status and financial protection against the cost of illness. Although growth translated into poverty reduction, the total head count of poor people depends significantly on historical levels of income distribution, policy choices, and institutional constraints (World Bank 2000). The best progress globally has been in the East Asia and the Pacific region. Sub-Saharan Africa and South Asia, where the majority of the world's poor live, have experienced the worst progress. Sub-Saharan Africa failed to grow during the 1990s, leaving a large part of the population in poverty. In Eastern Europe and Central Asia and the Middle East and North Africa, hunger increased during the 1990s.

FIGURE 11.1   Millennium Development Goals, Global Aggregate

a.   **Eradicate Poverty and Hunger**

People living on less than $1 a day

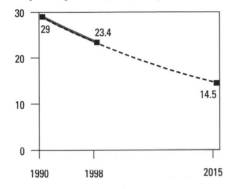

Ensure Environmental Sustainability

Improved water source
(% of population with access)

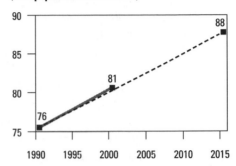

b.   **Universal Primary Education**

Net primary enrollment

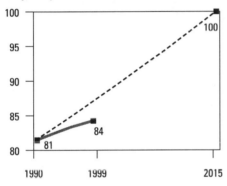

Promote Gender Equality

Ratio of girls to boys in primary and
secondary school (% of school age children)

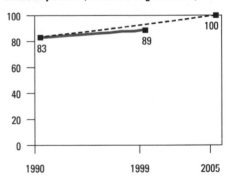

c.   **Improve Maternal Health**

Births attended by skilled
health personnel (% total)

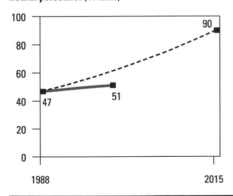

Reduce Child Mortality

Under five mortality
(per 1,000 live births)

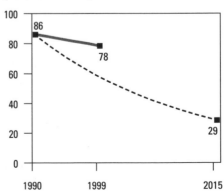

During this time period, people without access to water decreased from 27 percent to 21 percent of the population (first component of Goal 7; see figure 11.1a). This still left 900 million without access to clean water. Those without access to sanitation systems dropped from 56 to 48 percent of the population (second component of Goal 7). Improved policies and significant additional financial resources are required to address these problems.

Data for the global indicator on education and gender equality (Goals 2 and 3) are not complete. Based on the available data, both goals appear to be modestly off target (see figure 11.1b). Net primary enrollment rates increased only from 81 percent to 84 percent, and the ratio of girls to boys education increased only from 82 percent to 86 percent in 1990–99. Improved policies and significant additional financial resources are needed to address these problems.

Among all the MDGs, the health goals—maternal and child health—are the most seriously off track (see figure 11.1c). The MDG for maternal and child health calls for reducing maternal mortality by three-quarters and the under-five child mortality rates by two-thirds of their 1990 levels by 2015. Tracking progress in reducing maternal mortality is difficult. Deaths related to pregnancy and childbirth occur infrequently when compared with other health problems and are often outside the formal health system. This leads to a small sample size made more unreliable by underreporting. According to the last estimate of maternal mortality, for 1995, 500,000 women die annually during pregnancy and childbirth, most of them from conditions that could be prevented or treated in equipped medical facilities. Not surprisingly, maternal mortality is low in the Latin American and East European regions, where skilled attendants and equipped medical facilities are readily available, while high maternal mortality occurs in the African and South Asian regions where they are not.

Tracking progress in reducing infant and child mortality is more reliable. Global progress toward this goal is seriously off track. This is particularly vexing because so much is known about the causes of infant and child mortality. Furthermore, progress already made in some countries, even at very low income levels, indicates that effective interventions are both readily available and affordable to most countries.

Part of the problem is that progress in achieving under-five mortality targets relies significantly on both nonspecific intersectoral actions and specific health care interventions (preventive and curative services). The nonspecific activities include, for example, poverty reduction, nutrition, education, and gender equality programs, improvements in access to clean water and sanitation systems, and usage of insecticide-treated bed nets. Many of these activities require focused government policies across different sectors, coordination, and ongoing monitoring and evaluation of progress. This is often lacking at low-income levels and in settings with severely constrained management and institutional capacity.

But even with good general hygiene and other preventive and health promotion measures, children get sick and need medical interventions. Many interventions are as simple as vaccination, oral hydration during diarrhea, and use of antibiotics to treat complicated upper respiratory infections. Health providers with only basic skills are able deal with most of the conditions of childhood using simple protocols such as those available through integrated management of childhood illness. Other interventions, however, require skilled birth attendants, inpatient care during complicated pregnancies, and knowledge about appropriate treatment and referral at the time of trauma and other more serious illnesses.

Many of the old, and a few of the new, scourges of poverty are still ravaging low- and middle-income countries, threatening both human welfare and the potential for medium-term growth (see figure 11.2). In 2000, 34.7 million adults and 1.4 million children had HIV/AIDS, 300 million to 500 million cases of malaria resulted in 1 million to 2 million deaths, mainly in children under five years of age; and 8.4 million new TB cases were reported, between 10 and 15 percent of them in children. As measured by new cases reported, the incidence of HIV/AIDS and TB infections is still increasing, and the MDG global targets are far off track. Sub-Saharan Africa and South Asia are the regions most severely affected.

If they are to be effective, health sector-specific programs need to be underpinned by well-functioning health systems. These include strong government stewardship (policymaking, coordination, regulations, contracting, information dissemination, and monitoring and evaluation systems), health care financing (prepaid revenue collection, risk pooling, and resource allocation and purchasing

FIGURE 11.2 Strong Correlation between Wealth and Health across Time

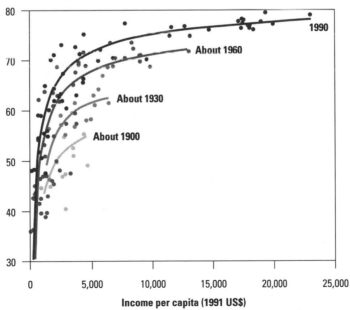

mechanisms), input generation and management (human resources, research, pharmaceuticals, medical technology, consumables, and capital), effective and responsive service delivery systems (public health and curative services), and the market forces created by demand for service by individuals and households. Many interventions known to be effective and affordable do not get to the children or households that need them due to failures in the health system. Once again, improved policies and significant additional financial resources are needed to address these problems in the underlying health systems.

KEY DRIVERS OF ACCELERATED PROGRESS TOWARD ACHIEVING THE MDGS

Increased Income from Economic Growth Is Necessary

Richer countries do better across a wide range of health indicators. As a result of complex synergies among income levels and expenditure on education, health-seeking behavior, public policy, and health services, people all over the world live almost 25 years longer today than they did at similar income levels in 1900 (see figure 11.2). This relationship between income, health spending, and health outcomes in developing countries is now well-established (World Bank 1993, 1997; Pritchett and Summers 1996; WHO 2000).

This story is as true for maternal and child mortality as it is for the major disease challenges facing low-income countries (see figure 11.3). Child mortality decreases as incomes increase, a relationship some analysts have used as a performance indicator for a country's overall development policy (Wang and others 1999). The "black box" assumptions is that income mediates through a variety of intermediate factors, including nonhealth sector determinants of better health outcomes (such as education, nutrition, safe water, roads, and sanitation systems), health-enhancing policies (maintaining health and preventing disease), and health services (treating disease, palliative care, and preventing death).

But recent work indicates that even at very high economic growth during the next few years, most countries will not reach the MDG targets of two-thirds reduction in under-five mortality rate (U5MR), a three-quarters reduction in maternal mortality (MMR), and a halving of the prevalence of underweight (UW) among children (Devarajan, Miller, and Swanson 2002; Alderman and others 2000). By projecting the current level of several health-related MDG indicators to 2015, using the historical elasticity of U5MR, MMR, and UW with respect to income, Wagstaff (2002a) demonstrates that even an unlikely 8 percent growth in income between 1990 and 2015 would reduce U5MR by only 20 percent, MMR by only 30 percent, and UW by only 40 percent, compared with the target reductions of 67 percent, 75 percent, and 30 percent, respectively.

Furthermore, in another paper, Wagstaff (2002b) argues that the importance of extrasectoral programs may mislead because they often act by improving the effectiveness of more specific health programs. For example, investment in roads allows pregnant mothers to get to delivery services on time, receive vaccines,

FIGURE 11.3   Income and Child Mortality

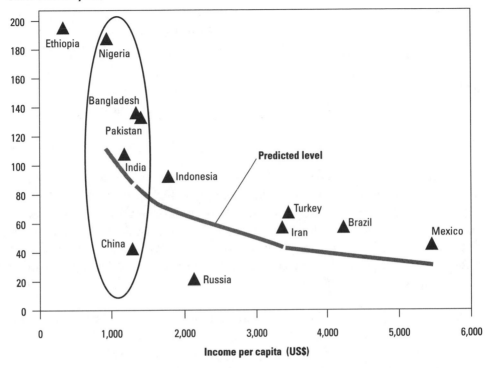

and reach health centers without having the cold chain broken. Education allows mothers to make the right choices when faced with illness episodes.

The advantages of investments across sectors are therefore likely to have important synergies and complementarities across sectors that specific investments in the health sector alone would fail to achieve. A disadvantage of this approach is that it may still fail to correct known constraints in the health sector that could be addressed effectively and at lower cost by focusing directly on the specific problems and their solutions. It is also a leap of faith to think that the marginal, untargeted dollar would always be spent on health-enhancing activities related to the MDGs. The alternative choices, some of which might even shunt resources away from priority activities, are almost limitless.

Income from Economic Growth Alone Is Not Enough to Achieve the MDGs

As seen in figures 11.2 and 11.3, at any given income level, there is a wide range of performance in terms of child health outcomes. Furthermore, the high performers in absolute terms are not always the best performers in relative terms. For example, both China and Singapore do well in terms of absolute performance but lag behind progress made during the 1980s (Wang and others 1999).

The variability in performance at any given income level is thought to be the result of a combined effect produced by several factors that include differences in both the effectiveness of interventions and the health systems delivering them (WHO 2000; Anell and Willis 2000; OECD 2001).

Increased Total and Public Spending on Health Care

A second driver of accelerated progress toward achieving the MDG targets is increased public and total spending on health or nutrition services—without increases in income.[2] Past work has shown a positive, though modest, correlation between health spending and health outcomes even when controlling for income and possible confounding factors (Filmer and Pritchett 1999). However, caution should be used when attributing improvements in health outcomes to nontargeted health spending since it is very hard to fully isolate all the confounding factors.

Notwithstanding this constraint, the current level of several health-related MDG indicators can be projected to 2015 using the historical elasticity of U5MR, MMR, and UW with respect to health expenditure. Wagstaff (2002a) demonstrated that between 1990 and 2015, U5MR would drop by an additional 40 percent, MMR by 30 percent, and UW by 35 percent, compared with the target reductions of 67 percent, 75 percent, and 30 percent, respectively. A sustained health expenditure growth rate of more than 15 percent would be needed to reach the U5MR target of 75 percent.

These findings refute earlier work that suggested health care services are not significant contributors to health status relative to other measures such as sanitation, income, and education (Newhouse and Friedlander 1980).

An advantage of such broad, systemwide expenditure increases on health services is that it allows policymakers and managers to exercise decision rights over the allocation and use of funds in areas they think are most effective and where there is the greatest demand. This is likely to be highly context specific and not readily specified under a blueprint.

A disadvantage of this approach is that it may fail to correct known constraints in financing, inputs, and service delivery, and deliver programs and interventions that could be addressed more effectively and at lower cost through a more direct targeting of scarce public resources in priority areas. It is a leap of faith to think that, without some strategic priority setting and targeting, the marginal dollars spent on the health sector will always be spent in areas that will have the greatest impact on accelerating progress toward the MDGs.

Increased Spending on Priority Populations, Priority Interventions, and Priority Health Programs

A third driver of improved outcomes is knowledge about the determinants of poverty and poor health related to the MDG targets (for example, the links between hygiene and infections, maternal nutrition and low birth weight, diet and malnutrition, and poverty and health) and the implementation of effective health programs and interventions.

Researchers have a much better understanding today of the determinants of poverty (World Bank 2000), the intersectoral synergies needed to achieve good health outcomes (Wagstaff 2002b), and the role health, prevention, and curative health services play in this story (World Bank 1993; WHO 2000; Van Doorslaer and others 2000; Wagstaff 2002c). Extensive work has been done in the area of targeting health programs to benefit the poor (Claeson and Waldman 2000; Gwatkin 2000; Gwatkin and Heuveline 1997).

During the past few years, a considerable body of knowledge has also accumulated on the cost and effectiveness of alternative interventions for specific health conditions (Murray, Evans and others 2000; Evans 1990b). Early work using such techniques in developing countries looked mainly at the cost-effectiveness of specific interventions (Barnum 1986), disease control programs (Barnum, Tarantola, and Setiady 1980), and investment projects (Barnum 1987; Prescott and De Ferranti 1985; Mills 1985a, 1985b). This type of work exploded following publication of the *World Development Report 1993: Investing in Health* (World Bank 1993; Jamison and others 1993) and subsequent extensive work by the World Health Organization in this area. Figure 11.4 provides a few examples of specific interventions that, if implemented well, would have a large impact on reducing the burden of disease, especially among the poor (World Bank 1997; Gwatkin and Heuveline 1997; Claeson, Mawji, and Walker 2000).

FIGURE 11.4   Cost-Effective and Affordable Public Health and Clinical Services

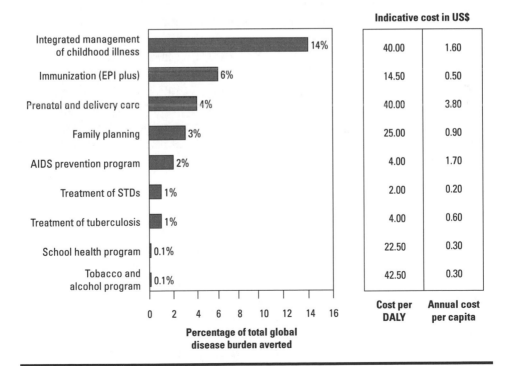

These interventions rank high in terms of their (a) potential to avert a large percentage of the global disease burden, (b) low cost per DALY averted, (c) low annual cost per capita, (d) potential impact on socially excluded and poverty groups, and (e) relevance to the MDGs.

At the heart of the broadened policy use of cost effectiveness is a belief among health professionals that resources in the health sector should be allocated across interventions and population groups to generate the highest possible overall level of population health. Stated in other terms, allocative efficiency of the health sector could be enhanced by moving resources from cost-ineffective to more cost-effective interventions (World Bank 1993).

Musgrove (1999) provides a decision tree for rational use of public financing in the health sector. It starts with the overarching issue of allocative efficiency by asking if the proposed expenditure is for public goods, generally population-based services. If the answer is "yes," the next step is to rank such expenditures in terms of cost-effectiveness—or even better, benefit-cost analysis—to decide what will be funded. If proposed expenditures do not meet public goods criteria, the tree asks whether significant externalities are involved, whether risks of catastrophic costs are involved, and whether the proposed beneficiaries are poor. Thus allocative efficiency, risk, equity, and cost-effectiveness interact to determine public financing decisions in health. Economic principles govern each decision point, but many other factors are often weighed, so the outcomes will vary considerably from country to country. The over-riding principle is maximizing the potential impact on people, especially the poor.

Several challenges to this wider use of cost-effectiveness analysis (CEA) have emerged, especially when it is used as a basis for priority setting or allocative efficiency within a given budget envelope or when it is used to undertake "bottom-up" costing to estimate marginal extra dollars spent on the health sector (M. Williams 1997; Filmer, Hammer, and Pritchett 2000, 2002; Jack 2000). Proponents of CEA defend their position with equal vigor (Musgrove 2000a, 2000b; Rivlin 2000).

First, analysts and decisionmakers have correctly noted that resource allocation decisions affecting the entire health sector must also take into account social concerns for the sick, reducing social inequities in health, the well-being of future generations, the insurance effect (spreading the cost of infrequent but expensive care across population groups), and the political economy of the middle classes who pay taxes (Hauck, Smith, and Goddard 2002). Second, current CEA practice often fails to identify existing misallocation of resources by focusing on the evaluation of new technologies or strategies. Third, for all but the richest societies, the cost and time needed to evaluate the large set of interventions required to use CEA to identify opportunities to enhance allocative efficiency may be prohibitive. Fourth, the difficulties of generalizing context-specific CEA studies have been institutionalized by the proliferation of multiple national and subnational guidelines for CEA practice, all using slightly different methods.

For example, costs can vary greatly from one country, context, and intervention modality to another. A naive generalization of the finding from one study to another can lead to serious mistakes in the planning and implementing of otherwise effective interventions. For example, in the management of malaria, it is suggested that at low-income levels one would choose case management and prophylaxis for pregnant women. At middle-income levels, one would add spraying. At higher income levels, one would add bed nets. A single estimate of the cost-effectiveness of malaria treatment could lead to the wrong conclusion that malaria programs are unaffordable if the estimate was based on a multitherapy program in a low-income country. Or it could lead to a serious underestimate of the actual cost of the program if the estimate was based on single therapy calculations but implementation of a multitherapy program in a middle-income country.

Factors other than income may also alter a program's actual cost during implementation. Major overlooked factors include availability, mix, and quality of inputs (especially trained personnel, drugs, equipment, and consumables); local prices, especially labor costs; implementation capacity; underlying organizational structures; incentives; and supporting institutional framework. Other confounding factors include poor quality of data; confusion between marginal, average, and shared costs; competing risks and synergies; failure to include non-monetary costs such as time and lost income; and miscalculation of discount rates (Hammer 1996; Peabody 1999).

The counterargument often used by proponents of cost-effectiveness analysis is that, although international estimates may not fully reflect local circumstances, there is a risk that excessive contextualized analyses will be too complex and resource-intensive for most low-income countries (Murray and others 2000). A move in this direction could ultimately lead to less use of evidence-based policy dialogue. This school of thought recommends an alternative approach: focusing on a general assessment of the different interventions' costs and health benefits based on general league tables of the cost-effectiveness of interventions for a group of populations with comparable health systems and epidemiological profiles. Such information on generalized cost-effectiveness can then be used alongside consideration of the effects of different resource allocations on other important social goals.

Spending on Management Capacity, Organizational Structures, and Institutional Environment

Several systemic factors in the health system may also act as drivers of improved outcomes. These include: management capacity, organizational incentives, and institutional environment (see figure 11.5).

Many countries currently failing to make progress toward the MDGs are plagued by, for example, weak management capacity, negative organizational incentives, and lack of a strong regulatory environment to ensure quality control and deal with the private sector (see figure 11.6). Often these countries ignore the demand side of utilization of health services. Critical supply chains, such as those involving pharmaceuticals and vaccines, are broken. In addition, top-down centralized control over public services excludes participation by the private sector, communities, and households in the care that they receive.

FIGURE 11.5   Three Nonfinancial Determinants of Good Outcomes

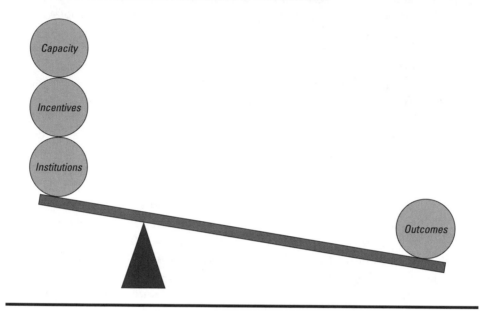

FIGURE 11.6   Lack of Management Capacity, Adverse Incentives, and Weak Institutions Break the Fulcrum

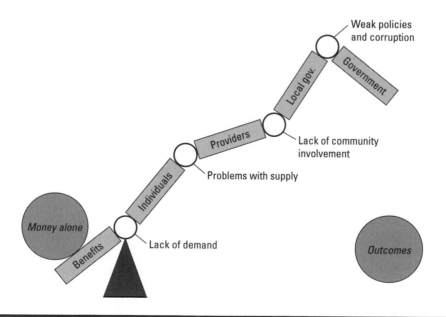

Notably the strategic use of stable and pooled revenue flows remains a critical factor in a country's ability to achieve good overall health outcomes (including those related to the MDGs) and protect its people against the impoverishing effects of illness (Preker and others 2002, 2001; WHO 2000; Carrin and others 2001). Countries and communities that channel health care financing through risk-sharing and collective-purchasing arrangements do significantly better on outcome indicators than countries that rely more heavily on out-of-pocket spending (Jakab and others 2001; Preker and others 2001).

The exact contribution of management, organizational, and institutional variables to the MDGs has not yet been quantified. The cost of reforms in this area is highly context sensitive, making it risky to apply estimates from one setting to another. An early attempt has been made by WHO (2000) to quantify the benefits of health systems in terms of the level and distribution of health outcomes, financial fairness, and responsiveness to patient expectations in terms of the quality and ethical dimensions of care. Unfortunately, as in the case of cost effectiveness, this initiative has met with great resistance from the international development community and countries themselves (A. Williams 2001; Murray and others 2001; Wagstaff 2001, 2002d; Navarro 2000, 2001; Blendon, Kim, and Benson 2001; Murray, Kawabata, and Valentine 2001).

ESTIMATING THE COST OF ACHIEVING THE MDGS

These caveats notwithstanding, several traditional approaches have been used to estimate the cost of accelerated progress toward achieving the MDGs. They include:

- Estimates of the cost of achieving the MDG goals based on known expenditure elasticities of health outcomes (Wagstaff 2002b; Devarajan, Miller, and Swanson 2002)

- Estimates of additional public expenditure needed to achieve outcome-based production frontiers

- Estimates of the total cost of introducing new programs using bottom-up costing (Evans 1990a; WHO 2001, 2002b; Kumaranayake, Kurowski, and Conteh 2001).

- Estimates of the marginal cost of addressing major constraints (Soucat and others 1992)

- Specific estimates of scaling up child heath and other interventions and treatment for priority diseases (Tulloch 1999; Lambrechts, Bryce, and Orinda 1999; Weissman 2001; Weissman and others 2001; Garrison and Mccall 1990).

The Use of Production Frontiers

In this chapter, we used production frontiers to estimate the costs of accelerated progress toward achieving the MDGs. Production frontiers have been the subject of a great deal of research on inefficiency (Farrel 1957). The *production function* shows the maximum output (for example, real observed outcome in terms of health) that can be obtained from a given level of input mix, such as factors of production (for example, capital, human resources, drugs, equipment, and consumables), product market (for example, hospital services, ambulatory services, and diagnostic clinics), and prevailing technology. Alternatively, production functions can also be used to describe the minimum amount of inputs required to achieve various specific outputs (MDG targets). The *production frontier* describes the limits to the outputs (outcome) that can be achieved using different combinations of inputs.

Variations in maximum output can occur either as a result of stochastic effects (for example, random events, unpredictable economic shocks, or bad weather), or it can occur from the fact that firms (health care providers) may operate at various levels of inefficiency due to suboptimal use of existing technology (input mix, throughput processes, outputs), mismanagement, inefficient organizational structures (for example, lack of economy of scope or scale, compromised decision rights, and adverse incentives), or dysfunctional institutional environment (for example, lack of an appropriate legal framework to deal with market failure or to promote efficient competition). Outputs (such as health outcomes) that fall short of a given target can sometimes be brought up to the production frontier by changing one or more of these critical variables.

Recently, stochastic production frontiers have been widely applied to assess firm inefficiencies in various settings (Aigner, Lovell, and Schmidt 1977; Battese and Coelli 1995). In theoretical models, a wide range of input and output variables can be specified. In real life, observable output levels and available data on the inputs impose constraints. Thus an initial challenge is to construct an empirical production function or frontier, based on the observable data (Lewin and Knox 1990; Coelli, Prasada-Rao, and Battese 1998).

Past Use of Production Frontiers in the Health Sector

The use of production frontiers in the health sector in developing countries is not new. Production frontiers have been used for many years to study efficiency in the heath sector of the Organisation for Economic Co-operation and Development (OECD). Production frontiers based on cost-effectiveness data were used in the 1993 *World Development Report* to select from among alternative cost-effective treatments that would be most effective and affordable at low-income levels (World Bank 1993). Production frontiers have been used to examine hospital performance issues (Wagstaff 1989; Wagstaff and Lopez 1996). Expenditures linked with inputs (such as beds and staff), intermediate measures (such as average lengths of hospital stays, waiting times), and outcomes (such as infant mortality) can begin to provide some relative notions of health system efficiency (Schieber, Poullier, and Greenwald 1991; OECD 1992, 1994; Anderson and Poullier 1999). They have been used to compare different levels of input mix (Anell and Willis 2000). Production frontiers have been used to examine efficiency issues related to public-private mix in service delivery and financing (Musgrove 1996).

Production frontiers have also been used to assess the overall country performance in achieving good health outcomes and more specifically U5MR (Wang and others 1999). WHO (2000) used production frontiers to rank the performance of health systems in different countries, using the relationship between health expenditure and three outcome indicators—financial fairness, patient responsiveness, and outcomes. The OECD (2002) also made use of production frontiers but employed a different set of indicators.

Application of Production Frontier Analysis in Estimating the Global Expenditure Gap

As described earlier, the production function for health and the determinants of U5MR, MMR, and UW are complex and multisectoral. A number of different production frontier models could be constructed that would shed some light on various dimensions of the input and product mix needed to attain maximum outcomes in terms of the MDG-related indicators.

The production frontier approach was one of the methodologies used to estimate the global expenditure gap for the Macroeconomic Commission on Health (WHO 2002c). To establish a production frontier relative to health spending and the MDGs, two assumptions were made (Preker, Langenbrunner, and Suzuki 2001). First, the maximum level of total resources for health care that a country can mobilize (if it could) is likely to be less than, or equal to, the current highest spender at similar income levels. Although there is some variation within income bands, the income versus health spending elasticity is well-known and research documented (Schieber and Maeda 1997). Second, although countries already spending much more than the best performers in outcomes at similar income levels may still benefit from additional spending (based on spending-outcome elasticities), there is probably also considerable scope for improving their efficiency of spending since other countries are able to do much better with fewer resources.

Source of Data

We examined 135 countries where gross domestic product (GDP) per capita is less than, or equal to, US$7,000. This cut-off point was chosen so that the analysis would correspond to low- and middle-income. The analysis was done for both total and public expenditure on health care. We used the most recent data on health expenditure available in the WHO health expenditure database (usually 1998 data) and GDP per capita from the World Bank SIMA database (matching as closely as possible the 1998 health data). For most of the health indicators, we also matched as closely as possible the date of the health expenditure (HIV prevalence 1999, incidence of tuberculosis 1999, life expectancy 1997, adult male mortality 1997, adult female mortality 1997, maternal mortality 1995). To assess relative performance in improving U5MR, we used the 1990 to 2000 trend.

Establishing the Production Frontier for Health Expenditure per Capita

To establish the production frontier, we used the health expenditure (total and public) for the 20 percent of countries that performed the best in absolute terms on several health indicators (most, but not all, related to the MDGs). The health indicators used to select the best performers in absolute terms included: U5MR, MMR, HIV prevalence rate between the ages of 15 and 49, incidence rate of tuberculosis, life expectancy at birth, adult male mortality rate, and adult female mortality rate (World Bank 2002c). For the U5MR, we also created a second production frontier, based on the health expenditure level for the 20 percent of countries that performed the best in relative improvement between the years 1990 and 2000.

An exponential regression on a double log scale was employed to construct the production frontier using the health expenditure (total and public) per GDP per capita data points for the high performers under each of the selected health indicators. Given the small size of the resulting dataset for the production frontier countries, the application of more refined statistical techniques, such as stochastic analysis, was not relevant.

Once the production frontier was established, the gap between the target health expenditure corresponding to the best performers and the observed health expenditure for any given country (adjusting for the population size) could be calculated. Figures 11.7a and 11.7b provide an example of the expenditure gap using the absolute level of spending in countries that performed the best on U5M compared with the expenditure for the production frontier countries. The figures illustrate the expenditure gap that would have to be filled in the case of six countries used as case study examples on scaling up for the September 2002 Development Committee Report (World Bank 2002a).

For China and India, where over 90 percent of the world's poor live, total expenditure on health care is already higher than in the corresponding production frontier countries. Public spending on health in India is, however, well below the best performance expenditure frontier, while public spending on health in China is slightly above expenditure in the production frontier countries for U5M. Table 11.1 provides the numerical estimate of the expenditure gap for these six countries, using different outcome indicators to establish the production frontier.

The production frontier trend lines for total expenditure on health care using best performance on various health outcomes—under-five mortality, maternal mortality, life expectancy, adult male mortality, adult female mortality, TB prevalence, HIV/AIDs prevalence—are shown in figure 11.8. Both the countries used to determine the frontier (large circles) and the nonfrontier countries (small circles) are indicated on each graph. The production frontier trend lines for public expenditure on health care, using best performance on various health outcomes, are shown in figure 11.9.

The total and public expenditure gap for countries with a per capita income of less than US$7,000 was estimated by summing the gap for each of the countries

FIGURE 11.7   Expenditure Frontier and Six Countries

a.

GDP per Capita and Total Health Expenditure
(frontiers = under-5 mortality)

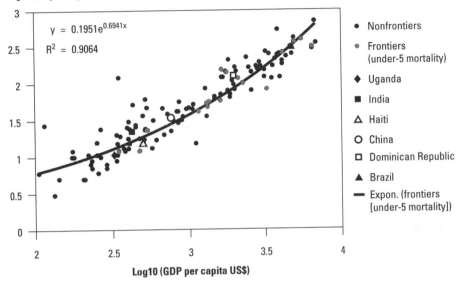

b.

GDP per Capita and Public Health Expenditure
(frontiers = under-5 mortality)

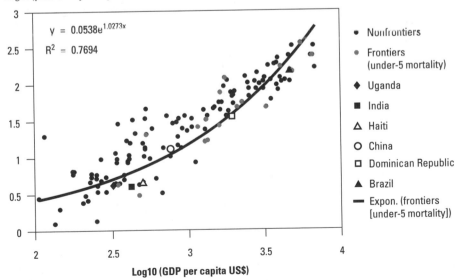

TABLE 11.1 Public Expenditure on Health Needed to Be More Like Frontiers (US$, Using Exponential Regressions, and log10 for HE and GDP)

Frontiers are the Best 20 Percent Performers of

Country	Public expenditure on health per capita (US$)	Under-5 mortality % change between 1990 and 2000			HIV prevalence 1999			TB incidence 1999			Life expectancy 1997		
		Needed/ capita	Gap/ capita	Gap as total public exp.	Needed/ capita	Gap/ capita	Gap as total public exp.	Needed/ capita	Gap/ capita	Gap as total public exp.	Needed/ capita	Gap/ capita	Gap as total public exp.
Uganda	4	6	2	31,600,000	8	4	75,000,000	11	7	144,000,000	6	2	47,300,000
India	4	7	3	2,740,000,000	9	5	5,350,000,000	13	9.2	8,970,000,000	8	4	3,600,000,000
Haiti	5	8	3	22,000,000	11	6	46,300,000	15	10	76,600,000	9	4	29,500,000
China	13	12	0	0	17	4	4,690,000,000	21	8	10,200,000,000	13	0	5,381,798
Dominican Republic	36	40	4	36,300,000	58	22	177,000,000	55	19	155,000,000	41	5	39,000,000
Brazil	154	224	70	11,600,000,000	301	147	24,300,000,000	177	23	3,820,000,000	189	35	5,780,000,000

Frontiers are the Best 20 Percent Performers of

Country	Public expenditure on health per capita (US$)	Adult male mortality 1997			Adult female mortality 1997			Maternal mortality 1995		
		Needed/ capita	Gap/ capita	Gap as total public exp.	Needed/ capita	Gap/ capita	Gap as total public exp.	Needed/ capita	Gap/ capita	Gap as total public exp.
Uganda	4	9	5	110,000,000	6	2	39,600,000	7	3	62,400,000
India	4	11	7	7,130,000,000	7	3	3,210,000,000	9	5	4,500,000,000
Haiti	5	13	8	60,600,000	8	3	26,400,000	10	5	37,800,000
China	13	19	6	6,850,000,000	13	0	0	15	2	2,140,000,000
Dominican Republic	36	51	15	121,000,000	43	7	59,400,000	47	11	87,100,000
Brazil	154	181	27	4,460,000,000	234	80	13,300,000,000	216	62	10,300,000,000

FIGURE 11.8   Production Frontiers for Total Expenditure on Health Care (Using Best Performance on Various Health Outcomes)

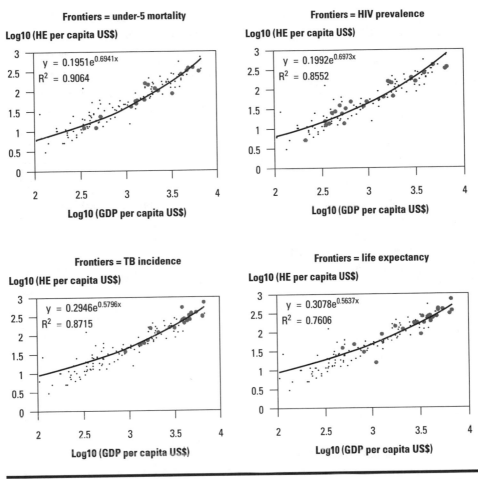

(continued)

within several income bands (tables 11.2 and 11.3).[3] Countries spending more than the expenditure frontier were assigned a value of zero even though they might still benefit from additional spending in terms of reaching the target outcome indicator.

(11.1)   Country gap = $Y - y$, where $Y = ce^{bx}$ (if $Y > y$) and gap = 0 where $Y < y$

where:

c and b are constants
e is the base of the natural logarithm
y is observed log10 (HE per capita US$) of all countries
Y is the estimated log10 (HE per capita US$) from frontiers
x is observed log10 (GDP per capita US$) of frontiers.

FIGURE 11.8   Continued

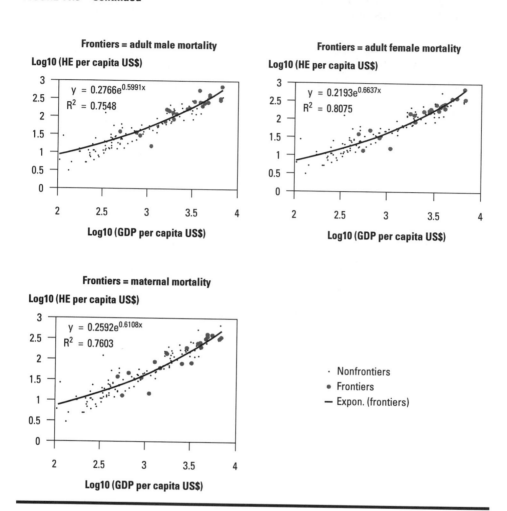

The use of production frontiers to estimate the cost of scaling up provides some insights that can be used to supplement other insights gained from work on elasticities of health spending and outcomes, bottom-up costing, and marginal constraints costing. Notably:

- For the 135 countries where GDP per capita is less than US$7,000, around $25 billion to $70 billion of additional spending would be needed to bring the low spenders up to the level of the high performers, depending on the outcome indicator used to establish the frontier.

- The best performers on health outcome are not always the highest spenders. Both India and China, where the largest share of the world's poor live, already spend more in terms of total expenditure on health than the frontier spending in the best performing countries.

FIGURE 11.9   Production Frontiers for Public Expenditure on Health Care Using Best Performance on Various Health Outcomes

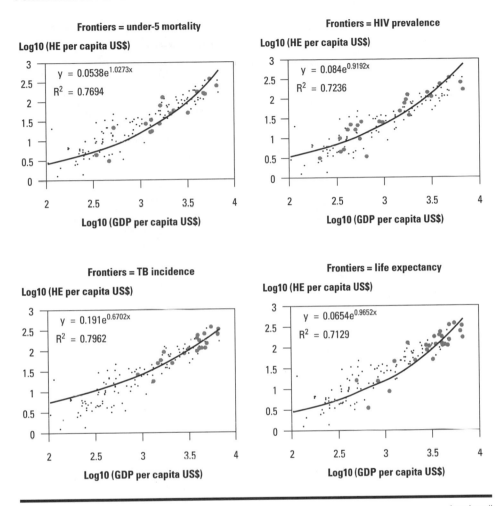

(continued)

- The best performers are not evenly distributed across income groups. The best performers for HIV prevalence rates are seen across all GDP levels, while the best performers for tuberculosis are seen only at higher GDP levels (log10 [GDP per capita > 2.9] or GDP per capita > $900). Other health outcomes start having best performers around the GDP levels of log10 (GDP per capita < 2.7) or GDP per capita < $500, Armenia, Azerbaijan, Georgia, and so on.

More than anything, the use of production frontiers indicates the developing countries' constraints in scaling up spending needed to accelerate progress toward the MDGs. Since the limit is not the "sky" and since developing countries have to live within realistic budget constraints, this analysis points to a

FIGURE 11.9   Continued

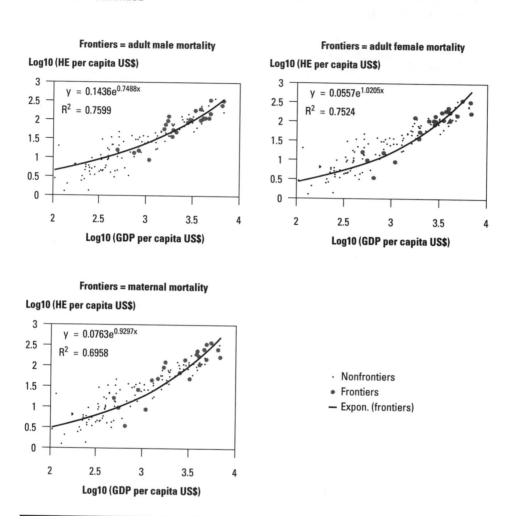

need for significant targeting and selectivity in additional spending. One way to reduce the total gap in needed spending would be to target specific income ground where the needs might be deemed the greatest. For example:

- For the 22 countries where GDP per capita is less than $300, around $350 million to $1.4 billion of additional spending would be needed to bring the low spenders up to the level of the high performers, depending on the outcome indicator used to establish the frontier. For public expenditure on health, the additional amount would be $150 million to $1 billion.

- For the 47 countries where GDP per capita is between $300 and $1,000, around $2 billion to $15 billion of additional spending would be needed to

TABLE 11.2   Total Health Expenditure Gap in US$ (in Millions) to Achieve Frontier Expenditure Levels (Countries with GDP < US$7,000 per Capita)

		Frontiers are the Best 20 Percent Performers of						
GDP per capita	*(N)*	*Under-5 mortality % change 1990–2000*	*HIV prevalence 1999*	*TB incidence 1999*	*Life expectancy 1997*	*Adult male mortality 1997*	*Adult female mortality 1997*	*Maternal mortality 1995*
$0–300	22	$345	$505	$1,137	$1,356	$1,133	$654	$916
$300–1,000	47	$1,947	$3,462	$10,875	$14,670	$11,731	$3,992	$5,134
$1,000–3,000	40	$1,472	$3,891	$4,475	$4,322	$5,110	$2,905	$2,562
$3,000–7,000	26	$28,488	$60,986	$20,958	$13,882	$25,731	$29,728	$15,003
Total	135	$32,252	$68,844	$37,445	$34,230	$43,705	$37,279	$23,615

TABLE 11.3   Public Health Expenditure Gap in US$ (in Millions) to Achieve Frontier Expenditure Levels (Countries with GDP < US$7,000 per Capita)

		Frontiers are the Best 20 Percent Performers of						
GDP per capita	*(N)*	*Under-5 mortality % change 1990–2000*	*HIV prevalence 1999*	*TB incidence 1999*	*Life expectancy 1997*	*Adult male mortality 1997*	*Adult female mortality 1997*	*Maternal mortality 1995*
$0–300	22	$154	$407	$1,079	$241	$725	$186	$337
$300–1,000	47	$4,606	$14,211	$26,414	$6,125	$19,537	$5,478	$9,954
$1,000–3,000	40	$675	$3,901	$3,617	$823	$2,613	$972	$1,547
$3,000–7,000	26	$47,864	$86,565	$19,280	$28,657	$21,859	$51,968	$40,807
Total	135	$53,299	$105,084	$50,390	$35,846	$44,734	$58,604	$52,645

bring the low spenders up to the level of the high performers, depending on the outcome indicator used to establish the frontier. For public expenditure on health, the additional amount would be around $5 billion to $26 billion.

- For the 40 countries where GDP per capita is between $1,000 and $3,000, around $1.5 billion to $5 billion of additional spending would be needed to bring the low spenders up to the level of the high performers, depending on the outcome indicator used to establish the frontier. For public expenditure on health, the additional amount would be $700 million to $4 billion.

- For the 26 countries where GDP per capita is between $3,000 and $7,000, around $14 billion to $61 billion of additional spending would be needed to bring the low spenders up to the level of the high performers, depending on the outcome indicator used to establish the frontier. For public expenditure on health, the additional amount would be $19 billion to $87 billion.

The use of efficiency frontiers for this type of analysis has several significant constraints. Unlike the work using elasticities of health spending and outcomes, production frontiers do not provide any insights into the potential impact of additional spending. The lagging countries could spend up to, and even beyond, the efficiency frontier without improving health outcomes. Although the frontier approach sheds some light on the limits to spending, like elasticities using aggregate spending levels, it does not inform the policymaker about the contents of those reforms. To understand the policy contents and implementation issues, other tools of investigation are needed.

FINANCING THE EXPENDITURE GAP

Although the various costing methods provide different estimates for the global funding gap, all of them indicate that additional funding will be needed to accelerate progress toward the health-related MDGs. Without additional funding, many countries are likely to continue tracking along the path of the past few years, significantly missing the 2015 outcome targets. Other management, organizational, and institutional reforms are necessary as well, but they will not be sufficient without additional funding. Prospects for significant increases in health spending, however, are grim for several reasons.

Potential Sources of Funding

Several potential sources of additional funding can be identified. They include:

- Increase in total health expenditure that will accompany economic growth, even if the share of GDP remains constant

- Increase in health expenditure as a share of GDP (that is, reallocation of some public funds from other spending programs toward health and an increase in private health care consumption)

- Reallocation of part of the health budget toward priority programs

- Donor aid from multilaterals, bilaterals, and nongovernmental organizations

- Private sector donation and differential pricing.

GDP Growth

Health care behaves as a superior good in economic terms—the share of expenditure increases with GDP—and pubic expenditure on health as a share of GDP also increases with income (World Bank 1993; Schieber and Maeda 1997; WHO 2000; OECD 2001). These trends are demonstrated in figure 11.10. Economic growth is therefore good for health spending.

FIGURE 11.10   Income and Health Spending

Total spending as share of GDP

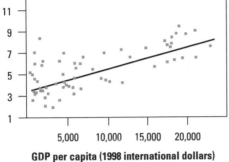

GDP per capita (1998 international dollars)

Public share of total spending

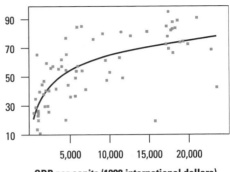

GDP per capita (1998 international dollars)

Unfortunately, the sluggish global economic outlook, with slower growth in the next 12 to 18 months than previously anticipated, will impede poverty reduction and health spending in many developing countries (World Bank 2002b). According to the latest forecasts, global GDP is expected to rise by 2.5 percent. This is higher than during the previous two years but significantly below previous long-term growth rates. High-income countries are expected to grow at about 2.1 percent in 2003. On average, developing countries will grow considerably faster, at 3.9 percent.

Health spending in low- and middle-income countries is currently around US$280 billion. Since the elasticity of health spending to income is just over one in low-income countries, annual GDP growth of 3.9 percent would yield US$11 billion in additional funding for the health sector.

But such averages mask wide regional differences, with East Asia leading the pack at 6.1 percent, followed by South Asia at 5.4 percent. Other regions are expected to grow less than 4 percent, with Latin America managing a mere 1.8 percent. Outside Asia and Eastern Europe, growth rates in most developing countries are too low to generate any significant increase in health expenditure in the immediate future.

Even though global spending increased dramatically during the 20th century, many of the world's poor did not benefit from this increase in overall spending. This is reflected in the large differences in the proportion of national GDP spent on health—from under 1 percent in some countries to 15 percent in the United States. Per capita health expenditures (public and private) vary almost 1,000-fold among countries—from around US$3 to $5 per capita per year in some low-income countries such as Mali to $3,600 in the United States (the ratio would be 225 using PPP-adjusted dollars). Once again, Sub-Saharan Africa and South Asia are the hardest hit in terms of both current spending and dismal prospects for increased spending due to economic growth (see figure 11.11).

FIGURE 11.11   Only 11 Percent of Global Spending for 90 Percent of the World's Population

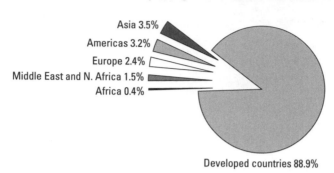

Asia 3.5%
Americas 3.2%
Europe 2.4%
Middle East and N. Africa 1.5%
Africa 0.4%

Developed countries 88.9%

Increase in Health Expenditure as a Share of GDP

Domestic funds can be raised for the health sector through a number of different mechanisms: general revenues, earmarked social health insurance premiums, community financing, private insurance, and direct user charges. Many low-income countries spend less than 2 percent of GDP, and some even less than 1 percent, on health care. The production frontier for health spending at different income levels indicates that, with good public polices and taxation practices, even poor countries can mobilize and allocate enough financial resources through public channels to reach spending levels of up to 7 percent of GDP.

A small increase in the share of health spending in GDP would yield huge gains (a 0.5 to 1.0 percent increase would yield US$25 billion to $50 billion in additional resources for the health sector). But once again the poorest countries in Africa and South Asia would benefit the least for several reasons. Weak taxation capacity prevents many low-income countries from mobilizing more than 5 to 10 percent of GDP through the public sector (Dror and Preker 2002; Preker and others 2002). Private spending is much greater than public spending at low-income levels (for example, in India, Bangladesh, and many other low-income countries, private spending composes more than 80 percent of total spending). As a result of these factors, low-income countries have little protection against the financial burden of illness even when, as in India, they spend a significant part of their income on health care—6 percent of GDP (Peters and others 2002). As seen in figure 11.12, a large share of the population in some of the world's poorest countries do not benefit from insurance protection against the cost of illness.

Reallocation of Health Budget toward Priority Programs

One frequently hears rhetoric about mobilizing additional resources through efficiency gains or channeling health expenditure from within the existing health budget toward priority health programs such as child and maternal care or the priority infectious diseases. In reality, this is not an easy policy to imple-

FIGURE 11.12   Low-Income Countries Have Less Pooling of Revenues

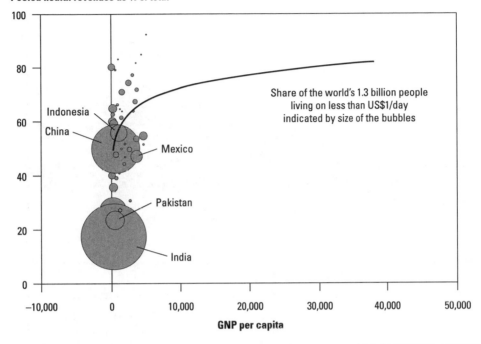

ment. For example, existing budget categories are often rigid, allowing for little fungibility among spending programs. Strong vested stakeholders will resist having their budgets channeled to other programs. Any resources that might be freed up through efficiency gains are better absorbed by expanding the scope and activities of the programs in which the gains were made: "Why scrimp and save if you cannot keep the results of your frugality?" (Wilson 1989). It is therefore prudent not to anticipate additional resources mobilized in this manner.

Donor Aid from Multilaterals, Bilaterals, and Nongovernmental Organizations

Total Overseas Development Assistance (ODA) on health was estimated at US$6 billion to $7 billion by Working Group 6 of the Macroeconomic Commission on Health. Additional funding from the international donor community is unlikely (WHO 2002a).

Annual World Bank lending has remained around US$1 billion to $1.5 billion despite efforts to increase this during the past few years. Although there was much posturing about increasing donor aid for the health sector during creation of the Global Trust Fund for HIV/AIDs, Tuberculosis, and Malaria, replenishment of the fund has been slower than expected and disbursement so far almost nonexistent.

FIGURE 11.13   Types of Private Financial Flows

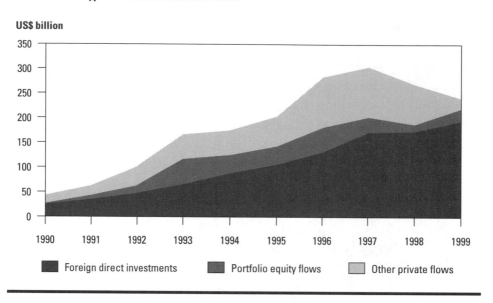

Hence donor aid has "hit the wall" in terms of both additional commitments and ability by developing countries to absorb such aid under existing procedures. Even an unrealistically optimistic scenario of a 15 percent increase would yield only an additional US$1 billion in donor assistance.

Direct Private Sector Investment and Differential Pricing Policies

The sagging global economy has also reduced private capital flows to developing countries (see figure 11.13). Net commercial bank lending has turned negative, and foreign direct investment (FDI) flows to developing countries have fallen since their peak in 1999. FDI flows to developing countries peaked at $180 billion in 1999 and have fallen back to the $160 billion range (World Bank 2002b). Although only a small amount of these resources benefit the health sector directly, they often contribute significantly to the health-enhancing environment of a country (for example, roads, clean water, and telecommunications systems).

Rising global risk premiums have led to a reversal in debt capital flows. The precarious market conditions have also reduced infrastructure investment sharply. Besides the fall in investment in absolute terms, investors are becoming more selective in choosing their investment destinations. As a result, investment is flowing to countries with better domestic investment climates: good governance, sound institutions, and a system of property rights. These are precisely the conditions that are often lacking in some of the poorest countries in Sub-Saharan Africa and South Asia, making future private sector engagement in those regions less attractive.

Adopting policies that promote competition is central to raising productivity. Policy barriers to competition in developing countries are common—legal restrictions prevent entry of foreign participants, trade barriers limit import competition, state monopolies protect domestic firms from private sector competition, and poorly designed regulatory regimes in privatized industries shun competitors—stifling productivity growth. The same is true in the health sector of developing countries (Harding and Preker 2003). Health care providers in Korea, Malaysia, and Thailand are more productive than in India and China partly because of lower trade restrictions and administrative barriers to entry.

Introduction of competition in corporatized and privatized industries is helpful as well. Private restraints on competition can also have adverse effects on prices for consumers and producers in developing countries and impair their ability to compete in global markets. For example, international cartels such as those in the pharmaceutical industry can tax consumers in developing countries. Ending exemptions to antitrust laws can help reduce private anticompetitive practices (Preker and Harding 2003).

Corporate social responsibility has also been evoked recently as a way to engage the private sector in helping developing countries (European Commission 2002). Assistance ranges from direct donations in cash and kind by the pharmaceutical industry to differential pricing of products that gives low-income countries access to vaccines, medicines, and supplies at a reduced price. Gross annual revenues in the pharmaceutical industry are currently around US$300 billion. Even a modest 1 to 2 percent "Robin Hood" tax on their revenues or differential reduction in prices would yield significant marginal additional resources (US$3 billion to $6 billion). Other industries such as the private health insurance industry, medical equipment industry, and health service providers could be called upon to make an equally modest contribution.

CONCLUSIONS

The Millennium Development Goals have become a quantitative set of targets for poverty reduction and improvements in health, education, gender equality, the environment, and other aspects of human development. The selected health-related goals and targets were limited in number to help focus national and international attention on a few priority areas: reducing the number of children who die before their fifth birthday and women who die from complications of childbirth and reversing the spread of HIV/AIDS, malaria, tuberculosis, and other major diseases.

This chapter has reviewed several approaches that have been used to estimate the cost of accelerating progress toward achieving the MDGs—the elasticity of outcomes with respect to health spending, health spending production frontiers with respect to outcomes, bottom-up costing, and marginal benefit costing. The chapter concludes that improvements in clinical effectiveness, management capacity, organizational incentives, and institutional environment are necessary elements but are not sufficient in themselves to make progress toward achieving the health-related MDGs. In many low- and middle-income countries, additional money is also necessary.

The level of aid needed might be more than the US$25 billion to $50 billion estimated by the research done for the Macroeconomic Commission on Health (WHO 2002a, 2002b, 2002c). The expenditure gap increases dramatically when the scenarios include countries with a GDP above US$1,000. The gap could be almost three times previous estimates, especially if middle-income countries and counties that are already high spenders are included in this aid effort.

The additional funding could come from growth in income (which would be automatically translated into higher health spending), a shift of some public spending toward the health sector, increased private consumption of effective care, increased international aid (public and private), and direct foreign investment in the health sector of developing countries. Unfortunately, in many of the worst performing countries, the needed additional resources outstrip both potential domestic and international sources of revenues, especially in the case of South Asia and Sub-Saharan Africa.

National governments, households, the international development community, and the private sector could do better in mobilizing these additional resources and provide some estimates of the order of such action. In many low-income countries, however, the targets appear unattainable. Caution should be exercised not to discourage countries that could make modest progress toward better health outcomes through the fervor of the current debate on achieving the MDGs.

The argument that health levels are always "lower than they need be" could be said of every country in the world. The diseases would be different, but even in the United States, there are diseases for which technology is available to improve health but whose cost is considered prohibitive for parts of the population, given competing claims on scarce resources.

Donor aid is also unlikely to be a solution by itself but may be important at the margins if it is well targeted to the poor and if it contributes to systemic reforms. This suggests that any analysis should not assume away the problem of governments' inability to allocate resources and deliver services effectively. Indeed, donor support should tie in with government performance in terms of resource allocation and outcomes. Much more work is needed to fully understand the variation in performance of different countries and their health systems in achieving maximum value for money.

Acknowledgments: The authors are grateful to Flavia Bustreo, Mariam Claeson, Shantayanan Devarajan, Dean Jamison, Margaret Miller, Philip Musgrove, Juan Rovira, Eric V. Swanson, and Adam Wagstaff for their reviews and helpful guidance. The findings, interpretations, and conclusions expressed in the chapter are entirely those of the authors and do not represent the views of the World Bank, its Executive Directors, or the countries they represent.

NOTES

1. The proposal to develop such a set of goals was first made by the Ministers of Development from the Development Assistance Committee (DAC) of the Organisation for Economic Co-operation and Development (OECD) in 1995 (OECD 1996). The General Assembly of the United Nations incorporated these goals in the Millennium Declaration in September 2000, while setting new targets for reducing the proportion of people suffering from hunger, increasing access to improved water sources, improving the lives of slum dwellers, and reversing the spread of HIV/AIDS, malaria, tuberculosis, and other major diseases (United Nations 2000, 2001).

2. Other outcome measures such as birthrate and population composition (for example, proportion of the population under 15 years) are not significantly associated with health spending (Gbesemete and Gerdtham 1992).

3. We ultimately used exponential regressions in log scale for both health expenditure and GDP, after observing patterns of relative fit for simple linear regressions, power regressions, polynomial regressions, as well as in ordinary scale for both health expenditure and GDP. Log scale for both GDP and health expenditure was used because converting them into log scale gave a higher R-squared than the one in ordinary scale. Exponential regressions were chosen because the fitted line showed higher R-squared (0.91) than R-squared of power regression line (0.87) and polynomial regression line (0.83). They were also chosen because the exponential regressions gave a higher intercept than simple linear regressions, where the values of R-squared of these two regressions were almost the same (0.91). In addition, we fitted the exponential regression line by controlling for levels of female primary education, but this did not produce a significantly different result.

REFERENCES

Aigner, D. J., C. A. Lovell, and P. Schmidt. 1977. "Formation and Estimation of Stochastic Frontier Production Function Models." *Journal of Econometrics* 6: 21–37.

Alderman, H., H. Appleton, L. Haddad, L. Song, and Y. Yohannes. 2000. *Reducing Child Malnutrition: How Far Does Income Growth Take Us?* Washington, D.C.: World Bank.

Anderson, G., and J.-P. Poullier. 1999. "Health Spending, Access, and Outcomes: Trends in Industrialized Countries." *Health Affairs* 18(3): 172–92.

Anell, A., and M. Willis. 2000. "International Comparisons of Health Care Systems Using Resource Profiles." *Bulletin of the World Health Organization* 78(6): 770–78.

Barnum, H. 1987. "Evaluating Healthy Days of Life Gained from Health Projects." *Social Science and Medicine* 24(10): 833–41.

Barnum, H. N. 1986. "Cost Savings from Alternative Treatments for Tuberculosis." *Social Science and Medicine* 23(9): 847–50.

Barnum, H. N., D. Tarantola, and I. F. Setiady. 1980. "Cost-Effectiveness of an Immunization Programme in Indonesia." *Bulletin of the World Health Organization* 58(3): 499–503.

Battese, G. E., and T. J. Coelli. 1995. "A Model of Technical Inefficiency Effects in a Stochastic Frontier Production for Panal Data." *Empirical Economics* 20: 325–32.

Blendon, R. J., M. Kim, and J. M. Benson. 2001. "The Public Versus the World Health Organization on Health System Performance." *Health Affairs* 20(3): 10–20.

Carrin, G., R. Zeramdini, P. Musgrove, J-P. Poullier, N. Valentine, and K. Xu. 2001. *The Impact of the Degree of Risk-Sharing in Health Financing on Health System Attainment.* Report submitted to Working Group 3 of the Commission on Macroeconomics and Health, Jeffrey D. Sachs (Chairman). WHO, Geneva.

Claeson, M., and R. J. Waldman. 2000. "The Evolution of Child Health Programmes in Developing Countries: From Targeting Diseases to Targeting People." *Bulletin of the World Health Organization* 78(10): 1234–45.

Claeson, M., T. Mawji, and C. Walker. 2000. *Investing in the Best Buys: A Review of the Health, Nutrition, and Population Portfolio, FY1993–99.* Washington, D.C.: World Bank.

Coelli, T. J., D. S. Prasada-Rao, and G. E. Battese. 1998. *An Introduction to Efficiency and Productivity Analysis.* Boston: Kluwer.

Devarajan S., M. J. Miller, and E. V. Swanson. 2002. *Goals for Development: History, Prospects, and Costs.* Washington, D.C.: World Bank.

Dror, D., and A. S. Preker, eds. 2002. *Social Re-Insurance: A New Approach to Sustainable Community Health Financing.* World Bank, HNP Discussion Paper. Washington, D.C.

European Commission. 2002. *Promoting a European Framework for Corporate Social Responsibility: Green Paper.* Brussels.

Evans, D. B. 1990a. "Principles Involved in Costing." *Medical Journal of Australia* 153(suppl.): S10–2.

———. 1990b. "What Is Cost-Effectiveness Analysis?" *Medical Journal of Australia* 153(suppl.): S7–9.

Farrel, M. J. 1957. "The Measurement of Production Efficiency." *Journal of Royal Society,* Series A, 120: 253–90.

Filmer, D., and L. Pritchett. 1999. "The Impact of Public Spending on Health: Does Money Matter?" *Social Science and Medicine* 49(10): 1309–23.

Filmer D., J. Hammer, and L. Pritchett. 2000. "Weak Links in the Chain: A Diagnosis of Health Policy in Poor Countries." *World Bank Observer* 15(2): 199–224.

———. 2002. "Weak Links in the Chain: A Prescription for Health Policy in Poor Countries." *World Bank Observer* 17(1): 47–66.

Garrison, L., and N. Mccall. 1990. *Measuring the Impact of Medical Technology on Health Care Costs: Report for the Prospective Payment Assessment Commission.* Washington, D.C.: U.S. Congress.

Gbesemete, K. P., and U. G. Gerdtham. 1992. "Determinants of Health Care Expenditure in Africa: A Cross-Sectional Study." *World Development* 20(2): 303–8.

Gwatkin, D. R. 2000. "Health Inequalities and the Health of the Poor: What Do We Know? What Can We Do?" *Bulletin of the World Health Organization* 78(1): 3–18.

Gwatkin, D. R., and P. Heuveline. 1997. "Improving the Health of the World's Poor." *BMJ* (London) 315(7107): 497–98.

Hammer, J. 1996. *Economic Analysis for Health Projects.* World Bank, HNP Discussion Paper. Washington, D.C.

Harding, A., and A .S. Preker, eds. 2003. *Private Participation in Health Services*. World Bank, HNP Discussion Paper. Washington, D.C.

Hauck, K., P. C. Smith, and M. Goddard. 2002. *Priority Setting for Health*. Washington, D.C.: World Bank.

Jack,W. 2000. "Public Spending on Health Care: How Are Different Criteria Related? A Second Opinion." *Health Policy* 53(1): 61–67.

Jakab, M., A. S. Preker, C. Krishnan, P. Schneider, F. Diop, J. Jütting, A. Gumber, K. Ranson, and S. Supakankunti. 2001. *Social Inclusion and Financial Protection through Community Financing: Initial Results from Five Household Surveys*. Report submitted to Working Group 3 of the Commission on Macroeconomics and Health, Jeffrey D. Sachs (Chairman). WHO, Geneva.

Jamison, D. T., W. H. Mosley, A. Measham, and J. L. Bobadilla, eds. 1993. *Disease Control Priorities in Developing Countries*. Washington, D.C.: World Bank.

Kumaranayake, L., C. Kurowski, and L. Conteh. 2001. *Costs of Scaling-up Priority Health Interventions in Low and Selected Middle Income Countries: Methodology and Estimates*. Geneva: World Health Organization.

Lambrechts, T., J. Bryce, and V. Orinda. 1999. "Integrated Management of Childhood Illness: A Summary of First Experiences." *Bulletin of the World Health Organization* 77(7): 582–94.

Lewin, A. Y., and C. A. Knox. 1990. "Frontier Analysis: Parametric and Nonparametric Approaches." *Journal of Econometrics* (Netherlands) 46: 3–245.

Mills, A. 1985a. "Economic Evaluation of Health Programmes: Application of the Principles in Developing Countries." *World Health Statistics Quarterly* 38(4): 368–82.

———. 1985b. "Survey and Examples of Economic Evaluation of Health Programmes in Developing Countries." *World Health Statistics Quarterly* 38(4): 402–31.

Murray C. J., K. Kawabata, and N. Valentine. 2001. "People's Experience Versus People's Expectations." *Health Affairs* 20(3): 21–24.

Murray, C. J., D. B. Evans, A. Acharya, and R. M. P. M. Baltussen. 2000. "Development of WHO Guidelines on Generalized Cost-Effectiveness Analysis." *Health Economics* 9(3): 235–51.

Murray, C. J., J. Frenk, D. Evans, K. Kawabata, A. Lopez, and O. Adams. 2001. "Science or Marketing at WHO? A Response to Williams." *Health Economics* 10(4): 277–82; discussion 283–85.

Musgrove, P. 1996. *Public and Private Roles in Health: Theory and Financing Patterns*. Washington, D.C.: World Bank.

———. 1999. "Public Spending on Health Care: How Are Different Criteria Related?" *Health Policy* 47(3): 207–23.

———. 2000a. "Cost-Effectiveness as a Criterion for Public Spending on Health: A Reply to William Jack's 'Second Opinion.'" *Health Policy* 54(3): 229–33.

———. 2000b. "A Critical Review of 'A Critical Review': The Methodology of the 1993 World Development Report, 'Investing in Health.'" *Health Policy Plan* 15(1): 110–15.

Navarro, V. 2000. "Assessment of the World Health Report 2000." *The Lancet* 356(9241): 1598–601.

————. 2001. "Science or Ideology? A Response to Murray and Frenk." *International Journal of Health Services* 31(4): 875–80.

Newhouse, J. P., and L. J. Friedlander. 1980. "The Relationship between Medical Resources and Measures of Health: Some Additional Evidence." *Journal of Human Resouces* 15(2): 200–18.

OECD (Organisation for Economic Co-operation and Development). 1992. *The Reform of Health Care: A Comparative Analysis of Seven OECD Countries.* Paris.

————. 1994. *The Reform of Health Care Systems: A Review of Seventeen OECD Countries.* Paris.

————. 1996. *Shaping the 21st Century: The Contribution of Development Co-operation.* Paris.

————. 2001. *OECD Health Data, 2000.* Paris.

————. 2002. *Measuring Up: Improving Health Systems Performance in the OECD.* Paris.

Peabody, J., ed. 1999. *Policy and Health: Implications for Development in Asia.* Cambridge: Cambridge University Press.

Peters, D. H., A. S. Yazbeck, R. R. Sharma, G. N. V. Ramana, L. Pritchett, and A. Wagstaff, eds. 2002. *Better Health Systems for India's Poor: Finding, Analysis, and Options.* World Bank, HNP Discussion Paper. Washington, D.C.

Preker, A. S., and A. Harding, eds. 2003. *Innovations in Health Service Delivery: The Corporatization of Public Hospitals.* World Bank, HNP Discussion Paper. Washington, D.C.

Preker A. S., J Langenbrunner, and E Suzuki. 2001. *The Global Expenditure Gap: Securing Financial Protection and Access to Health Care for the Poor.* Report submitted to Working Group 3 of the Commission on Macroeconomics and Health, Jeffrey D. Sachs (Chairman). WHO, Geneva.

Preker, A. S., J. Langenbrunner, M. Jakab, and C. Baeza. 2001. *Resource Allocation and Purchasing (RAP) Arrangements that Benefit the Poor and Excluded Groups.* World Bank, HNP Discussion Paper. Washington, D.C.

Preker, A. S., G. Carrrin, D. Dror, M. Jakab, W. Hsiao, and D. Arhin-Tenkorang. 2001. *Role of Communities in Resource Mobilization and Risk Sharing: A Synthesis Report.* Geneva: World Health Organization.

————. 2002. "Effectiveness of Community Health Financing in Meeting the Cost of Illness." *Bulletin of the World Health Organization* 8(2): 143–50.

Prescott, N., and D. De Ferranti. 1985. "The Analysis and Assessment of Health Programs." *Social Science and Medicine* 20(12): 1235–40.

Pritchett, L., and L. H. Summers. 1996. "Wealthier Is Healthier." *Journal of Human Resources* 31(4): 841–68.

Rivlin, M. M. 2000. "Why the Fair Innings Argument Is Not Persuasive." *BMC Medical Ethics* 1(1): 1.

Schieber, G., and A. Maeda. 1997. "A Curmudgeon's Guide to Health Care Financing in Developing Countries." In G. Schieber, ed., *Innovations in Health Care Financing.* Washington D.C.: World Bank. (Proceedings of a World Bank Conference, March 10–11, 1997.)

Schieber G., J.-P. Poullier, and L. Greenwald. 1991. "Health Systems in Twenty-Four Countries." *Health Affairs* 10(3): 22–38.

Soucat A., W. Lerberghe, F. Diop, and R. Knippenberg. 1992. *Buying Results, Budgeting for Bottlenecks: The New Performance Frontier.* World Bank, HNP Discussion Paper. Washington, D.C.

Tulloch, J. 1999. "Integrated Approach to Child Health in Developing Countries." *The Lancet* 354(suppl. 2): 16–20.

United Nations. 2000. *A Better World for All: Progress toward the International Development Goals.* New York: United Nations.

––––––. 2001. *Road Map towards the Implementation of the United Nations Millennium Declaration.* New York.

Van Doorslaer, E., A. Wagstaff, H. Van Der Burg, T. Christiansen, D. De Graeve, I. Duchesne, U. G. Gerdtham, M. Gerfin, J. Geurts, L. Gross, U. Hakkinen, J. John, J. Klavus, R. E. Leu, B. Nolan, O. O'Donnell, C. Propper, F. Puffer, M. Schellhorn, G. Sundberg, and O. Winkelhake. 2000. "Equity in the Delivery of Health Care in Europe and the U.S." *Journal of Health Economics* 19(5): 553–83.

Wagstaff, A. 1989. "Estimating Efficiency in the Hospital Sector: A Comparison of Three Statistical Cost Frontier Models." *Applied Economics* 21: 659–72.

––––––. 2001. "Economics, Health, and Development: Some Ethical Dilemmas Facing the World Bank and the International Community." *Journal of Medical Ethics* 27(4): 262–67.

––––––. 2002a. *Economic Growth and Government Health Spending: How Far Will They Take Us towards the Health MDGs?* Washington, D.C.: World Bank.

––––––. 2002b. *Intersectoral Synergies and the Health MDGs: Preliminary Cross-Country Findings, Collaboration, and Policy Simulations.* Washington, D.C.: World Bank.

––––––. 2002c. "Poverty and Health Sector Inequalities." *Bulletin of the World Health Organization* 80(2): 97–105.

––––––. 2002d. "Reflections on and Alternatives to WHO's Fairness of Financial Contribution Index." *Health Economics* 11(2): 103–15.

Wagstaff, A., and G. Lopez. 1996. "Hospital Costs in Catalonia: A Stochastic Frontier Analysis." *Applied Economics* 3: 471–74.

Wang, J., D. T. Jamison, E. Bos, A. S. Preker, and J. Peabody. 1999. *Measuring Country Performance on Health: Selected Indicators for 115 Countries.* Washington, D.C.: World Bank.

Weissman, E. 2001. *IMCI Costing Tool.* Geneva: World Health Organization.

Weissman, E., F. Bustreo, K. Krasovec, M. Claeson, and H. Troedson 2001. *Estimating the Cost of Basic Health Services for Children: The Experience from Nepal and Nigeria.* New York and Geneva: UNICEF and World Health Organization.

Williams, A. 2001. "Science or Marketing at WHO? A Commentary on 'World Health 2000.'" *Health Economics* 10(2): 93–100.

Williams, M. 1997. "Rationing Health Care: Can a 'Fair Innings' Ever Be Fair?" *BMJ* (London) 314(7079): 514.

Wilson, J. Q. 1989. *Bureaucracy: What Government Agencies Do and Why They Do It.* New York: Basic Books.

World Bank. 1993. *World Development Report 1993: Investing in Health.* New York: Oxford University Press.

————. 1997. *Sector Strategy for HNP.* Washington, D.C.

————. 2000. *World Development Report 2000/2001: Attacking Poverty.* New York: Oxford University Press.

————. 2002a. *Development Effectiveness and Scaling Up: Lessons and Challenges from Case Studies.* Washington, D.C.

————. 2002b. *Global Economic Prospects and the Developing Countries 2003.* Washington, D.C.

————. 2002c. *World Development Indicators.* Washington, D.C.

WHO (World Health Organization). 2000. *World Health Report 2000: Health Systems—Improving Performance.* Geneva.

————. 2001. *Macroeconomics and Health: Investing in Health for Economic Development.* Geneva.

————. 2002a. *Development Assistance and Health.* Geneva.

————. 2002b. *Improving Health Outcomes of the Poor.* Geneva.

————. 2002c. *Mobilisation of Domestic Resources for Health.* Geneva.

CHAPTER 12

Impact of Risk Sharing on the Attainment of Health System Goals

Guy Carrin, Riadh Zeramdini, Philip Musgrove, Jean-Pierre Poullier, Nicole Valentine, Ke Xu

Abstract: A simple econometric analysis is undertaken concerning the impact of the degree of risk sharing in countries' health-financing organizations on the goals of the health system. Those goals are defined in the *World Health Report 2000*—the level of health and its distribution across the population, the level of responsiveness and its distribution across the population, and fair financing. The degree of risk sharing varies according to whether countries have a universal coverage system, financed via social health insurance or general taxation, or systems with less-developed coverage. We undertook a classification of countries according to the degree of risk sharing, based primarily on the health-financing legislation of the World Health Organization's 191 member states and on its database of Health System Profiles. The results obtained give empirical support to the hypothesis that the degree of risk sharing in health-financing organizations positively affects health system attainment, as measured by the five goals indicators.

There are important linkages between what health systems can achieve in terms of preset goals and the functions that they undertake. *The World Health Report (WHR) 2000* has designed a coherent framework for analyzing these linkages (WHO 2000; see also Murray and Frenk 2000). In this chapter, we specifically address the health-financing function of pooling of resources and how it influences health systems attainment. One essential question is whether health-financing organizations provide sufficient financial risk protection for the population. People's access to health services depends on this protection. Health-financing organizations that do not include the low-income population groups, for instance, will lead to many individuals' being unable to pay for care. The extent to which these population groups are effectively included in risk-sharing arrangements is therefore likely to affect a goal such as the equality of health status. Health-financing organizations may also be more or less engaged in purchasing an adequate package of health services for the entire population. In this sense, they may affect the average level of access to good care and therefore indirectly have an impact upon the average level of health. Apart from the level and distribution of health status, other goals may be considered. In the next section, we give an overview of the goals of health systems as proposed by the *WHR 2000* and discuss how they relate to the functions of these systems.

This chapter's main purpose is to undertake a simple econometric analysis of the impact of the degree of risk sharing in countries' health-financing organization on the goals of the health system. The degree of risk sharing will vary according to whether countries have a universal coverage system, financed via social health insurance or general taxation, or systems with less-developed coverage. For the latter, specific population groups may be covered by variants of social health insurance and general taxation. Risk sharing via community health-financing schemes could not be considered for lack of data at the national level.

In preparation of the econometric analysis, we turn to the specific linkage between the goals and the health-financing function. Then we classify the health-financing organization of 191 countries by the degree of risk sharing. This classification will help in defining the variables that measure risk sharing and will be used in the econometric analysis. A descriptive data analysis of the endogenous variables is provided further. Finally, the specification of the econometric models and estimation results are presented.

HEALTH SYSTEM GOALS AND FUNCTIONS IN A NUTSHELL

The framework, as presented in the *WHR 2000*, defines a set of goals or objectives and includes ways to measure the achievement toward these goals. Of course, to obtain these achievements, health systems do need to carry out a number of functions. Below we address both goals and functions.

The goals considered are good health, responsiveness, and fair financing. Good health is approached in two ways. One is by striving for the best attainable average level for the entire population. The other is by minimizing the differences in health status among individuals and groups. In other words, the distribution of health as well as the level of health matters. Note that health is measured via disability-adjusted life expectancy,[1] whereby account is taken of time lived with a disability. Responsiveness measures how the health system performs relative to nonhealth aspects of provided health services. Responsiveness captures the extent to which the health system is client-oriented and treats people with respect. Respect for people includes the following aspects: respect for the dignity of the person, confidentiality, and autonomy. Within client orientation, we consider prompt attention, the quality of the amenities, the access to social support networks, and the choice of provider. Note that the distinction between overall level and distribution across the population also applies to responsiveness. Fair financing requires that the health expenditure of households be distributed according to an individual's ability to pay rather than his or her risk of illness. In a fairly financed system, everyone should be financially protected. It is crucial therefore that health systems rely as fully as possible on prepaid contributions that are unrelated to individual illness or utilization. It is clear that when analyzing fair financing, we are concerned with distributive aspects only. We thus obtain five objectives: the level and distribution of health, the level and distribution of responsiveness, and fair financing. Measurements have been designed so as to quantify the achievement with respect to each of these objectives. (See WHO 2000 for a summary of the methods.)[2]

We further consider four main functions of the health system: the delivery of health services, the creation of resources for health (investment in people, buildings, and equipment), health financing (raising, pooling, and allocating the revenues to purchase health services), and stewardship. The latter refers to a government's responsibility for the general health of its population. The stewardship function is of special importance as it has an impact on the way the other three functions are carried out.

Work is currently underway at the World Health Organization (WHO) to define indicators for the various functions so their possible impact on goal achievement can be measured. This chapter can be seen as an element of this particular work in that it focuses on the nature of risk sharing in the world's different health-financing systems and its possible impact on the goals as defined above.

THE ORGANIZATIONAL FORM OF HEALTH FINANCING AND ITS LINK TO THE ATTAINMENT OF HEALTH SYSTEM GOALS

A crucial concept in health financing is that of pooling. Pooling is defined as the "accumulation and management of revenues in such a way as to ensure that the risk of having to pay for health care is borne by all members of the pool and not by each contributor individually" (WHO 2000, p. 96). The larger the degree of pooling, the less people will have to bear the financial consequences of their own health risks.

Health-financing systems encompass various degrees of risk sharing. There are two major ways to ensure financial risk protection for a nation's entire population. One is a system whereby general taxation (GT) is the main source of financing health services. Services are usually provided by a network of public and contracted private providers, often referred to as a national health service. The second is social health insurance (SHI), whereby workers, enterprises, and government pay financial contributions. The base for workers' and enterprises' contributions is usually a worker's salary. Social health insurance either owns its own provider networks, works with accredited private providers, or combines the approaches. In principle, both systems pool all of the population's risks, with contributions that are delinked from individual risks. This approach theoretically avoids exposing individuals to insufficient or no access to the health care they need. These systems are often denoted as universal coverage systems, but financial protection may still be judged inadequate in a number of these systems.

There are also systems with no explicit reference to overall coverage of the population. These include mixed health-financing systems, in which some part of the population is partially covered via general taxation and another part is covered by health insurance schemes. The latter may address specific groups only. Still, they may practice full pooling among their members and define health insurance contributions according to capacity to pay rather than individual health risks. In other words, these schemes may apply a community rating (as a social health insurance scheme does) but for specific groups only. Such schemes may include voluntary private insurance arrangements, mutual health funds, and enterprise-based and community health insurance. Finally, some countries do finance health services via GT but offer only incomplete coverage.

For the purpose of this chapter, we will say that countries that have achieved or are near to universal coverage, and use either general taxation or social health insurance, enjoy systems with *advanced risk-sharing*. Such schemes allow for more equal access to health services among individuals. In addition, such schemes generally better define an adequate package of health services to which citizens are entitled. Countries with mixed health-financing systems will be associated with *medium risk-sharing*. The countries with general taxation systems that incompletely cover the population are then associated with *low risk-sharing*. In this chapter, we will investigate whether larger degrees of risk sharing have a beneficial impact on the five indicators of goal achievement.

ORGANIZATION OF HEALTH FINANCING IN THE WORLD

In table 12.3 (see appendix), countries are classified according to the criterion of risk sharing as defined above, based on the health care-financing legislation of WHO's 191 member states. Our main source for this revision was the publication *Social Security Programs throughout the World*, provided by the U.S. Social Security Administration (1999). However, for 52 countries, insufficient information or none was given. For the latter group, and in order to identify the category of health-financing system, WHO's database of Health System Profiles (http://www.who.int/country_profiles/main.cfm) and other selected publications were used (Nolan and Turbat 1995; see also the Web site of the Center for International Health Information http://www.cihi.com).

In table 12.3, approximately 40 percent of the countries are characterized as advanced risk-sharing systems, having either a general taxation system (50 countries) or a social health insurance scheme (30 countries) that covers nearly the entire population. The 61 countries with medium risk-sharing are further classified into three main variants. In the first variant, health insurance covers all employees and the self-employed, though subject to a number of exclusions.[3] The second variant covers only employees. The third covers specific groups only, using, for instance, mutual health funds and enterprise-based health insurance for particular categories of workers. In these three variants, there are 9, 20, and 32 countries, respectively. Finally, 50 countries are classified among those with low risk-sharing. These countries are generally characterized by underfinanced health systems as compared with the health needs of the population. It is admitted, however, that for a number of countries, the proposed classification is not final, due to incomplete or absent information on the size and structure of the eligible population effectively covered by the health-financing system.

We can also rank countries according to the category of risk sharing and the percentage share of public health expenditure in total health expenditure.[4] The three categories considered are shares between 75 and 100 percent, between 50 and 75 percent, and below 50 percent. We use the latter ratio as a simple quantitative indicator of the system's degree of financial risk protection. In fact, of the countries with advanced risk-sharing, 74 out of 80 have a ratio above 50 percent and 41 have a ratio above 75 percent. Of the countries with medium risk-sharing, only 3 out of 61 have a ratio above 75 percent. For countries with low risk-sharing, a tilt toward low ratios would be expected. However, for 9 out of 50 countries with low risk-sharing, ratios above 75 percent are reported, which is surprising. However, it is recognized in the *WHR 2000* that quite a number of countries have incomplete data and mixed degrees of reliability,[5] which may partly explain this finding.

In addition, it is interesting to rank countries according to the category of risk sharing and to the income level, as measured by the 1998 gross domestic product (GDP) per capita (in U.S. dollars). Of the 80 countries with advanced risk-sharing, 20 belong to the category of upper middle-income countries, and 34 to the high-income category. Most countries with low to medium risk-sharing belong to the low-income and lower middle-income categories. In this set of countries, only Andorra and the United States belong to the upper middle-income or high-income category.

MODELING THE IMPACT OF THE ORGANIZATIONAL FORM OF HEALTH FINANCING ON HEALTH SYSTEM ATTAINMENT INDICATORS

Descriptive Data Analysis

As a prelude to the econometric analysis, descriptive statistics for the five health attainment indexes are computed. The health attainment indexes are the disability-adjusted life expectancy (DALE), the index of level of responsiveness (IR), the index of fairness of financial contribution (IFFC), the index of distribution of responsiveness (IRD), and the index of equality of child survival (IECS). All data used originate from the Statistical Appendix of *WHR 2000*. In table 12.1, statistics related to all countries that have observations on the indexes are presented. In table 12.2, however, countries whose risk sharing classification is uncertain are removed from the samples.

The indexes are classified according to the category of risk sharing of countries' health-financing organizations. We present the mean, coefficient of variation, minimum, and maximum. First, a general tendency is that the means of the indicators are larger the greater the degree of risk sharing. One exception is in table 12.1, in which the mean fair-financing index for countries with advanced and medium risk-sharing is smaller than that of the countries with low risk-sharing.

TABLE 12.1   Descriptive Statistics (Full Samples)

Statistics	Disability adjusted life-expectancy (DALE)	Index of level of responsiveness (IR)	Index of fairness of financial contribution (IFFC)	Index of distribution of responsiveness (IRD)	Index of equality of child survival (IECS)
Total sample					
Mean	56.8262	0.5165	0.8730	0.8967	0.6659
CV[a]	0.2165	0.1542	0.1203	0.0969	0.2878
Min	25.9000	0.3740	0.6230	0.7230	0.2450
Max	74.5000	0.6880	0.9920	0.9999	0.9990
Number of observations	191	30	21	33	58
Countries with advanced risk-sharing					
Mean	66.0725	0.5849	0.8732	0.9772	0.9296
CV	0.0755	0.1272	0.0643	0.0252	0.1490
Min	52.3000	0.4430	0.8020	0.9180	0.6320
Max	74.5000	0.6880	0.9390	0.9999	0.9990
Number of observations	80	8	5	9	7
Of which countries with social health insurance					
Mean	68.5267	0.5452	0.8945	0.9715	0.9990
CV	0.0552	0.1150	0.0704	0.0290	0
Min	62.2000	0.4430	0.8500	0.9180	0.9990
Max	74.5000	0.6120	0.9390	0.9960	0.9990
Number of observations	30	5	2	6	4
Of which countries with general taxation					
Mean	64.6000	0.6510	0.8590	0.9886	0.8370
CV	0.0785	0.0492	0.0694	0.0128	0.2237
Min	52.3000	0.6320	0.8020	0.9750	0.6320
Max	73.0000	0.6880	0.9210	0.9999	0.9990
Number of observations	50	3	3	3	3
Countries with medium risk-sharing					
Mean	52.9033	0.5153	0.8623	0.8846	0.6792
CV	0.2152	0.1109	0.1463	0.0932	0.2320
Min	29.1000	0.4180	0.6230	0.7230	0.2610
Max	72.3000	0.6230	0.9920	0.9860	0.9660
Number of observations	61	16	11	17	34
Countries with low risk-sharing					
Mean	46.8180	0.4285	0.8962	0.8227	0.5309
CV	0.2411	0.1165	0.1183	0.0847	0.2816
Min	25.9000	0.3740	0.7140	0.7280	0.2450
Max	66.7000	0.4940	0.9610	0.9490	0.7850
Number of observations	50	6	5	7	17

a. CV is the coefficient of variation.

However, in table 12.2, the mean IFFC for countries with advanced risk-sharing exceeds that for countries with low risk-sharing. Second, using the restricted samples (table 12.2), the coefficients of variation (CV) indicate that, except in the case of IR, there is a lower relative dispersion around the mean in countries with advanced risk-sharing than in countries with medium risk-sharing. The latter is consistent with the fact that we have defined three subgroups with different degrees of risk sharing *within* the set of countries with medium risk-sharing. Notice also that in three cases (fair financing, distribution of responsiveness, and distribution of health), countries in the low risk-sharing category show lower coefficients of variation than those for the countries with medium risk-sharing. It stands to reason that the low risk-sharing category of countries is likely to be more homogeneous than the group of countries with medium risk-sharing. Except for the value related to IR, the coefficients of variation are higher, however, when compared with the CV of countries with advanced risk-sharing.

Specification of the Basic Model

A basic model is constructed, with the main objective to examine the degree to which risk sharing has a beneficial impact on five indicators of health systems attainment. These are the indexes of DALE, IR, IFFC, IRD, and IECS. Only the observed data for these indicators were included in the analysis (WHO 2000).

The independent variables were divided into three groups based on the degree to which they provided risk-sharing arrangements. As discussed above, countries belong either to the *advanced risk-sharing* category, or to the *medium risk-sharing* or *low-risk-sharing* category. This classification allows us to define the three main organizational dummy variables: DARS = 1 when a country belongs to the set of advanced risk-sharing systems and 0 otherwise; DMRS = 1 when a country belongs to the set of medium risk-sharing systems and 0 otherwise; DSHI = 1 when an country belonging to the advanced risk-sharing category has a social health insurance system and 0 otherwise.

We used the following basic specification for the impact of risk sharing on the *level of health:*

(12.1) $\text{Ln} (80 - \text{DALE}) = a_1 + b_1 \, \text{Ln HEC} + c_1 \, \text{Ln EDU} + d_1 \, \text{DARS}.$

The dependent variable is the logarithm of the difference between the observed DALE and a maximum. HEC refers to the health expenditure per capita (in US$). EDU refers to the educational attainment in society and is measured by the primary enrollment. Both HEC and EDU are expected to raise DALE and so to be negatively related to the distance of DALE from the maximum of 80. In other words, the higher HEC and EDU, the closer one gets to the maximum DALE. The hypothesis is further that advanced risk-sharing (DARS = 1) is associated with a more comprehensive definition of the benefit package of health services to which citizens are entitled, which translates into increased overall level of health.

TABLE 12.2   Descriptive Statistics (Restricted Samples)

Statistics	Disability adjusted life-expectancy (DALE)	Index of level of responsiveness (IR)	Index of fairness of financial contribution (IFFC)	Index of distribution of responsiveness (IRD)	Index of equality of child survival (IECS)
Total sample					
Mean	58.0588	0.5165	0.8721	0.8967	0.6843
CV[a]	0.20840	0.1542	0.1233	0.0969	0.2636
Min	25.9000	0.3740	0.6230	0.7230	0.2610
Max	74.5000	0.6880	0.9920	0.9999	0.9990
Number of observations	160	30	19	33	52
Countries with advanced risk-sharing					
Mean	67.1179	0.5849	0.8910	0.9772	0.9378
CV	0.0645	0.1272	0.0513	0.0252	0.1598
Min	56.3000	0.4430	0.8500	0.9180	0.6320
Max	74.5000	0.6880	0.9390	0.9999	0.9990
Number of observations	67	8	4	9	6
Of which countries with social health insurance					
Mean	68.5267	0.5452	0.8945	0.9715	0.9990
CV	0.0646	0.1150	0.0703	0.0290	0
Min	62.2000	0.4430	0.8500	0.9180	0.9990
Max	74.5000	0.6120	0.9390	0.9960	0.9990
Number of observations	30	5	2	6	4
Of which countries with general taxation					
Mean	65.9757	0.6510	0.8875	0.9886	0.8155
CV	0.0674	0.0492	0.0534	0.0128	0.3183
Min	56.3000	0.6320	0.8540	0.9750	0.6320
Max	73.0000	0.6880	0.9210	0.9990	0.9990
Number of observations	37	3	2	3	2
Countries with medium risk-sharing					
Mean	53.7596	0.5153	0.8623	0.8846	0.6849
CV	0.2081	0.1109	0.1464	0.0932	0.2282
Min	29.1000	0.4180	0.6230	0.7230	0.2610
Max	72.3000	0.6230	0.9920	0.9860	0.9660
Number of observations	57	16	11	17	33
Countries with low risk-sharing					
Mean	48.0056	0.4285	0.8800	0.8227	0.5655
CV	0.2452	0.1165	0.1307	0.0847	0.2258
Min	25.9000	0.3740	0.7140	0.7280	0.3360
Max	66.7000	0.4940	0.9590	0.9490	0.7850
Number of observations	36	6	4	7	13

a. CV is the coefficient of variation.

Variants of the basic model are also tested. One tests whether social health insurance has a specific impact on the health level. A dummy variable DSHI, equal to 1 when the country has a social health insurance scheme and 0 otherwise, will be added to the explanatory variables of equation 12.1. If we reason that, on average, general taxation and social health insurance schemes cover similar population groups with similar health interventions, social health insurance should not do better or worse than general taxation; hence we expect an effect that is not statistically different from 0.

The second alternative model studies the marginal impact of a mixed health-financing scheme. A dummy variable DMRS, equal to 1 when the country has a mixed health-financing system and 0 otherwise, is included next to DARS. Mixed health-financing schemes also include health insurance schemes applying risk sharing and therefore should have a beneficial impact on health-level attainment. Therefore, our hypothesis is that the marginal impact of DMRS on Ln (80 – DALE) is negative.

In a third alternative model, we test whether certain groups of schemes within the overall set of mixed health-financing systems would have an additional net effect on the level of health. We select the group of mixed systems that encompass health insurance schemes in which only employees are covered (DMRS1 = 1 and 0 otherwise) and health insurance schemes that cover other specific groups only (DMRS2 = 1 and 0 otherwise). As these health insurance schemes offer a lower degree of financial risk protection, as compared with schemes that cover all employees and the self-employed, the hypothesis is that the impact of DMRS1 and DMRS2 on DALE is negative; hence, the expected sign of the impact on the dependent variable is positive.

These alternative models are combined further. Namely, we add both DSHI and DMRS to the explanatory variables of equation 12.1. Finally, we bring DSHI, DMRS, DMRS1, and DMRS2 together into the equation.

The level of responsiveness is measured by an index (IR) that varies between 0 and 1, with 1 being the maximum. We adopted a logistic specification, implying that predicted values for IR stay within the 0–1 interval:

$$(12.2) \quad \text{Ln} \left[IR/(1 - IR) \right] = a_{21} + b_{21} \, HEC + c_{21} \, EDU + d_{21} \, DARS.$$

The impact of HEC is presumed to be positive as more resources are likely to facilitate the responsiveness of the health system. EDU can be understood as capturing the positive effect of a literate and more developed society on responsiveness. The hypothesis to be tested further is that advanced risk-sharing systems are associated with a larger degree of stewardship. The latter in turn is likely to positively influence the mechanisms and incentives that entail a greater responsiveness.

As in the case of the health level, alternative models can be estimated. DSHI is expected to be neutral vis-à-vis responsiveness; we therefore expect a coefficient that is not statistically different from 0. Medium risk-sharing schemes are expected to do better than low risk-sharing schemes in terms of responsiveness;

hence the marginal impact of DMRS is expected to be positive. However, a negative impact is expected to be associated with DMRS1 and DMRS2.

The basic model further comprises the analysis of three measures for distributional impact: an index of IECS, IFFC, and IRD. Equations are developed that examine the impact of the dummy variable (DARS) on these distributional variables. We have adopted the same functional form as in equation 12.2:

(12.3) $\text{Ln} [I_j/(1 - I_j)] = a_{31} + b_{31} \text{ DARS},$

where I_j (j = 1,...,3) refers to the three above-mentioned indexes, respectively.

The effect of DARS on the indicator of fair financing is expected to be positive when using the logit form of the equation. The hypothesis to be tested is that in countries with advanced risk-sharing, more so than in other systems, people pay financial contributions according to their capacity to pay. This would be associated with a higher IFFC. Second, systems with universal coverage generally pay more attention to the objective of equal treatment for equal need. It is therefore assumed that such systems also respond to people's expectations as to the nonmedical aspects of health care in a more equal way. Hence the effect of DARS on the distribution of responsiveness is anticipated to be positive as well. Third, it is assumed that universal coverage systems are more likely to provide people with a similar benefit package than are other systems, irrespective of their socioeconomic background, with a resulting positive impact on the distributional aspects of child health.

For alternative models, we first include DSHI as an additional dummy variable in the equation. The sign of the coefficients of DSHI is uncertain, however. Whether social health insurance is inferior or superior to general taxation in terms of fair financing depends on a host of factors. Those factors include the way health insurance contributions are levied (with an earnings ceiling or without), the progressivity of income taxes, the level of copayments, user fees, or both, and the types of health services that are excluded from coverage and their prices. In general, when adding DMRS to the explanatory variables, we expect it to have an additional positive effect. The effects of DMRS1 and DMRS2 are anticipated to be negative.

Specification of Enlarged Models

We also studied enlarged models, adding other potentially significant explanatory variables to the specification of the equations. In one enlarged model, the GINI index measuring the distribution of income is included:

(12.4) $\text{Ln} [I_j/(1 - I_j)] = a_{41} + b_{41} \text{ GINI} + c_{41} \text{ DARS},$

where I_j (j = 1,...,3) refers again to the three indexes, respectively.

Income inequality in society, as measured by the GINI, is expected to be mirrored, at least partially, in the distribution of the health-financing burden on the various households. For instance, it is expected, other things being held constant, that the larger the income inequality, the lower the degree of fair financ-

ing. The coefficient b_{41} is therefore expected to be negative. We further anticipate that countries with advanced risk-sharing are apt to counteract the initial
effect of overall income inequality by introducing better financial risk protection
for all the population. Hence we expect that the impact of DARS is maintained.

Further variants of equation 12.4 are investigated via the inclusion of DSHI,
DMRS, DMRS1, and DMRS2. In principle, there should be no change in the supposed direction of the effects already commented upon earlier. In addition, the
impact of interaction variables, combining the GINI index with the organizational dummy variables, can be studied. The coefficients of the interaction variables are expected to show that the larger the degree of risk sharing, the more
the impact of the GINI index is offset. For instance, the coefficient of the interaction term between GINI and DARS is anticipated to be positive.

The various models considered so far measure the "average" impact of the different risk-sharing schemes on the attainment indicators. Enlarged models with
the inclusion of interaction variables between the ratio of public health expenditure to total health expenditure (PHE%) and the organizational dummy variables
among the determinants can also be considered. The equations are the following:

$$(12.5) \quad \text{Ln}\,(80 - \text{DALE}) = a_{51} + b_{51}\,\text{Ln}\,\text{HEC} + c_{51}\,\text{Ln}\,\text{EDU}$$
$$+\, d_{51}\,\text{DARS} + e_{51}\,\text{DARS*PHE\%}$$

$$\text{Ln}\,[\text{IR}/(1 - \text{IR})] = a_{52} + b_{52}\,\text{HEC} + c_{52}\,\text{EDU} + d_{52}\,\text{DARS} + e_{52}\,\text{DARS*PHE\%}$$

$$\text{Ln}\,[\text{I}_j/(1 - \text{I}_j)] = a_{53} + b_{53}\,\text{DARS} + c_{53}\,\text{DARS*PHE\%},$$

where I_j (j = 1,...,3) refers to the three equality indexes, respectively.

We expect that a higher PHE% would reinforce the effect of the organizational variables in the earlier models. This means that coefficient e_{51} is expected
to be negative, whereas we expect e_{52} to be positive. The more health expenditure is managed through the public sector, and thus the higher the degree of risk
pooling, the larger the equality of people within the health system is presumed
to be. Coefficient c_{53} is therefore anticipated to have a positive sign. Note that in
alternative equations, we also investigate the interaction of PHE% with DSHI,
DMRS, DMRS1, and DMRS2.

Estimation Results

For a comprehensive account and discussion of all estimation results, we refer to
Carrin and others 2001. In this chapter, we only present the "best" regressions[6]
of both the basic and enlarged models in tables 12.4 and 12.5 (see appendix). In
addition, only the results using restricted samples or restricted samples with
additional deletion of influential data are presented.

The estimation results for the basic model are presented in table 12.4. First,
concerning the **level of health (DALE),** the coefficients of DARS, HEC, and
EDU are negative as expected and are statistically significant at the 1 percent significance level.

Second, from the equation for the **level of responsiveness (IR),** we see that HEC and EDU do not have a statistically significant impact. One major reason is likely to be that the index of responsiveness contains both elements of respect for persons and client orientation and that these are influenced differently by HEC and EDU. For instance, HEC may be important in explaining client orientation, whereas it may not be in explaining respect for persons. Therefore, when analyzing the determinants of the overall index of responsiveness, the effect of HEC may disappear. The coefficient of DSHI is also not statistically significant, as expected. Notice, however, that the coefficients of both DARS and DMRS have the expected sign and are statistically significant.

Third, the explanatory power of the regression for the **index of fair financing (IFFC)** is minimal; DARS does not have a statistically significant impact on the IFFC. We submit that the major reason for this unsatisfactory result is the relatively small sample size. Moreover, the sample did not include sufficient data on countries with advanced and with low risk-sharing. For instance, the (full sample) data on advanced risk-sharing are those of Bulgaria, Jamaica, Kyrgyz Republic, Romania, and Russia and inadequately reflect the experience of high-income countries with either social health insurance or general taxation financing.

Fourth, in the equation for the **distribution of responsiveness (IRD)** the coefficient of DARS is statistically significant. The impact of DSHI is statistically insignificant. Fifth, the results for the **index of equality of child survival (IECS)** show that both DARS and DMRS have statistically significant impacts.

We next present an overview of the estimation results for the enlarged models with the GINI index as an explanatory variable in the equations for the distributional measures. The results are presented in table 12.5. In the **fair-financing equation (IFFC),** which has very low explanatory power, the coefficient of the GINI index has the anticipated sign but is not statistically significant. The coefficient of DARS is also not statistically significant.

Related to the **distribution of responsiveness (IRD),** the result shows significant impacts of both DARS and DMRS, as well as of the GINI index. All coefficients have the expected sign. One can conclude that these risk-sharing arrangements are efficient in counterbalancing the overall effect of income inequality. A threshold for the GINI indexes can be computed, indicating the value above which risk sharing is no longer able to counteract the effect of overall income inequality. In the case of a country with an advanced risk-sharing scheme, the threshold value is 57.9. In the case of medium risk-sharing schemes, the threshold is 26.3. From these estimates, one can infer that advanced risk-sharing schemes are more effective in counteracting the effects of overall income inequality in society.

In the regression result related to the **inequality of child survival (IECS),** the sign of the GINI coefficients is against our expectations. Surprisingly, the coefficient of GINI is also statistically significant at the 10 percent level. The coefficient of DARS has the anticipated sign, however, and is statistically significant at the 1 percent level.

Inclusion of the interaction variables with PHE% in the equations did not result in a general improvement of the estimation results. For instance, in a number of cases, the coefficients of DARS have the correct sign but are statistically insignificant. In other instances, the coefficient of DARS has a negative sign. Further estimations were done with transformed interaction variables. In the case of the interaction between DARS and PHE%, the variable constructed was DARS*(PHE% – 0.5). The coefficient associated with this variable reveals the impact of the difference between PHE% and a threshold of 50 percent. The results for IR, IFFC, IRD, and IECS are not satisfactory: the coefficient of the new interaction variable has a wrong sign, is not statistically significant, or both. Only in the case of DALE did we obtain a satisfactory result: both the coefficients of DARS and the interaction variable have the expected sign and are statistically significant. This result is presented in summary table 12.5. In other words, for those advanced risk-sharing systems with a PHE% above 50 percent, the level of PHE% reinforces the "average" effect of DARS.

Key Conclusions

A first conclusion is that the degree of advanced risk-sharing, as measured by the dummy variable DARS, is significant in the equations for four of the five goal measurements. No impact could be found in the case of the index of fair financing, but we submit this is due to the small sample size. In addition, in at least two of these measurements (level of responsiveness, distribution of health), the variable DMRS also has been shown to have a statistically significant impact.

Second, when enlarging the set of explanatory variables in the models for the distributional measures with the GINI index, DARS remains statistically significant in the equations for IRD and IECS. In addition, DMRS has a statistically significant impact in the equations for IRD. An additional interpretation emerges from the results, namely that risk sharing corrects for, or may even outweigh, the negative effect of overall income inequality on the fair-financing index and the index of distribution of responsiveness.

Third, using interaction terms with PHE% leads to plausible results for DALE only: the level of PHE% reinforces the average positive effect of advanced risk-sharing.

An analysis with preliminary updated data was also undertaken; since publication of the *WHR 2000*, WHO has developed updated estimates for the level (HEC) and share of public health expenditure in total health expenditure (PHE%). When using updated data for HEC in the equations for DALE and IR, similar results (in terms of explanatory power, sign and statistical significance of coefficients) are obtained as those presented here. The use of the updated PHE% does not significantly change the estimates for the equations with the interaction terms. Estimates of the index of fair financing were also obtained for an additional 30 countries. Reestimation of the equations using an enlarged sample of 50 now leads to two interesting results: (1) the advanced risk-sharing dummy variable DARS exerts a statistically significant effect on the fair-financing index; and (2) the GINI index has a statistically significant impact on IFFC but is counterbalanced by a health-financing system characterized by advanced risk-sharing. These preliminary results prove to be more in line with those obtained for the other distributional measures.

COMMUNITY RISK-SHARING ARRANGEMENTS: FURTHER NEED TO MEASURE THEIR IMPACT

Community risk-sharing arrangements are increasingly recognized as an intermediate response to the constraints many countries experience in rapidly extending financial risk protection to the national population. A body of research exists with respect to community-financing arrangements and their functioning within communities, districts, or regions. Information at the national level is clearly lacking. We have made an attempt to scan the literature and other sources (especially, Atim 1998; Bennett, Creese, and Monasch 1998; Carrin, De Graeve, and Devillé 1999; ILO and PAHO 1999; and Ginneken 1999) to see whether community risk-sharing organizations exist at country level. Only countries with low to medium risk-sharing will be considered, as countries with advanced risk-sharing in principle do not need to be complemented by community risk-sharing schemes.

We recorded that in the set of countries with a public health expenditure ratio of 50 to 75 percent, 25 out of 44 countries have community risk-sharing schemes operating. In the countries with a ratio below 50 percent, 42 out of 58 are reported to have such schemes. This is not unexpected, as we would expect community risk-sharing schemes to be established where governments are not able to make sufficient advancement in risk protection. However, these data are insufficient for econometric analysis. Further work concerning the quantitative importance of community risk-sharing arrangements at the country level is needed. This could be measured by the number of risk-sharing schemes and the percentage of population covered by such schemes. Alternatively, one could measure the ratio of the expenditures incurred by such schemes to overall private health expenditure. The higher this ratio, the greater is the effort to share risks. Current work on National Health Accounts at WHO goes in this direction by attempting to collect data on expenditure by nongovernmental institutions and communities. Further work is needed on identifying the part of this expenditure that is spent within the framework of risk-sharing arrangements.

CONCLUDING REMARKS

The results presented here give empirical support for the hypothesis that the degree of risk sharing in health-financing organizations matters for health system attainment, as measured by the five indicators. The categorical variables indicating whether a country has a health-financing organization with advanced or medium risk-sharing categories are especially seen to have significant impact. These effects prove to be quite robust after the GINI index is introduced among the explanatory variables in the models for the distributional measures.

We noted that the plausibility of the results improves when using the restricted samples, deleting data for those countries whose classification was considered uncertain. Further information will be necessary to address this uncertainty. In general, final data for larger samples of countries are welcome for four of the health system attainment indexes, especially for the index of fair-financing contribution, so that these will better reflect the patterns of risk sharing in the world. In the current samples, some of the risk-sharing schemes are underrepresented, which has entailed sensitivity of the results to specific data points.

Further work could also be done on designing much more refined quantitative measures for the degree of risk sharing. Indeed, within each of the categories of health-financing organization that we considered, a further variety in the degree of financial protection of different population subgroups may well be present.

In addition, more work needs to be undertaken to measure the quantitative importance of risk-sharing schemes for communities and the informal sector at the country level as well as the depth of risk sharing of these schemes. Only then can further econometric analysis be undertaken. In the meantime, given the empirical results obtained so far, one can clearly hypothesize beneficial impacts of these schemes on the health system attainment indicators.

See page 415 for acknowledgments, notes, and references.

TABLE 12.3 Classification of Countries by Degree of Risk Sharing in the Health-Financing System

Advanced Risk-Sharing		Medium Risk-Sharing			Low Risk-Sharing
Social health insurance (SHI)	General taxation	All employees and self-employed (with some exclusions) covered by health insurance	All employees covered by health insurance	Specific groups only covered by health insurance	
Australia	Albania	Colombia	Algeria	Botswana	Afghanistan
Austria	Antigua and	Ecuador	Andorra	Brazil	Angola
Belgium	Barbuda	El Salvador	Argentina	Burkina Faso	Armenia
Bulgaria	Azerbaijan	Equatorial Guinea	Bolivia	Burundi	Bahamas, The
Chile	Bahrain	Libya	Cape Verde	Cameroon	Bangladesh
Costa Rica	Barbados	Mongolia	Congo, Rep. of	China	Benin
Croatia	Belarus	Peru	Egypt, Arab Rep.	Côte d'Ivoire	Bhutan
Czech Republic	Belize	Tunisia	Gabon	Dominican	Cambodia
Estonia	Bosnia and	Uruguay	Guinea	Republic	Central African
France	Herzegovina		Honduras	Guatemala	Republic
Germany	Brunei Darussalam		Lebanon	Guinea-Bissau	Chad
Greece	Canada		Mali	Haiti	Comoros
Hungary	Cook Islands		Mexico	India	Congo, Dem.
Israel	Cuba		Namibia	Indonesia	Rep. of
Japan	Cyprus		Panama	Iran, Islamic	Djibouti
Korea, Rep. of	Denmark		Paraguay	Rep. of	Eritrea
Latvia	Dominica		Philippines	Iraq	Ethiopia
Lithuania	Finland		Senegal	Jordan	Fiji
Luxembourg	Iceland		Turkey	Kenya	Gambia, The
Macedonia, FYR	Ireland		Venezuela	Lesotho	Georgia
Monaco	Italy			Madagascar	Ghana
Netherlands	Jamaica			Mauritania	Grenada
Norway	Kazakhstan			Morocco	Guyana
Poland	Korea, DPR			Mozambique	Kiribati
Romania	Kuwait			Myanmar	Lao PDR
San Marino	Kyrgyz Republic			Nicaragua	Liberia
Slovak Republic	Malaysia			Niger	Malawi
Slovenia	Malta			Pakistan	Maldives
Switzerland	Mauritius			South Africa	Marshall Islands
Yugoslavia,	Moldova			Thailand	Micronesia
Fed. Rep.	New Zealand			Trinidad and	Nauru
(Serbia/	Niue			Tobago	Nepal
Montenegro)	Oman			United States	Nigeria
	Palau			Vietnam	Papua New Guinea
	Portugal			Yemen, Rep. of	Rwanda
	Qatar				São Tomé and
	Russian Federation				Principe
	St. Kitts and Nevis				Sierra Leone
	St. Lucia				Solomon Islands
	St. Vincent				Somalia
	Samoa				Sri Lanka
	Saudi Arabia				Sudan
	Seychelles				Suriname
	Singapore				Swaziland
	Spain				Syrian Arab Rep.
	Sweden				Tanzania
	Tajikistan				Togo
	Turkmenistan				Tonga
	Ukraine				Tuvalu
	United Arab				Uganda
	Emirates				Vanuatu
	United Kingdom				Zambia
	Uzbekistan				Zimbabwe

TABLE 12.4   Estimation Results[a] for the Basic Model

Explanatory variables	DALE[b] Ln (80- DALE)	IR[c]	IFFC[b]	IRD[d]	IECS[e]
Constant	4.9423 (0.3328) (14.8493)	−0.4896 (0.2160) (−2.2663)	2.2874 (0.2786) (8.2099)	1.6327 (0.4507) (3.6228)	0.2798 (0.2038) (1.3329)
HEC	−0.1919 (0.0197) (−9.7498)	0.0000 (0.0003) (0.1150)			
EDU	−0.2141 (0.0834) (−2.5684)	0.0032 (0.0026) (1.2540)			
DARS	−0.2963 (0.0654) (−4.5321)	0.7244 (0.2244) (3.2275)	−0.1146 (0.6072) (−0.1888)	4.2257 (0.8228) (5.1355)	6.6269 (0.3868) (17.1343)
DSHI		−0.2521 (0.1987) (−1.2688)		−1.4049 (0.9107) (−1.5427)	
DMRS		0.2673 (0.1148) (2.3294)		0.7217 (0.5355) (1.3478)	1.0737 (0.4202) (2.5550)
DMRS1					−0.1079 (0.4607) (−0.2343)
DMRS2					−0.6458 (0.3995) (−1.6165)
R-squared	0.7874	0.5678	0.0021	0.5749	0.8778
Adjusted R-squared	0.7821	0.4597	−0.0566	0.5276	0.8671
S.E. of regression	0.2639	0.2134	1.0791	1.1924	0.7350
Ak. info criterion	0.2049	−0.0525	3.0894	3.3097	2.3149
Sample size	124	26	19	31	51

a. The first and second coefficients in the parentheses refer to the standard error and t-statistic, respectively.
b. Restricted samples.
c. Bulgaria excluded from the sample.
d. Chile and Poland excluded from the full sample.
e. Uzbekistan excluded from the restricted sample.

TABLE 12.5 **Estimation Results[a] for the Enlarged Models (Summary)**

Explanatory variables	IFFC[b] Ln(80- DALE)	IRD	IECS[b]	DALE[b]
Constant	2.8260 (1.3698) (2.0630)	3.0610 (0.7956) (3.8539)	−0.7471 (0.9164) (−0.8153)	4.9446 (0.3306) (14.9580)
GINI	−0.0119 (0.0296) (−0.4020)	−0.0375 (0.0180) (−2.0853)	0.0355 (0.0206) (1.7240)	
DARS	−0.2568 (0.7162) (−0.3586)	2.1713 (0.5222) (4.1577)	5.3537 (0.5531) (9.6789)	−0.2088 (0.0843) (−2.4774)
DARS*[PHE%- 0.5]				−0.4556 (0.2798) (−1.6284)
DMRS		0.9873 (0.4637) (2.1291)		
HEC				−0.1897 (0.0196) (−9.6837)
EDU				−0.2166 (0.0828) (−2.6155)
R-squared	0.0121	0.5191	0.7053	0.7920
Adjusted R-squared	−0.1114	0.4590	0.6906	0.7850
S.E. of regression	1.1067	0.9320	1.1912	0.2621
Ak. info criterion	3.1846	2.8286	3.2550	0.1990
Sample size	19	28	43	124

a. The first and second coefficients in the parentheses refer to the standard error and t-statistic, respectively.
b. Restricted samples.

Acknowledgments: The authors of this chapter are grateful to the World Health Organization for having provided an opportunity to contribute to the work of the Commission on Macroeconomics and Health and to the World Bank for having published the material in this chapter as an HNP Discussion Paper. Discussions with and suggestions from Alex Preker, Melitta Jakab, David Evans, Kei Kawabata, and Ajay Tandon are gratefully acknowledged. Thanks also to Chris James for a thorough review of an earlier draft of this chapter. During the writing, Philip Musgrove was on secondment to the World Health Organization. The views expressed in this document are solely the responsibility of the authors.

NOTES

1. This summary-measure of population health adjusts life expectancy at birth for the burden of disability. Disability weights are used to convert years lived in disability into equivalent years lived in good health. (See further Mathers and others 2000.)

2. For further details, we refer to http://www3.who.int/whosis/discussion_papers/ discussion_papers.cfm?path=whosis,evidence,discussion_papers&language=english.

3. For instance, the agricultural self-employed population may not be covered. Workers in small enterprises with fewer than 10 workers may not be insured either.

4. Note that social insurance expenditure is included in public health expenditure.

5. For these nine countries, the data are either incomplete with low reliability (two countries out of nine) or are incomplete with high to medium reliability.

6. "Best" according to the adjusted R-square, the Akaike criterion, or both, as well as the theoretical consistency of the model.

REFERENCES

Atim, C. 1998. *Contribution of Mutual Health Organizations to Financing, Delivery, and Access to Health Care: Synthesis of Research in Nine West and Central African Countries.* Technical Report No. 18. Partnerships for Health Reform Project. Abt Associates Inc., Bethesda, Md.

Bennett S., A. Creese, and R. Monasch. 1998. *Health Insurance Schemes for People Outside Formal Sector Employment.* ARA Paper 16. World Health Organization (WHO), Geneva.

Carrin, G., D. De Graeve, and L. Devillé, eds. 1999. "The Economics of Health Insurance in Low- and Middle-Income Countries." *Social Science and Medicine* 48(special issue): 859–64.

Carrin G., R. Zeramdini, P. Musgrove, J-P. Pouillier, N. Valentine, and K. Xu. 2001. *The Impact of the Degree of Risk-Sharing in Health Financing on Health System Attainment.* World Bank, HNP Discussion Paper. Washington, D.C.

ILO (International Labour Office) and PAHO (Pan American Health Organization). 1999. *Synthesis of Case Studies of Micro-Insurance and Other Forms of Extending Social Protection in Health in Latin America and the Caribbean.* Paper presented at the meeting on extension of social protection in health to excluded groups in Latin America and the Caribbean. Mexico, November 29–December 1; http://oitopsmexico99.org.pe.

Mathers, C., R. Sadana, J. Salomon, C. J. L. Murray, and A. D. Lopez. 2000. *Estimates of DALE for 191 Countries: Methods and Results*. GPE Discussion Paper 16. WHO, Geneva.

Murray, C. J. L., and J. Frenk. 2000. "A Framework for Assessing the Performance of Health Systems." *Bulletin of the World Health Organization* 78 (6): 717–31.

Nolan, B., and V. Turbat. 1995. *Cost Recovery in Public Health Services in Sub-Saharan Africa*. Washington, D.C.: Economic Development Institute of the World Bank.

SSA (Social Security Administration). 1999. *Social Security Programs throughout the World, 1999*. Washington, D.C.: U.S. Government Printing Office.

van Ginneken, W., ed. 1999. *Social Security for the Excluded Majority: Case Studies of Developing Countries*. Geneva: International Labour Office.

WHO (World Health Organization). 2000. *The World Health Report 2000. Health Systems— Improving Performance*. Geneva.

About the Coeditors and Contributors

THE COEDITORS

Alexander S. Preker, lead economist and editor of the Health, Nutrition, and Population (HNP) Publication Series, is responsible for overseeing the World Bank's analytical work on public policy in the health sector, market dynamics, health financing, service delivery, pharmaceuticals, and health labor markets, focusing on ways to help developing countries accelerate progress toward achieving the U.N. Millennium Development Goals by 2015. He is a member of a team of researchers currently undertaking a major review of disease control priorities in developing countries, with support from the Gates Foundation and the Fogarthy International Center of the U.S. National Institutes of Health. Recently, he has worked closely on a number of projects with the World Health Organization (WHO), the International Labour Organization (ILO), the Rockefeller Foundation, the International Federation of Pharmaceutical Manufacturers Associations, the International Hospital Federation, the International Federation of Health Plans, and several leading academic centers involved in health and financial protection in developing countries.

Preker has published extensively and is a frequent speaker at major international events. He is on the editorial committee of the Bank's Publications Department, is the chief editor of its HNP publications, and is a member of the editorial committees of several international journals. Preker also is on the External Advisory Board of the London School of Economics Health Group and is a member of the teaching faculty for the Harvard/World Bank Institute Flagship Course on Health Sector Reform and Sustainable Financing. He has an appointment as adjunct associate professor at the George Washington University School of Public Health.

His training includes a Ph.D. in economics from the London School of Economics and Political Science, a fellowship in medicine from University College London, a diploma in medical law and ethics from King's College London, and an M.D. from the University of British Columbia/McGill.

Guy Carrin is senior health economist in the Department of Health Financing and Stewardship at the WHO in Geneva, Switzerland. His current work deals with issues of community and social health insurance. He has published extensively in the areas of social security, macroeconomic modeling and simulation, and health economics.

In the field of health economics, he is the author of the books *Economic Evaluation of Health Care in Developing Countries* and *Strategies for Health Care Finance in Developing Countries;* and coeditor of *Macroeconomic Environment and Health* and a special issue of *Social Science and Medicine* on "The Economics of Health Insurance in Low- and Middle-Income Countries."

Carrin was a member of Working Group 3 of the WHO Commission on Macroeconomics and Health and is currently a member of the editorial committee of the *Bulletin of the World Health Organization*. He is associated with the University of Antwerp (Belgium) and with Boston University.

He holds an M.A. and a Ph.D. in economics from the University of New Hampshire (United States) and the University of Leuven (Belgium), respectively. He held a Canada Council Fellowship at the University of Toronto and was visiting research fellow at the University of Michigan and Brandeis University. He was econometrician at the Ministry of Planning in Tunis (Tunisia), researcher at the Center for Operations Research and Econometrics in Leuven, fellow in international health at the Harvard School of Public Health, and economic adviser to the Minister of Public Health of the federal government of Belgium in 1987–88.

OTHER CONTRIBUTING AUTHORS

Dyna Arhin-Tenkorang is a public health physician and health economist and holds a clinical lectureship position in health economics at the London School of Hygiene and Tropical Medicine (LSHTM). The London School is Britain's national school of public health and a leading postgraduate institution in Europe for public health and tropical medicine. In 2000–02, Arhin-Tenkorang held the position of senior economist of the WHO Commission on Macroeconomics and Health (CMH), which was established to assess the place of health in global economic development.

At LSHTM, Arhin-Tenkorang has managed several health economics research projects focusing on the equity of access to health care and the role of fees and risk-sharing mechanisms and has published extensively on the findings of her empirical work. She was also a contributor to the *World Health Report 2000: Health Systems—Improving Performance* and the editorial manager of the report of the WHO Commission on Macroeconomics and Health, released in December 2001.

Her recent publications include: *Health Insurance for the Informal Sector in Africa: Design Features, Risk Protection, and Resource Mobilization,* a World Bank HNP Discussion Paper; "Mobilizing Resources for Health: The Case for User Fees Revisited," CMH Working Paper Series WG3; and "Beyond Communicable Disease Control: Health in the Age of Globalization," a chapter in a United Nations Development Programme (UNDP) publication on global public goods (2002).

Arhin-Tenkorang's qualifications in health economics and health planning include a Ph.D. from the London School of Economics and Political Science, an M.Sc. from the University of York, and a postgraduate diploma from the Nuffield Center, University of Leeds. She is a member of the West African College of Physicians and has a medical degree from the University of Ghana Medical School.

François Diop is a senior health economist who has extensive experience in health financing, demography, and survey research. Currently, he serves as one of the Partnerships for Health Reform (PHR) advisers in Senegal and PRIME II in Rwanda. Diop has extensive experience in health sector reform and health care financing, with a focus on Africa. He specializes in conducting applied research on alternative health-financing mechanisms for primary health care, including community-based financing schemes, demand surveys, facilities surveys (such as cost studies), analyses of means testing policies, and studies on quality of health services.

Under the Health Finance and Sustainability Project, he served as the resident adviser to the Ministry of Health in Niger. He played a major role in the design, implementation, and analysis of large-scale pilot tests in three districts in which cost-recovery mechanisms and quality improvements were introduced in public primary health facilities, which led to the development of a national policy of cost recovery for primary health care. Diop placed special emphasis on building the institutional capabilities of the Ministry of Health in formulating and assessing policy and in conducting applied research. Under the PHR project, he played a key role in the design and evaluation of the Rwanda prepayment schemes and community-based health insurance experiment; he is currently providing technical support to Rwanda for scaling up community-based health insurance nationwide. Diop designed and initiated the experimentation of a multilevel integrated health-planning and financing scheme to support the coordination of health interventions within the devolved health sector in Senegal. While employed at the World Bank, Diop worked on the implementation of country status reports on poverty and health in African countries to support the elaboration of the health component of the poverty reduction strategy papers. He has also worked with the Ministry of Finance of Senegal and has conducted research and provided technical assistance in demography and family planning in Côte d'Ivoire, Liberia, Nigeria, and Senegal. He has worked as a consultant to many other organizations, including the Population Council, Centers for Disease Control, the World Bank, and the WHO.

Diop received his B.A. in geography from the University of Dakar in Senegal, an M.S. in demography from the Institute for Demographic Training and Research in Cameroon, and a Ph.D. in demography and economics from the Johns Hopkins University. He is fluent in English and French.

David Dror is associate director of research at the Laboratoire d'Analyse de Systèmes de Santé (UMR 5823, CNRS), University of Lyon 1, France (ongoing, since 2002). From January 1998 to April 2003, he served as senior health insurance specialist within the International Labour Organization's Social Protection Sector, with special interest in development and stabilization of microinsurance schemes. During this period, he was the project leader for an ILO–World Bank project on social reinsurance for health care. This project developed the conceptual framework for, and piloted the reinsurance of, community-funded health schemes in developing countries. From 1989 to 1997, he served as chief of staff, Health Insurance Fund of the ILO-ITU (International Telecommunication Union), an in-house health insurance plan providing coverage in more than 100 countries and operating a full multicurrency financial system. He was an official of the ILO from 1982 to 2003. Prior to working at the international level, he held several posts at the national level, notably with the Israeli Employers' Federation (1977–81), where he was responsible for a national occupational pension agreement for the private sector (1979); negotiated innovative solutions for COLA wage indexation, which were applied nationwide during Israel's years of hyper-inflation (1975–81); served as lead representative on the Council of the National Insurance Institute of Israel; and was appointed delegate to the International Labour Conference (1977–81) and a member of the ILO Committee of Experts on Social Security Questions (1980–82).

Dror has a Ph.D., with highest distinction (University of Lyon 1, France), a D.B.A., magna cum laude (St. George University), an M.A. (Hebrew University of Jerusalem), and degrees in liberal arts, business administration, health services, and economics (as well as a teaching diploma). He earned a Fulbright Scholarship (1965).

Anil Gumber is a senior research fellow at the Centre for Health Services Studies, Warwick Business School (United Kingdom). Gumber was previously senior economist at the National Council of Applied Economic Research, New Delhi. He was awarded a Ph.D. in economics from Gujarat University, Ahmedabad. He has also held the Takemi Fellowship at the Harvard School of Public Health, Boston.

Gumber, trained in international health, has specifically addressed health issues of the poor, disadvantaged, and vulnerable. He has undertaken several consultation projects funded by the World Bank, the UNDP, UNICEF, the United Nations Population Fund, the WHO, the U.K. international development agency (DFID), and the Ford Foundation. He is a specialist in econometrics, management, and analysis of large data sets as well as in designing survey instruments and sampling frames for primary data collection. Gumber is currently undertaking research activities sponsored by the Economic and Social Research Council in the areas of ethnicity, health, and population diversity in the United Kingdom. His research interests are ethnicity and health; equity and international health; health care financing and insurance in developing countries; cost and efficiency issues in health; child health and nutrition; injury prevention and control; migration and resettlement; and poverty, welfare, and social policy issues.

Gumber's most recent papers include: "Economic Reforms and Health Equity"; "External Assistance to the Health Sector"; and "Health Insurance for the Poor." He is the author of *Displaced by Development: Oustees of an Irrigation Project;* coauthor of *Inter-Village Differences in Social Overheads and Their Correlates in Matar Taluka;* coauthor of *Health Insurance for Workers in the Informal Sector: Detailed Results from a Pilot Study;* and coauthor of *Who Benefits from Public Health Spending in India: Results of a Benefit Incidence Analysis for India.*

William C. Hsiao is the K. T. Li Professor of Economics and director of the program in health care financing at the Harvard School of Public Health. He received his Ph.D. in economics from Harvard University and is a qualified actuary with extensive experience in insurance. His current research focuses on developing a theory of health system economics that could provide an analytical framework in diagnosing the causes of the successes or failures of a system and on advising governments on their health sector reforms, including China, Colombia, Cyprus, Hong Kong, Poland, South Africa, Sweden, Taiwan, Uganda, and Vietnam. His research has also concentrated on payment for hospital and physician services, social and private insurance, and competition in managed care markets. Hsiao developed a rational fee schedule for physician services, the resource-based relative value scale (RBRVS) adopted by Australia, Canada, France, and the United States. He was named the Man of the Year in Medicine for his work on the RBRVS.

Hsiao has published more than a hundred papers and several books. He was elected to the Institute of Medicine, National Academy of Sciences, and National Academy of Social Insurance. He has served on the boards of directors of a number of professional organizations, including the National Academy of Social Insurance and the Society of Actuaries. He has also served as an adviser to three U.S. presidents and to the U.S. Congress, the World Bank, the International Monetary Fund, and the WHO. He is a recipient of honorary professorships from several leading Chinese universities.

Melitta Jakab, a Hungarian national, is completing her Ph.D. in health economics at Harvard University. Previously, she worked at the World Bank's Health, Nutrition, and Population Network. Her research interests include assessing alternative health-financing options for the poor, the operation of hospital markets, and health system reform in transition economies. Jakab is a member of the teaching faculty of the Harvard/World Bank Institute Flagship Course on Health Sector Reform and Sustainable Financing. She is codirector of international training programs at the Health Services Management Training Centre in Budapest.

Johannes Paul Jütting is affiliated with the OECD Development Centre in Paris, where he works as a senior economist. He is in charge of the research project on Social Institutions and Development, a main activity of the center's work program in 2003–04. He was previously research fellow at the Center for Development Research (ZEF) in Bonn, where he directed the Research Group on Poverty. In that position, he coordinated ZEF's research on Innovative Health Insurance Schemes for the Poor. He is also a scientific adviser of a joint program of the World Bank, the WHO, and the ILO—Resource Mobilization and Risk Pooling in Low-Income Environments.

Jütting holds a Ph.D. in agricultural economics awarded by Humboldt University of Berlin and received his postgraduate habilitation degree from the University of Bonn.

Chitra Krishnan has a master's degree in public health from the Johns Hopkins School of Public Health. At the time of this research, she was working as a junior researcher at the World Bank's Health, Nutrition, and Population Network.

John C. (Jack) Langenbrunner is a senior health economist with both research and operations experience. He is currently working in the World Bank's Europe and Central Asia region. He has worked on health-financing issues in Azerbaijan, Croatia, Kazakhstan, Kyrgyz Republic, Poland, Russia, and Uzbekistan as well as in several countries in the Middle East and North Africa region.

In 2001, Langenbrunner led a Bank study on introducing health insurance in the Kingdom of Bahrain. Before joining the Bank, he worked in several countries in the South Asia and East Asia and Pacific regions. He is currently based in Moscow. Langenbrunner is leading the World Bank's work in Resource Allocation and Purchasing (RAP) and has authored or coauthored a number of papers related to this initiative. He is also leading the Bank's work on a manual for National Health Accounts for low- and middle-income countries, the "NHA Producers Guide," which is now in draft and is available upon request.

Before working at the Bank, Langenbrunner was with the U.S. Health Care Financing Administration, a health insurance program for more than 80 million Americans. There he worked on case-mix payment systems for hospitals and physician relative value scales. Later, in the U.S. Office of Management and Budget, he served on the Clinton Health Care Reform Task Force.

Langenbrunner holds master's and doctoral degrees in economics and public health from the University of Michigan (United States). He is an occasional lecturer on health-financing topics at both the Johns Hopkins University and the George Washington University.

Philip Musgrove is chief economist of the Disease Control Priorities Project at the Fogarty International Center of NIH. He is also adjunct professor in the Department of Health Policy, School of Public Health and Health Services, George Washington University, having previously taught at American University and the University of Florida. Until 2002, he was a principal economist at the World Bank. In 1982–90, he was an adviser in health economics, Pan American Health Organization. He served from 1996 to 1998 at the Bank's Resident Mission in Brasilia, Brazil, and in 1999–2001 was seconded by the Bank to the World Health Organization in Geneva.

Musgrove has worked on health reform projects in Argentina, Brazil, Chile, and Colombia, in addition to dealing with a variety of issues in health economics, financing, equity, and nutrition. His publications include more than fifty articles in economics and health journals; he has also authored, edited, or contributed chapters to more than twenty books.

Jean-Pierre Poullier is a former research associate at the Brookings Institution, Washington, D.C., for *Why Growth Rates Differ* (E. F. Denison with J-P. Poullier,

1967). He was a consultant for the European Commission (on the competitive capacity of the European economy), the European Commission Statistical Office (on purchasing power parities), the Peruvian and the Algerian governments (on productivity and on industrial development), and the International Institute of the Management of Technology. He worked for the Organisation for Economic Co-operation and Development between 1972 and 1998, where he created and directed the Health Policy Unit; between 1999 and 2003, he headed the National Health Accounts Unit of the World Health Organization. He is the author of more than a hundred publications and articles on public finance and health systems. He has been a consultant to the World Bank on the construction of National Health Accounts in Iran, Saudi Arabia, and other countries in the Middle East.

M. Kent Ranson is a lecturer in the Health Policy Unit at the London School of Hygiene and Tropical Medicine, and a research coordinator for the Self-Employed Women's Association Insurance (Vimo SEWA). Ranson has degrees in clinical medicine (M.D., McMaster University), public health epidemiology and biostatistics (M.P.D., Harvard University), and health economics and financing (Ph.D., University of London). He currently heads a three-year research project that will assess the impact of several interventions to optimize the equity impact of Vimo SEWA. His other research interests include the cost-effectiveness of public health interventions (antitobacco, antimalaria, and antitrachoma-blindness) and the identification and measurement of characteristics of health systems that prevent implementation of the (theoretically) most cost-effective interventions.

Pia Schneider worked for Abt Associates Inc. in Kigali, Rwanda, for two years, until September 2000. She was the head of the Rwanda office of the Partnerships for Health Reform, financed by the U.S. Agency for International Development and provided technical assistance to the Rwandan Ministry of Health. The main activities included the development, implementation, and evaluation of a community-based prepayment-insurance scheme for primary care in three health districts; and the implementation and analysis of the first Rwandan National Health Accounts with a disease-specific HIV/AIDS component. In addition, she managed and implemented a series of country activities to improve cost recovery and assess impacts on equity. She trained local staff in health care financing and health sector reform and responded to health sector reform needs as they arose during the transition period at the Ministry of Health. As a faculty member of the Abt Training Institute, she has designed and delivered training in health economics and in policy analysis and formulation to local counterparts from various countries.

Schneider has an extensive background in health economics, international economics, and nursing. Prior to joining Abt Associates Inc., she served as an applied health research analyst–health economist for HMO Oregon at Blue-Cross/BlueShield of Oregon. In this position, Schneider designed clinical quality improvement studies and analyzed access, quality, effectiveness, costs, outcome, health behavior, satisfaction, and treatment measures. She was also involved with financial analysis of HMO provider groups. Schneider has worked as a delegate for the International Committee of the Red Cross, where she collaborated with public health projects and local governmental and nongovernmental organizations in Dem. Rep. of Congo (former eastern Zaire) and South Africa. Schneider holds an R.N. degree from Lindenhof Hospital in Bern, Switzerland. She received her B.A. and M.A. in economics at the University of Basel in Switzerland. She is now working as a part-time employee for Abt on issues related to health financing and economics as she completes her Ph.D. in health economics at the London School of Hygiene and Tropical Medicine.

Siripen Supakankunti, Ph.D., is associate professor in economics and currently director of the WHO Collaborating Centre for Health Economics at the Faculty of Economics, Chulalongkorn University, Bangkok, Thailand. Since 1979, the Centre for Health Economics (CHE) has developed expertise in the field of health economics through a research, training, and teaching program. In late 1993, the center was designated a WHO Collaborating Centre for Health Economics, with regional and global responsibilities. The center's objectives are to develop expertise and commitment to the application of health economics in formulating health care policies, planning resource allocation, and refining health care delivery processes in the Southeast Asia region and Thailand; to strengthen health economics research capacity in Thailand and Southeast Asia, particularly with respect to economic analysis and evaluation in the control of tropical diseases; to encourage research in economic analysis and evaluation of disease control, with special attention to tropical diseases; and to provide advisory and information services, particularly in Southeast Asia and other regions, on health economics research. As a WHO Collaborating Centre for Health Economics, CHE has made some progress in accordance with the proposed strategy for strengthening health economics capability in the region and going well beyond that geographic area to form wider international linkages such as collaboration with the World Bank Institute at the World Bank, for organizing the Asia Flagship Training Program in Health Sector Reform and Sustainable Financing.

Supakankunti is responsible for overall activities of the center and for coordinating and organizing the Asia Flagship Training Program in Health Sector Reform and Sustainable Financing in Bangkok. She has published on various topics related to health economics.

Her area of specialized work and interests are specific components of health sector reform such as health care financing, health insurance, health policy and planning; impacts of structural change on the health sector; economic modeling; the pharmaceutical industry; and international trade in health services, economic analysis, and evaluation (malaria, HIV/AIDS, water pollution).

Emi Suzuki, a Japanese national, is a consultant to the World Bank's Health, Nutrition, and Population unit. With her strong statistical and demographic skills, she is working on compiling, updating, and analyzing Millennium Development Goals health indicators and time-series data on health expenditure and health service and utilization. She is also working with UNICEF and the WHO for data harmonization. Suzuki received her Ph.D. in public health from the Johns Hopkins Bloomberg School of Public Health. Prior to her work at the Bank, Suzuki worked in Japan for several NGOs that are implementing health, education, and environmental projects in developing countries.

Nicole Valentine is a health economist in the Global Program on Evidence for Health Policy at the WHO in Geneva, Switzerland. For the past three and a half years, she has worked at the WHO on interpersonal aspects of the quality of health systems (being treated with dignity, having personal information kept confidential, having clear communication, being attended to promptly). Prior to this appointment, she worked as a lecturer at the University of Cape Town and as a researcher, whose topics included patient satisfaction, national health accounts, and private, national, and local government health expenditure in South Africa.

In the field of interpersonal aspects of quality of care, Valentine has contributed several chapters to the book *Health Systems Performance Assessment: Debates, Methods, and Empiricism* (2003).

She holds an M.A. degree in economics from the University of Cape Town (South Africa) and an M.P.H. degree in health services from the University of Washington (Seattle, United States), where she studied as a Rotary Ambassadorial Scholar. She is currently a Ph.D. candidate at the Amsterdam Medical Centre, University of Amsterdam (Netherlands).

Ke Xu joined the WHO as a Global Health Leadership Fellow in 1999. Currently, she works as a health economist in the Global Program on Evidence for Health Policy at WHO headquarters in Geneva, Switzerland. Her focus is health payments distribution and the relation of catastrophic health costs to impoverishment. For the *World Health Report 2000: Health Systems—Improving Performance,* she worked on development of the concept and methodology of the index of fairness in financial contributions. In the field of inequality of health financing, she contributed several chapters to the book *Health Systems Performance Assessment: Debates, Methods, and Empiricism.* She is also associate editor of the electronic journal *Evidence for Health Policy.*

Xu holds an M.D. degree and a Ph.D. in health economics from Fudan University (formerly Shanghai Medical University). She has been a faculty member in the Department of Health Economics, Fudan University, teaching health economics, health insurance, survey design, and other economics courses. Her main research areas include: health financing and service originating; health financing for the elder population in Shanghai; improvement in access to health services for the urban poor; and sustainable development of a rural cooperative medical scheme in China. She was a visiting scholar at the RAND Corporation and the University of Southern California before joining the WHO.

Riadh Zeramdini worked as a health economist at the WHO headquarters in Geneva and as a trainee in the Consulting Cabinet (Sousse). He holds a Ph.D. in health economics and an M.S.E from the University of Lausanne (Switzerland), where he also worked as a research assistant in 1999–2000. He was awarded a license in management from the Faculty of Economic Sciences and Law of Sousse (Tunisia).

Index

Note: *f* indicates figures, *n* indicates notes (*nn* more than one note), and *t* indicates tables.